Davis's Manual of Psychosocial Nursing in General Patient Care

D0222110

Davis's Manual of Psychosocial Nursing in General Patient Care

Linda M. Gorman, RN, MN, CS, OCN, CRNH
Clinical Nurse Specialist, Hospice Program
Cedars Sinai Medical Center
Los Angeles, California

Assistant Clinical Professor
University of California, Los Angeles
Los Angeles, California

Certified Clinical Nurse Specialist
Adult Psychiatric/Mental Health Nursing

Donna F. Sultan, RN, MS
Mental Health Counselor, RN
West Valley Mental Health Center
Los Angeles County Department of Mental Health
Los Angeles, California

Marcia L. Raines, PhD, RN, MN, CS
Associate Professor
California State University, San Bernardino
San Bernardino, California

Lecturer, Statewide Nursing Program
California State University, Dominguez Hills
Carson, California

Formerly
Director of Education
San Bernardino County Medical Center
San Bernardino, California

 F. A. DAVIS COMPANY • Philadelphia

F. A. Davis Company
1915 Arch Street
Philadelphia, PA 19103

Printed in the United States of America

Last digit indicates print number: 10 9 8 7 6 5 4 3 2 1

Publisher, Nursing: Robert G. Martone
Nursing Acquisitions Editor: Joanne Patzek DaCunha, RN, MSN
Production Editor: Glenn L. Fechner
Cover Designer: Steven R. Morrone

As new scientific information becomes available through basic and clinical research, recommended treatments and drug therapies undergo changes. The authors and publisher have done everything possible to make this book accurate, up to date, and in accord with accepted standards at the time of publication. The authors, editors, and publisher are not responsible for errors or omissions or for consequences from application of the book, and make no warranty, expressed or implied, in regard to the contents of the book. Any practice described in this book should be applied by the reader in accordance with professional standards of care used in regard to the unique circumstances that may apply in each situation. The reader is advised always to check product information (package inserts) for changes and new information regarding dose and contraindications before administering any drug. Caution is especially urged when using new or infrequently ordered drugs.

Library of Congress Cataloging-in-Publication Data

Gorman, Linda M.
    Davis's manual of psychosocial nursing in general patient care / Linda M. Gorman, Donna F. Sultan, Marcia L. Raines.
      p. cm.
    Includes bibliographical references and index.
    ISBN 0-8036-0113-1
    1. Psychiatric nursing—Handbooks, manuals, etc. 2. Nursing—Social aspects—Handbooks, manuals, etc. I. Gorman, Linda M. II. Sultan, Donna. III. Luna-Raines, Marcia. IV. Title.
    [DNLM: 1. Nursing Care—psychology—handbooks. 2. Nursing Assessment—handbooks. 3. Nursing Diagnosis—handbooks. 4. Nurse-Patient Relations—handbooks. WY 39 G671d 1996]
RC440.G659 1996
610.73'68—dc20
DNLM/DLC
for Library of Congress
                                            95-48201
                                            CIP

Preface

Having worked in a variety of specialty areas over the years as staff nurses, clinical nurse specialists, educators, and managers, we realize that nurses aspire to become highly proficient in their area of practice but that psychological skills are often more difficult to perfect. Very often nurses feel inadequately prepared to deal with complex behavioral and psychiatric problems. Even nurses who practice in the psychiatric setting find themselves dealing with unique situations that challenge their level of expertise. And yet, a large percentage of nurses' time is spent dealing with these issues or more likely trying to compensate for them as they intervene with the underlying illness.

Davis's Manual of Psychosocial Nursing in General Patient Care bridges the gap between the information contained in large, comprehensive psychiatric nursing texts and the information that the clinician or student needs to function effectively in a variety of healthcare settings. The clinician can refer to this book to find the information to effectively handle specific patient problems. The nursing student can use this book as a review of basic psychosocial information which will be useful throughout nursing school curriculum. It can also supplement the psychiatric nursing text.

The concise, quick reference format used in this book allows the nurse to easily find information on the psychosocial problems commonly seen in practice. In addition to common psychosocial problems, psychiatric disorders are explained and discussed using less technical language. The nurse can look up a specific behavior problem and find information on etiology, assessment, pediatric, adult and geriatric implications, nursing diagnosis and interventions, patient education, discharge planning, documentation, and other important information.

Today's fast paced healthcare environment demands

quick assessment and treatment plans which are realistic, cost-effective, and outcome oriented. The information contained in this book is readily applicable to the inpatient, outpatient, home care, and long term care settings.

Each psychosocial problem includes a section on common nurse's reactions to these patient behaviors. Nurses often think that they should only have "acceptable" and "proper" emotional reactions. They needlessly deny certain feelings, have unrealistic expectations of patients, and consequently, may have an impaired ability to effectively address and resolve the patient's problem. The more aware the nurse becomes of how one reacts to patients' behaviors the easier it will be to accept one's own feelings and understand how those feelings affect the patient and influence interventions.

As a matter of convenience throughout this book, "family" describes people who play important roles in the patient's life and may include significant others who may or may not be legally related to the patient.

This is our second collaboration in book writing and we are still friends. We want to recognize the roles our families, friends, and colleagues have had in encouraging us through the preparation of this manuscript. We want to acknowledge our three contributors for the unique perspective each of them provided. We also want to recognize the nurses we have worked with over the years. They have taught us so much about the demands, pressures and rewards of nursing. That is the foundation of this book.

Linda M. Gorman
Donna F. Sultan
Marcia L. Raines

Contributors

Nancy Jo Bush, RN, MN, OCN
Lecturer and Assistant Clinical Professor
University of California, Los Angeles

Nurse Educator and Consultant
Oncology Education Associates
Los Angeles, California

James Espinoza, PharmD, MPA
Clinical Pharmacist
AIDS/Immune Disorders Center
Cedars Sinai Medical Center
Los Angeles, California

Margaret L. Mitchell, RN, MN, MDIV, MA, CNS
Senior Mental Health Counselor, RN
Treatment Authorization Request Unit
Los Angeles County Department of Mental Health
Los Angeles, California

Reviewers

Jeri Jaquis, RN, MSN
Assistant Professor of
   Nursing
Galveston College
Galveston, Texas

**Sharon L. Roberts, RN,
   PhD**
Professor of Nursing
California State University,
   Long Beach
Long Beach, California

**Daryl Sharp Minicucci,
   MSN, RN, CS**
Instructor
Syracuse University College
   of Nursing
Syracuse, New York

Carol J. Nelson, RN, MSN
Director of Nursing
   Education
Spokane Community
   College
Spokane, Washington

Jean Graves, RN, MSN
Instructor
Wallace Community College
Dothan, Alabama

**Judy A. Bourrand, RN,
   MSN**
Assistant Professor
Ida V. Moffett School of
   Nursing
Samford University
Birmingham, Alabama

**Sherly Jaroush, RN, MS,
   EdD**
Instructor
Lakeshore Technical
   College
Cleveland, Wisconsin

Betty Richardson, RN, PhD
Instructor
Austin Community College
Austin, Texas

Evelyn Wills, RN, PhD
Director of Research
University of Southwestern
   Louisiana
College of Nursing
Lafayette, Louisiana

Contents

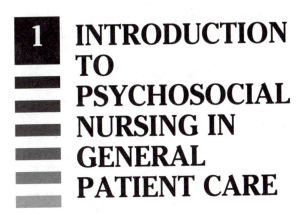

1 INTRODUCTION TO PSYCHOSOCIAL NURSING IN GENERAL PATIENT CARE

LEARNING OBJECTIVES

▼ *Define* psychosocial nursing care.
▼ *Describe the impact of patient behavior problems in a managed care setting.*
▼ *Describe how patient education is part of psychosocial care.*
▼ *Describe resources for discharge planning the nurse may use in psychosocial care.*

Every day nurses are confronted with and must find a way to deal with psychosocial patient problems and patient crises. Nurses are faced with caring for patients with:

- intense emotional responses to illness;
- personality styles that make caring for them difficult;
- psychiatric disorders;
- stresses and family problems that impact their reaction to illness or hospitalization.

While often proficient in managing the patient's physical health problems, the nurse may be less prepared to manage the emotional ones. Recognizing behaviors that suggest psychosocial problems exist and developing the ability to effectively manage them can improve the patient's chances of healing and reduce frustration for the nurse.

Psychosocial care emphasizes interventions focused on assisting individuals having difficulty coping with the emotional aspects of illness, life crises that affect health and health care, or psychiatric disorders. For example, problems with depression, anger, substance abuse, or grief can influence response to illness or to the healthcare system. Psychosocial care focuses on the effects of stress in psychologic and physiologic illness and on the intrapsychic and social functioning of the individual responding to stress.

The nurse has a responsibility to facilitate the patient's adaptations to his or her unique stresses by helping and supporting the person in his or her environment, level of wellness, and adjustment to the illness or condition. Identifying the patient's coping responses, maximizing strengths, and maintaining integrity will help the nurse meet this responsibility.

Possible Nurses' Reactions

A factor whose importance cannot be overlooked in psychosocial care is becoming aware of one's own reactions to patient behaviors. These reactions will influence the nurse-patient relationship, assessment findings, and selection of potential interventions. They can help or hinder the relationship. Recognizing the influence of these reactions:

- Increases the nurse's awareness of his or her own reactions that influence objectivity

- Helps the nurse identify reactions frequently experienced by other nurses to ease feelings of guilt and resentment
- Increases understanding of colleagues' reactions to enhance the work environment
- Facilitates support to oneself, reducing self-criticism and reinforcing one's own skills
- Helps the nurse select better assessment tools to identify patients' dilemmas and responses

The Role of Psychosocial Nursing in Managed Care Settings

Some patients require many more resources because of psychosocial and psychiatric problems. A patient's emotional reactions can increase lengths of stay, contribute to noncompliance, and drain physical and emotional resources. Once these patient problems are identified, the nurse needs to use skills to meet the patient's needs while making judicious use of available resources.

Managed care is a system whereby controls are exerted over access, use, quality, and effectiveness of health services. Managed care has led to shortened hospital stays and limitations in available resources. To work within this system, the nurse must quickly identify the patient's needs, establish a realistic plan of care, implement interventions, and evaluate the outcomes within a predetermined length of time. Psychosocial and psychiatric patient problems only complicate the demands made on the nurse in an already stretched healthcare environment and can negatively impact patient outcomes. When the nurse has skills readily at hand to identify and intervene effectively, better patient outcomes can be achieved, and nurse satisfaction will be enhanced.

Lifespan Issues

Though each individual is unique, there are patterns and common links we all share through the life cycle. Psychosocial development proceeds through a series of stages and developmental crises. Each phase of the lifespan presents new challenges, experiences, and problems. Many psychosocial problems have their origins in developmental crises that remain unresolved or that are resolved with negative outcomes. Problems such as depression and grief can affect individuals differently depending on the stage of their life. Childhood, adolescence, and old age are points of particular vulnerability.

Interventions in this book are geared to adults, though many of them can be adapted to children. To adapt to a pediatric population, the child's developmental and cognitive levels must be incorporated in the care plan. Seek out specialists in pediatrics, as needed.

Collaborative Interventions

Our complex healthcare system relies on a variety of professionals to meet patients' needs. Obviously, the nurse does not work in a vacuum. The nurse needs to participate in the multidisciplinary team and be aware of how other disciplines are resources for psychosocial intervention. The nurse also needs to know when the work needs to be shared or delegated through referrals. For example, social workers are often familiar with community support groups for emotional problems and psychotherapists. The nurse should be aware of agency policies regarding giving referrals for psychotherapists. Some may require a doctor's order. Other resources include the physician, pharmacist, clergy, dietitian, and others depending on the specialty and setting. Knowing when and how to access them and work effectively together will improve patient outcomes and enhance the working environment.

Patient Education

Patient education is another important component of psychosocial care. The nurse is required to incorporate appropriate patient education in one's practice. To provide adequate education, the nurse needs to be aware of how psychosocial issues influence learning. For example, assessing the patient's anxiety level or disturbed thoughts will influence timing of teaching and the type of information given. Inability to understand the language or customs also inhibits learning. Patient education will enhance independence and control, patient and family involvement in the treatment plan, preparation for possible emotional changes, coping skills, and responses to medications. Patient education takes on added importance with reduced lengths of stay and the need for patients to take on more responsibility for their care.

When to Call for Help

Many difficult, challenging situations require a number of complex skills. While continuing to gain knowledge in identifying and intervening in psychosocial care, the nurse also needs to recognize her limitations and be able to identify when patient behaviors are precursors to or are currently presenting a dangerous, emergency situation. Knowing when to call for help and how to use resources are essential in providing quality, cost-effective care.

Discharge Planning

For most patients, there is an end to the type of care currently being received, and he or she must move on to another care site or level of care. To ensure continuity of care, planning for the next phase must be begun as early as possible.

Discharge planning is essential to ensure that adequate resources are available to maintain coping skills and to diminish future problems. Discharge planning can include referrals to support groups, follow-up counseling, hotlines, and home health care. Home healthcare staff can evaluate the home environment, assess patient-family interactions and coping skills, and provide skilled nursing care. Evaluating home care needs early helps the patient and family to be prepared by the time the patient goes home.

Many home health agencies also have psychiatric nurses on staff. They can be helpful in evaluating suicidal risk, psychotic behavior, confusion, and response to psychotropic medications. Patients may also need referrals to other levels of care, such as psychiatric hospitalization or convalescent care, and assistance with financial support. Other professionals such as social workers, case managers, and counselors can help ensure that the patient can safely return home.

DSM-IV

The American Psychiatric Association (APA) has developed a classification system for mental disorders. It is the most widely accepted system in the United States today and is published and revised periodically as the *Diagnostic and Statistical Manual*. The current (fourth) edition was published in 1994 and is referred to as DSM-IV. This reference provides clinicians with guidelines, specific criteria, and accepted terminology. Throughout this book, you may see references to the criteria published in DSM-IV. The criteria are used to prevent negatively labeling or miscategorizing patient behaviors as psychiatric disorders.

Overview

Chapters 1 through 6 cover basic skills and emphasize the need for psychosocial assessment and culturally sensitive care. Chapters 7 through 19 each address specific problems commonly encountered. Nursing interventions are provided for the most outstanding nursing diagnoses. Chapter 20 reviews antipsychotic, antidepressant, antianxiety, and antimanic medications that the nurse will be administering.

2 PSYCHOSOCIAL RESPONSE TO ILLNESS

LEARNING OBJECTIVES

▼ Describe the role of self-esteem, body image, powerlessness, and guilt in the patient's emotional response to illness.
▼ Describe the role of Maslow's Hierarchy of Needs in explaining a patient's response to illness.
▼ Define defense mechanisms, and describe examples of each.
▼ Describe commonly used coping mechanisms.

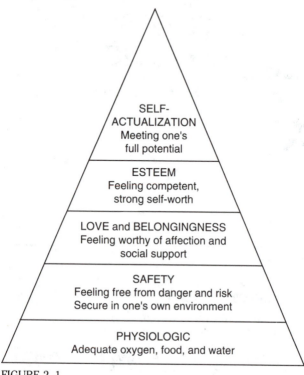

FIGURE 2–1.

Any illness will have some psychologic impact. Illness threatens the individual and evokes a wide array of emotions, such as fear, sadness, anger, depression, despair, and loss of control. Each individual who faces an illness responds differently based on personality, previous life experiences, and coping style. Denial, noncompliance, suicide, and aggression may be some of the more maladaptive responses that the nurse may face when caring for those who are ill. Most often these responses are temporary and subside as the threat lessens. But they can also be chronic maladaptive behavioral responses that the person uses whenever he or she experiences a stressful situation. There is often no way of knowing on first meeting a patient whether his or her response is temporary or habitual.

All behavior is an attempt to communicate needs. To determine underlying motivation, identifying the need the behavior fulfills can be a first step to understanding. Maslow's Hierarchy of Needs (1954) provides a framework within which to begin examining the motivation (Fig. 2–1). Maslow identified five levels of needs. Each level of need, starting at the most basic physiologic level, must be met before one can strive for the next level.

Professional nursing uses a holistic framework by which it views the individual and his or her environment in its entirety. The influence of the mind as well as the body is recognized in the development of and response to illness. It is known that the response to stress involves the immune and neuroendocrine systems. Emotional response to stress suppresses the immune system, stimulates the cardiovascular system, and alters secretions of hormones influencing the body's response to the illness.

Stress cannot be avoided. It is a normal part of living. It does not matter if a stressor is pleasant, such as an upcoming holiday, or unpleasant, such as illness, disability, and hospitalization. What is critical is the individual's perception of the intensity of the demand requiring readjustment and his or her capacity to adjust.

Key Issues in Response to Illness

ALTERED SELF-ESTEEM

Self-esteem is the personal judgment of the individual's own worth. The roots of self-esteem are in early parental and social relationships as well as personal perception of goal attainment and one's own ideal. Maslow places esteem at a very high level, indicating that this need can be accomplished only when the more basic needs are fulfilled. Self-esteem increases as the individual achieves personal goals. High self-esteem indicates that the individual has attained self-acceptance with his or her good and bad points. This person knows that he or she is loved and respected by others. High self-esteem also implies a sense of control over personal destiny. Feeling good about one's self influences many aspects of life including dealing with others, managing conflict, standing up for one's own beliefs, taking risks, and believing in one's ability to handle adversity.

Throughout life, both internal and external factors influence one's self-esteem. For instance, falling in love or graduating from school promotes positive self-esteem, while illness can represent a threat to self-esteem. Illness and disability often require a person to alter or even abandon personal goals strongly influencing one's view of oneself. Some people are able to adjust readily, creating new realistic goals with little impact on self-esteem. Others may struggle with the changes and are unable to regain previous levels of esteem. Serious illnesses like prostate or breast cancer, heart disease, or stroke not only require adaptation of personal goals but often distort a deeper sense of self. This is a major contributor to depression. But maintaining a strong sense of self is a powerful drive, and over time many people will make adaptations.

ALTERED BODY IMAGE

Body image is the mental picture a person has of his or her own body. It significantly influences the way a person thinks and feels about his or her body as a whole, body functions, and the internal and external sensations associated with it. It also includes perceptions of the way others see his or her body and is central to self-concept and self-esteem. Often a person's belief about one's own body mirrors self-concept. This is evident when an individual seeks out cosmetic surgery to alter his or her appearance. However, when self-concept is poor, even cosmetic surgery may not change the person's body image. This person may continue to struggle with low self-esteem even though the physical "imperfections" are changed.

A person's body image changes constantly. Illness, surgery, or weight loss can have a major influence on how one views one's self. Amputation, colostomy, and dependence on equipment such as dialysis are examples of obvious external changes that influence one's body image. Some conditions such as a myocardial infarction may cause no obvious external body changes, but the individual may now view his or her body as weak. Altered body image may contribute to lowered self-esteem and, possibly, depression.

POWERLESSNESS

Powerlessness is the perception of lack of personal control over certain events as well as oneself. Individuals need to maintain a sense of power and control over their destiny and environment. Loss of this sense of control can negatively affect how one views one's effectiveness as an individual. Illness consistently forces the individual to face his or her powerlessness over a situation.

Entry into the healthcare system adds to this sense of powerlessness. Now, in addition to facing the feeling of helplessness over the illness, the person is being subjected to following the orders of strangers, complying with other's schedules, and loss of privacy. As soon as the hospitalized patient gives up his or her clothes and puts on a hospital gown, the person is reminded of his or her powerlessness within the new role. Resisting a doctor's orders and even refusing pain medications can suggest that the patient is attempting to maintain some sense of control and fighting off feelings of powerlessness. Helping these patients to maintain some sense of power and control is an important nursing intervention. Individuals who chronically view themselves as helpless may be more prone to depression and vulnerable to being victimized by others who try to control them.

LOSS

Actual or potential loss is any situation where something valued is rendered or threatened to be rendered inaccessible. Loss occurs all through life as one experiences changes in relationships, inability to reach an expected goal, and disappointment in others. Any time we have an emotional investment in someone or something, we are vulnerable to losing it. This includes loss of a body part or body function. All losses in life can contribute to loss of hopes, dreams, and goals and require some period of grieving as the individual adapts to the new situation. The degree of response to the loss depends on the amount of value the individual has placed on it. Eventually, the individual will go on to develop new attachments and goals. Maladaptive responses to loss can include anger, guilt, depression, and, possibly, suicidal thoughts.

HOPELESSNESS

Hope is fundamental to life. No matter how bad the situation may be, the ability to hope for improvement will help an individual get through it. Hopelessness is the sustained subjective state in which an individual sees no alternatives or personal choices available to solve problems or to achieve desired goals. Lack of hope can develop from an overwhelming loss of control and is related to a sense of despair, helplessness, apathy, and depression.

The person without hope is unable to mobilize enough energy to even establish personal goals and may be unable to recognize or accept help or new ideas. Serious illness alone usually does not cause hopelessness. Usually deep personal feelings of loss, depleted emotional reserves, and an overwhelming sense of powerlessness also contribute. To regain a sense of hope, this individual needs to view the situation differently and to alter any negative goals and expectations and, possibly, to create new ones. For example, if a patient is terminally ill, rather than hoping to cure the illness, goals may need to be refocused on achieving a pain-free state or making contact with family members. For some individuals, hopelessness can lead to discovery of alternatives that will add meaning and purpose to life. Spiritual crises may be related to hopelessness as well.

GUILT

Guilt is self-blame and regrets for some real or perceived action. It is a painful emotion that can negatively influence feelings, behaviors, and relationships with others. Conflicts within relationships can occur when an individual feels guilty about feeling resentful because his or her needs are not being met.

Nurses frequently observe behavior in patients or their families that seem to be motivated by guilt. Examples may include the family who suddenly hovers over an ill patient, the family who makes numerous demands on the staff or unjustly accuses them of providing inadequate care, or the patient who won't ask for help. Self-blame is another frequent behavior motivated by guilt, for example, a wife who blames herself for not taking her husband to the doctor sooner or a patient who blames himself for the stress his illness is causing for his wife. Survivor guilt can be seen in people who survive traumatic events in which others are killed or injured.

ANXIETY

Anxiety is a universal primitive unpleasant feeling of tension and apprehension. It provides an early warning signal to the self for danger. Anxiety is an important motivator of behavior that makes people act or change to reduce the uncomfortable feelings of tension. Low to moderate levels of anxiety can enhance learning and action. More severe anxiety may be reduced by using defense or coping mechanisms as the unconscious tries to protect us from this discomfort.

Defense Mechanisms

Defense mechanisms protect the individual from threats, feelings of inadequacy, and/or unacceptable feelings or thoughts. Defense mechanisms are unconscious mental processes used to reduce anxiety and conflict by modifying, distorting, and rejecting reality (see Table 2–1). Because they are unconscious, the individual is not aware of how these mechanisms affect thoughts, feelings, and behavior. In some ways they are used to alter reality to make the situation more acceptable. Without these mechanisms, the threatening feelings might overwhelm and paralyze the individual and interfere with daily living. The essential, adaptive mechanisms help to lower anxiety so that goals can be achieved. We could not survive without them. However, if used too extensively, they can contribute to highly distorted perceptions and interfere with normal functioning and interpersonal relationships. Excessively distorted defense mechanisms can be characterized as psychiatric disorders.

An individual's repertoire of defense mechanisms is learned through childhood experiences. Each time a de-

TABLE 2–1. **Common Defense Mechanisms**

Defense Mechanism	Definition	Example
Denial	Attempt to remove an experience or a feeling from consciousness	After a diagnosis of terminal condition, the patient does not exhibit any expected emotional reaction and states that diagnosis is not true.
Displacement	The belief that one would be in great danger if true feelings about someone were known to that person, which causes the individual to discharge or displace feelings onto a third person or object	A family member is angry at the patient for not taking better care of himself and feels too guilty to express this to the ill person. Instead, he expresses anger at the nursing staff for giving inadequate care.
Identification	Accepting the other person's circumstances as though they were one's own	A man's wife died a very painful death from cancer. When he is diagnosed with cancer, he experiences extreme anxiety because he has accepted his wife's experiences as if he had lived them.
Intellectualization	Separating emotion from an idea or thought because emotionally it is too painful	A patient discusses the physiology of his leukemia at length without any emotional reaction.
Isolation	Blocking out feelings associated with an unpleasant or threatening situation or thought	A nurse caring for critically ill patient who is the same age provides care without experiencing the emotions related to tragedy of the patient's situation.

TABLE 2–1. **Common Defense Mechanisms**

Defense Mechanism	Definition	Example
Projection	Transferring or blaming others for one's own unacceptable ideas, impulses, wishes, or feelings	After a myocardial infarction, a patient relates how his wife is coping poorly with his condition. This patient's anxiety may be so great and too threatening to face so he places his own fears onto his wife.
Rationalization	Substituting acceptable reasons for the true reasons for personal behavior because admitting true reasons is too threatening	Smoker continues to smoke despite physician's warning because he knows many people who smoke and have no ill effects.
Reaction formation	Actions that are opposite of the true, unacceptable feelings that the person is experiencing	A woman has negative feelings about her pregnancy but then lavishes constant attention on her newborn.
Regression	Reverting to earlier patterns of development as a way to reduce anxiety and demands on one's self	During serious illness, a patient exhibits behavior more appropriate for a younger developmental age, such as excessive dependency.
Repression	Forcibly dismissing unacceptable thoughts, feelings, impulses, or memories from consciousness	A person is unable to recall feelings of hostility toward a sibling or specific memories from childhood.
Sublimation	Expressing repressed urges or desires in socially acceptable ways	An angry person writes a poem about his reactions to his feelings.

fense mechanism reduces uncomfortable anxiety feelings, it provides positive reinforcement.

Coping Mechanisms

Coping mechanisms are usually conscious methods used by the individual to overcome a problem or stressor. They are learned, adaptive or maladaptive responses to anxiety based on problem solving and lead to changed behavior. They involve higher levels of emotional and ego development than defense mechanisms; however, overuse can create problems such as overeating or smoking. In addition, unconscious mechanisms can also play a role in using or selecting a specific coping mechanism. Coping mechanisms are more readily changed if inappropriate since the patient is more aware of using them.

Some common coping mechanisms include:
- Talking problems out with others and gaining new insights on looking at or coping with the problem
- Expressing intense emotion by crying, yelling, or laughing
- Seeking comfort from friends, favorite foods, cigarettes, treasured objects, or mind-altering substances
- Using humor to discharge tension in a way that avoids fully acknowledging a difficult situation
- Exercising or performing manual labor
- Problem solving using a series of strategies and step-by-step approaches to the resolution of a problem
- Sleeping
- Avoiding upsetting situations, such as feigning illness to avoid an unpleasant situation

3 PSYCHOSOCIAL SKILLS

LEARNING OBJECTIVES

▼ *Describe the key components of a psychosocial assessment.*
▼ *Describe how and when a mental status examination is used.*
▼ *List the forms of therapeutic communication.*
▼ *Describe how culture will influence a psychosocial assessment.*
▼ *Describe the impact of the psychosocial skills of role modeling, role playing, and acceptance.*

Providing psychosocial care requires a combination of astute psychosocial assessment skills, experience in performing mental status examinations and using therapeutic communication and a sensitivity to the influence of culture on behaviors.

Psychosocial Nursing Assessment

Psychosocial information needs to be part of every patient assessment as psychosocial problems will influence the selection of a diagnosis and treatment of the illness. With a thorough assessment, the nurse can determine the patient's needs, problems and potential problems, and identify those patients who are at a higher risk for developing more serious problems.

To perform a thorough psychosocial assessment, the nurse uses many skills. First, the nurse must be able to establish a rapport with the patient. Showing an interest in what the patient is saying, asking appropriate questions, and making observations help to put the patient at ease and enable him or her to divulge personal information. To establish the best relationship for conducting a psychosocial assessment, use the following guidelines:

- Create a quiet, private environment.
- Minimize interruptions, if possible.
- Maintain appropriate eye contact.
- Sit at eye level with the patient.
- Ask open-ended questions to encourage the patient to talk (see Table 3–1).
- Avoid writing a lot of notes during the interview.
- Demonstrate an interest in the patient's concerns.
- Indicate acceptance of patient by avoiding criticism, frowning, or demonstrating shock.
- Avoid asking more personal questions than are actually needed.
- Determine whether the family can provide information if the patient is unable to communicate.
- Maintain confidentiality.
- Be aware of your own biases and discomforts that could influence the assessment.

The psychosocial assessment focuses on the effect that the illness has on the patient and family rather than on

TABLE 3–1. **Therapeutic Communication Techniques**

Technique	Definition	Example
Empathy	The helper becomes keenly attuned to the patient's feelings to understand them fully while maintaining a sense of one's own separateness	In response to a patient's recounting the recent loss of a baby, the nurse says, "You must have felt very disappointed."
Open-ended questions	Questions structured to encourage the patient to share information and feelings	"How did you feel when the doctor told you of your diagnosis?"
Closed-ended questions	Information-gathering questions that require only a one-word or very brief answer	"Where does it hurt?"
Active listening	Accepting what the speaker has said, analyzing it, and reflecting back your understanding of what was heard	"From what I understand, you are planning to stop coming to counseling."
Clarification	Increasing the understanding of what the patient is trying to communicate	"I'm not sure I understand what happened next. Could you go over it again?"
Silence	Allowing time for the patient to gather thoughts and ponder a topic without interruption (This can communicate acceptance and concern.)	

TABLE 3–1. **Therapeutic Communication Techniques** (*Continued*)

Technique	Definition	Example
Reflection	Verbally giving back the feeling part of the patient's communication to help focus on the feeling tone	"You sound very worried about the test results."
Nonverbal communication	Overt behavior that indicates listening and attention	Maintaining eye contact, leaning forward, keeping facial expressions appropriate for the emotions being expressed, keeping a comfortable distance.
Congruent communication	Body language, facial expression, and verbal content all expressing the same thing	Nurse's physical appearance, voice, and emotional reaction all communicate that she or he is listening, accepting, concerned, and understanding.

physical symptoms. This assessment will begin the process of identifying key nursing diagnoses. In addition, it gives important information for the patient's treatment plan. The assessment should include:

Lifestyle information: Determine with whom the patient lives, significant relationships, available support people, marital status, religion, occupation, and other important components of the patient's lifestyle.

Normal coping patterns: Identify which coping mechanisms the patient uses when under stress and in past illnesses or hospitalizations. What happened the last time the patient was under severe stress? How is the patient currently coping?

Understanding of current illness: Ask patient about his or her understanding of the diagnosis or reason for seeking medical attention. Determine how the patient views this problem affecting his or her life.

Personality style: After interacting with the patient, identify any important personality traits that may affect his or her care or compliance, such as the tendency to be dependent, hostile, dramatic, or critical.

History of psychiatric disorder: If the patient is currently taking psychiatric medications, make sure to ask the patient why they are being taken. Consider asking if he or she has experienced any psychiatric symptoms, such as depression. If the patient's behavior indicates a psychiatric disorder, explore this further.

Recent life changes or stressors: Determine if there has been any major changes or traumatic events recently. Keep in mind that these changes may be both positive or negative, such as moving to a new house or area, a death in the family, a job or role change, or recent birth of a child.

Major issues raised by current illness: Determine how this illness has affected his or her lifestyle or sense of self, including areas such as self-esteem, body image, loss of intimacy, role changes, and change in family dynamics.

Mental status examination: Perform the mental status examination to help identify dysfunctions in emotional, cognitive, or behavioral spheres.

The Mental Status Examination

The mental status examination is used in the determination of whether or not there are abnormalities in thinking and reasoning ability, feelings, or behavior of the patient. Often without realizing they are doing it, nurses perform quick mental status examinations every time they see their patients. Taking note of changes in a patient's appearance, memory, emotions, or thinking can be done while making quick rounds or having a social conversation with the patient. A more formal mental status examination can be part of a psychosocial assessment in a new patient, or it may be done when changes in the patient's condition are noted.

The mental status examination includes observations

and questions in the following categories: appearance, behavior, and speech; thoughts; mood and affect; ability to perform abstract reasoning; memory; intelligence; concentration; orientation; judgment; and insight (see Table 3–2 and Fig. 3–1).

To gather a comprehensive evaluation, review all the categories of the examination. Congruence or discrepancies between sections may reveal important information. Note inappropriate responses as well as the absence of the usual anticipated responses. For example, a patient relates that the physician says her cancer has metastasized too much to consider surgery (thought). This clear and coherent thought said in a droning, monotonous voice (speech) without any apparent intensity, distress, or expression of emotion (mood) may suggest that she is denying her illness. A patient who may be experiencing an extreme stress response to his illness may be unable to verbalize any expected concerns (thoughts), but may become increasingly anxious or depressed (mood and/or emotions) with increasing restlessness (behavior). Choosing an appropriate nursing diagnosis will depend on integrating all these observations along with knowledge of the patient's usual responses to stress.

Changes in mental status often result from alterations in psychologic or physical state. For example, behavioral changes such as confusion, depression, delirium, or even psychosis may be a sign of drug toxicity, electrolyte imbalance, or intracranial bleeding (see Table 3–3).

Therapeutic Communication

The essence of the helping relationship, therapeutic communication occurs when the nurse communicates with the patient in a manner that facilitates acquiring information and understanding the patient's concerns and problems. It is the art of reaching a person by means of verbal and nonverbal messages. Acceptance, respect, honesty, trust, concern, protection, and support must all be present for communication to be therapeutic. Therapeutic communication allows the patient to share feelings, feel accepted, and look at problems from a new perspective. It should not be con-

TABLE 3–2. **Mental Status Examination and Related Definitions**

Category	Description	Related Definitions
Appearance	Describe what patient looks like including dress, posture, grooming.	
Behavior	Describe behavior, motor activity, mannerisms.	*Catatonic:* Remaining totally immobile *Posturing:* Assuming inappropriate or bizarre positions *Compulsions:* Insistent, repetitive unwanted actions
Speech	Describe how patient speaks; list barriers to communication.	*Perseveration:* Mechanical repetition of words, thoughts *Pressured:* Highly accelerated rapid speech *Loose associations:* Absence of logical connections between thoughts *Flight of ideas:* Rapidly jumping from one thought to another with minimal links *Tangential:* Talking around main point *Word salad:* Unconnected words and phrases without meaning or logic *Thought blocking:* Stopping suddenly in the middle of verbalizing a thought and staring into space *Neologism:* Making up new words only speaker understands

TABLE 3–2. **Mental Status Examination and Related Definitions** (*Continued*)

Category	Description	Related Definitions
Mood/affect	Describe the emotions that are apparent by facial expressions, motor behavior, words used.	*Labile:* Emotions that change quickly and unpredictably *Flat affect:* No demonstration of any feeling *Blunted affect:* Constricted display of emotions *Anhedonia:* Absence of any pleasure *Inappropriate affect:* Emotions displayed not fitting with topic discussed *Ambivalence:* Contradictory feelings experienced simultaneously
Thoughts	What are themes in conversation? Does patient make sense? Is patient preoccupied with certain thoughts?	*Hallucinations:* Sensory perceptions (auditory, visual, gustatory, olfactory, tactile) without external stimuli, e.g., hearing nonexistent voices *Illusions:* Misinterpretations of real external sensory stimuli, e.g., seeing a ghost in a shadow *Delusions:* False, fixed beliefs not alterable by logical explanations *Obsessions:* Unwanted, distressing recurring thoughts *Phobia:* Irrational fear of a specific situation, accompanied by avoidance of the phenomenon feared

TABLE 3–2. **Mental Status Examination and Related Definitions**

Category	Description	Related Definitions
		Depersonalization: Sense of not being real; sense of being detached from one's body or self
		Magical thinking: Thinking about something happening is the same as doing it
		Grandiosity: Exaggerated beliefs in own worth and/or abilities
		Paranoia: Unwarranted belief that others have harmful intentions to person
Ability to abstract	Describe patient's ability to define similarities between objects or explain a proverb.	*Concrete description:* Sees objects in very definite simple ways, e.g., sees an apple and an orange as "round" rather than the overall category "fruit"
		Abstract ability: Can generalize the meaning of a concept and find meaning in symbols, e.g., "still water runs deep" means that quiet people have depth rather than lakes are deep bodies of water.)
Memory	Describe patient's ability to repeat the names of 3 objects immediately after being told and again in 5 minutes.	

TABLE 3–2. **Mental Status Examination and Related Definitions** (*Continued*)

Category	Description	Related Definitions
Intelligence	Describe patient's level of knowledge, language, understanding of instructions.	
Concentration	Describe patient's ability to focus on a single thought without becoming distracted.	*Serial 7s:* Test to determine the patient's ability to concentrate by having him or her continually subtract from 100 by 7 (93, 86, etc.)
Orientation	Describe patient's awareness of person and surroundings. A person is fully oriented when he or she is aware of person, place, time and situation.	*Orientation to person:* Knows his or her name *Orientation to place:* Knows where he or she is (Ask for specific location.) *Orientation to time:* Knows the date, day of week, year; most serious impairment is if the patient cannot identify year *Orientation to situation:* Knows what is wrong with him or her, why he or she is receiving care, the circumstances of current situation
Judgment	Describe patient's ability to use common sense to make reasonable decisions.	
Insight	Determine patient's understanding of factors contributing to his or her condition.	

Mental Status Examination Answer Sheet

Circle the correct words or fill in the blanks.

Appearance

Neat   clean   disheveled   poor grooming   erect posture   good eye contact

inappropriate makeup, _____

Behavior

Calm   appropriate   restless   agitated   compulsions   unusual actions

_____

Speech

Appropriate   pressured   loose association   loud   soft   mute

_____

Mood

Appropriate   labile   flat   depressed   worried   anxious   angry

hopeless _____

Thoughts

Appropriate   low self-esteem   suicidal ideations   hallucinations   delusions,

phobias _____

FIGURE 3–1.

Ability to abstract

Impaired   Yes   No

Memory

Impaired recent memory   Yes   No

Impaired past memory   Yes   No

Number of objects able to remember after 5 minutes_____

Estimated Intelligence

Below average   average   above average

Concentration

Able to focus,   easily distractible _____

Able to subtract backwards by 7's from 100 correctly until number_____

Orientation

Person_____Time_____

Place_____ Situation_____

Judgment

Realistic decision making   Yes   No

Insight

Good   fair   poor

Summary of Impressions:

FIGURE 3–1. *continued*

TABLE 3–3. **Mental Status Changes Caused by Electrolyte Imbalance**

Electrolyte Imbalance	Possible Cause	Mental Status Changes
Calcium (Blood Level: 8.5–10.5 mg/dL)		
Hyper-calcemia	Hyperparathyroidism Lung, breast cancer	Loss of energy Depression Confusion Irritability
Hypo-calcemia	Hypoparathyroidism due to calcium deficiency, lack of dietary vitamin D, or iatrogenic causes	Reduced concentration and intellectual function Emotional lability Depression Psychosis (if surgical excision of a parathyroid gland)
Sodium (Blood Level: 135–145 mEq/L)		
Hyper-natremia	Dehydration caused by excessive water loss (diarrhea, vomiting, diuresis) Restricted fluid intake Diabetes insipidus	Irritability Hyperactive intellectual function Stupor
Hypo-natremia	Severe dietary sodium restriction Addison's disease Excessive water intake	Depression Lethargy Withdrawal Anorexia
Phosphorus (Blood Level: 2.6–4.5mg/dL)		
Hypophos-phatemia	Gram-negative septicemia Alcohol withdrawal Intravenous hyperalimentation Low dietary intake	Apprehension Irritability Numbness Stupor
Potassium (Blood Level: 3.5–5 mEq/L)		
Hyper-kalemia	Renal disease Potassium-sparing diuretics Increased IV intake	Weakness Dysphagia
Hypo-kalemia	Renal disease Cushing's syndrome Potassium-wasting diuretics Vomiting Diarrhea	Mood and personality change Tearfulness Hopeless Helplessness

TABLE 3–3. **Mental Status Changes Caused by Electrolyte Imbalance** (*Continued*)

Electrolyte Imbalance	Possible Cause	Mental Status Changes
Base Bicarbonate (Blood Level: 24 mEq/L, pH 7.38)		
Alkalosis	Prolonged vomiting	Decreased intellectual function
	Large intake of sodium bicarbonate	Apathy
	Hyperventilation	Delirium
		Stupor
Acidosis	Severe emphysema	Decreased intellectual function
	Status asthmaticus	
	Renal failure	Drowsiness
	Diabetes mellitus with ketosis	Confusion
		Delirium

Adapted with permission from Barry, P: Psychosocial Nursing Assessment and Intervention. Philadelphia, JB Lippincott, 1989.

fused with counseling, which focuses on interpretation and the process of communication rather than the content.

Because nonverbal language is such a major part of any communication, the nurse needs to be aware of how his or her body language may enhance or inhibit therapeutic communication (see Tables 3–1 and 3–4). Studies consistently support that how we communicate is much more powerful than the content of our words. Nonverbal communication includes eye contact, body movements, facial expressions, gestures, and posture. Facial expressions are probably one of the most important sources of communication. Posture can communicate interest, tension, or boredom. One's walk can convey anxiety or confidence. Eye contact can be comforting and supportive or invasive and threatening. Gestures like a hand on the patient's arm during intense emotions can be very supportive as opposed to a nurse's standing away from the patient with her or his arms crossed in a judgmental way.

Other Psychosocial Skills

In addition to therapeutic communication, the nurse uses several other skills to the help the patient find new ways of

TABLE 3–4. **Barriers to Therapeutic Communication**

Technique	Possible Result	Example
Giving advice	Inhibits communication and sharing feelings. Patient may think you are not listening.	"You should go back to school."
False reassurances	May communicate that you do not fully understand the patient's feelings.	"I'm sure you'll do just fine."
Judgment	Patient will sense your disapproval	"How can you still smoke when your husband has lung cancer?"
Leading statements	Inhibits communication by possibly imposing feelings on the patient that he or she may not have.	"I'm sure you must have felt depressed after the divorce."
Multiple questions	Patient may not know what to answer first.	"Whom do you live with? Is that the way you want to live?"
Why question	May inhibit communication by threatening the patient. Often we may not know why we do the things we do or feel the way we do.	"Why do you feel that way?"
Parroting	Continually repeating what the patient says may appear to be too mechanical and frustrate the patient.	*Patient:* "I'm worried about the test results." *Nurse:* "You're worried about the test results?"

coping with his or her illness and the problems it causes. Many of these are used without the nurse's even being aware of using them. Perfecting these techniques can greatly enhance your ability to meet the psychosocial needs of your patients:

Acceptance: Demonstrating an interest in a patient's behavior and feelings communicates to the patient that he or she is valued. You can demonstrate acceptance of the patient by listening to him or her even if you disagree with the ideas being communicated. It is important to not criticize or judge the patient. Acceptance reinforces self-esteem.

Reassurance: Providing support by giving attention to matters that are important to the patient reinforces emotional security and helps reduce the patient's anxiety. When the patient has less anxiety to deal with, he or she can spend more time on effective problem solving and healing. However, avoid false reassurance because if events occur that were unexpected, it can reinforce a sense of distrust in the nurse.

Enhancing self-esteem: Increased self-esteem provides the patient with a sense of control and hope. This will help reduce anxiety and give the patient more time for problem solving and healing. Techniques to reinforce positive self-esteem include focusing on patient's positive traits and accomplishments, providing opportunities for the patient to demonstrate skills and abilities successfully, and emotional support and reassurance.

Expression of feelings: Providing an environment in which a patient can feel safe and comfortable to express emotions including crying or anger as well as verbalize disagreement, fears, disappointments is essential for both enhancing a therapeutic relationship and for allowing the patient to solve problems.

Role modeling: The nurse can exhibit more socially acceptable ways of performing a certain role or demonstrating a certain behavior. When the patient observes how effective these behaviors are, he or she can more easily understand how to use them and emulate the behaviors. For example, the nurse can communicate assertively to a family member who may be intimidating the patient. When the patient sees how that family member responds to assertive behavior, he or she may adopt that method of interaction. By eating healthy foods, not smoking, and exercising, the nurse also provides a role model for adopting a healthy lifestyle.

Role playing: Role playing is acting out other methods of response to a situation. It can be done to increase one's own or another's understanding of the other's point of view or to practice appropriate responses, such as assertiveness. This is done with a supportive person playing the part of someone you want to communicate with in a new way.

Stress management: Accepting stress as a fact of life and managing it using specific, tested techniques can reduce feelings of anxiety. The techniques are meant to promote a feeling of calm and a sense of control over the situation. Common stress management techniques include physical interventions, such as taking deep breaths, exercising, and avoiding caffeine, and psychological interventions, such as counting to 10, avoiding additional stressors, maintaining a positive attitude, and seeking out emotional support.

Assertiveness: Assertiveness is the use of behavioral techniques that allow the individual to stand up for his or her rights without infringing on the rights of others. To gain an expertise in using assertive behavior, role playing and practicing with others is useful. You may try role playing assertive responses to common situations in a supportive environment such as asking for a refund or telling a colleague that you are not satisfied with the quality of work performed.

Limit setting: Limit setting is a form of behavior modification rather than a punishment and is used for those times when accepting the patient's behavior is no longer appropriate. To set limits on behavior, you need to clearly define the desired behaviors and consequences for not conforming to them. Then you must be prepared to follow through with the stated consequences. By not using appropriate limits to control behavior, the patient's inappropriate behavior can escalate and possibly lead to injury and resentment from those who feel manipulated by the patient.

Deescalation: These techniques are also used to reduce anxiety and slow down the emotional response to it, such as aggressive behavior. Useful techniques include removing the patient from volatile situations, and using appropriate medication and physical restraints.

Confrontation: At times it will be necessary to make direct statements that challenge the patient's behavior or beliefs. Confrontation is a verbal message designed to help another recognize inconsistencies or inappropriate behavior. It can assist the patient in gaining insight. However, it can also be so threatening it could precipitate a crisis situation, so be sure to consult with specialists before using this method.

Cultural Considerations

INFLUENCE ON HEALTH BELIEFS

One's culture can significantly influence communication, particularly when the cultures of the nurse and patient are vastly different and not understood. *Culture* is defined as a configuration of learned behaviors that are shared and transmitted in a society and by a particular group of people. The values, beliefs, traditions, attitudes, and prejudices that each of us brings from our culture and past experiences influence all interactions with others. *Ethnocentrism* is defined as the belief that one's own cultural beliefs and healthcare practices are superior to those of other cultures. To provide quality care to all individuals, nurses must be sensitive to the patients' cultural differences.

Rather than stereotyping individuals into specific cultural classes, nurses should approach each patient as an individual who holds very personal attitudes, beliefs, and values that are influenced by his or her culture and environment. Keep the following points in mind to ensure that you remain sensitive to the cultural variations among your patients:

- Know your own attitudes, values, and beliefs.
- Be aware of your own ethnocentrism.
- Be aware of your own prejudices that may influence assessment.

- Maintain an open mind, and seek out more information about patients' culture, beliefs, and values.
- Communicate your interest about the patient's beliefs.
- Approach each patient as an individual. Avoid assuming people from one cultural background all hold the same beliefs.

Culture often influences what a patient believes about his or her illness, its causes, and when and from whom to seek care. Although you may not be able to be aware of the specific beliefs of every culture, having some general information about a culture of patients for whom you care for frequently is important. Incorporating some questions in the assessment on culture and observing for influences can help you become more familiar with these cultures. Questions to be included in the assessment may include "What do you believe caused your illness?" and "What other treatments have you pursued for the illness?" Recognize the impact of these beliefs on the patient's ability to accept the illness and his or her response to it. For example, in cultures that view the male as always being strong, even a mild illness could contribute to depression.

Be sensitive to each individual's belief, and design your care to incorporate these values. For example, in a culture where the oldest woman plays the pivotal role, the grandmother may be the one the patient consults on decisions about surgery, discharge planning, and follow-up care. She would need to be incorporated in the treatment plan for this patient to receive adequate care.

If a patient believes in folk healers or cures, don't ridicule or judge his beliefs. Rather, acknowledge the beliefs, and incorporate them in the treatment plan if possible. For example, if a Chinese patient is taking herbs to cure his diabetes, it is more beneficial to discuss the possible impact of these herbs on blood sugar rather than ignoring their use or forbidding the patient to use them.

Respect the role of the family. In some cultures, the family is responsible for protecting the patient, especially when the patient is the parent. In their role, family members may want to protect the patient from bad news. This may be contrary to your own belief in patient autonomy and may therefore lead to conflicts between the healthcare providers and the family. The patient must be in agreement with involving the family. Also be aware that in psychiatric settings, different approaches may be used in order to preserve patient autonomy and confidentiality.

Psychiatric professionals have recognized that some symptoms commonly seen in mental illness, such as delusions or hallucinations, could represent a culturally appropriate behavior. For example, being possessed by an evil spirit could be a delusion or a culturally sanctioned experience of an altered state of consciousness. Be careful not to judge individual cultural variations as psychopathology.

INFLUENCE ON COMMUNICATION

Verbal and nonverbal communication patterns are closely tied to cultural beliefs and practices. Eye contact, hand gestures, facial expressions, and personal space as well as how words or slang are used and what can be discussed are defined by our culture and environment.

For many people, *eye contact* indicates honesty, openness, and alertness. People in some cultures do not value eye contact and, in fact, even avoid it. For example, in Asian cultures eye contact is viewed as impolite and an invasion of privacy. It is especially inappropriate with authority figures, such as nurses. Judging a patient's response based on eye contact without understanding this point can lead to an invalid assessment finding.

Some nonverbal behaviors such as *facial expressions, hand gestures*, and *distance* vary among cultures. For example, it may be important to know that lack of facial expression in some Asian groups is not an indication of lack of feeling or that an Arab family member who stands very close is not threatening.

Addressing a patient, especially an elderly one, by his or her first name may suggest a lack of respect, or even seduction in many Asian and Latin cultures. And some patients may be extremely uncomfortable when asked intimate, highly personal questions, no matter how accepting and professional the nurse may be. If this information is vital to patient care, efforts need to be made to explain how it will be used.

Communicating With the Non-English-Speaking Patient

Caring for a patient who does not speak the same language as you can cause anxiety, frustration, fear, and a sense of helplessness. Or it may cause resentment because of the extra time and work that are needed. Some nurses try to compensate for their perceived deficiency by concentrating on performing tasks rather than on the patient's concerns. Although it usually isn't possible to learn the language of every potential patient, it would be beneficial to learn a language if a majority of the patients you care for speak it.

Use an interpreter as much as possible if you cannot speak the language. There may be a family member who can translate, and you may need to provide accommodations if this person needs to stay with the patient. When using a family member to translate, realize that because of the emotional ties to the patient, he or she may filter information before giving it to the patient. For example, if the family member does not want the patient to know about his or her condition, the interpreter may not relay the most accurate information to the patient. Using family as interpreters is probably best when basic communication is needed rather than when critical conversations are needed for diagnosis, treatment, and psychosocial assessments.

Check with your institution to see if an interpreter is available. The Civil Rights Act of 1964, the 1973 Rehabilitation Act, and the more recent Americans with Disabilities Act (ADA) have established the federal standards that ensure that communication does not interfere with equal access to health care for all people. Therefore, all healthcare institutions must establish systems for identifying available language interpreters, as well as interpreters trained in sign language, TDDs (telecommunication device for the deaf), closed-caption decoders for the televisions, and amplifiers on the phones.

Interpreters can be professional interpreters or employees of the institution who have other duties. If you are using employees, evaluate their abilities to understand the information you wish to have translated. If the interpreter has limited medical knowledge or knowledge of the patient, it may be difficult to ensure effective communication. In the home, family members and neighbors are usually the only resource unless nurses who speak their language are available. In addition to being aware of agency resources for interpreters, the nurse should become knowledgeable of key words that can be useful in assessing patients who speak another language.

When using an interpreter, keep the following points in mind:

- Address the patient directly rather than speaking to the interpreter. Maintain eye contact with the patient to ensure the patient's involvement.
- Avoid interrupting the patient and interpreter. At times their interaction may take longer because of the need to clarify, and descriptions may require more time due to dialect differences or the interpreter's awareness that the patient needs more preparation before being asked a particular question. Teach the interpreter to give you verbatim translations.
- Avoid using medical jargon that interpreter may not understand.
- Avoid talking or commenting to interpreter at length; the patient may feel left out and distrustful.
- Be aware that asking intimate or emotionally laden questions may be difficult for the patient as well as the interpreter. Lead up to these questions slowly. Always ask for permission to discuss these topics first, and prepare the interpreter for the content of the interview.
- If possible, allow the patient and interpreter to meet each other ahead of time to establish some rapport. If possible, try to use the same interpreter for succeeding interviews with the patient.

If an interpreter is not available, using picture charts or flash cards can help the patient communicate some basic needs such as degree of pain or needs for elimination. Some patients with limited English may tend to appear agreeable and nod yes even though they do not understand. Be sure to determine the patient's understanding by asking questions that require more than a yes or no answer.

4 NURSES' RESPONSES TO DIFFICULT PATIENT BEHAVIORS

LEARNING OBJECTIVES

▼ List qualities expected in a "good" patient.
▼ Describe how the concept of "difficult patient" reflects both the patient's behavior and the nurse's interpretation of that behavior.
▼ Identify the process of evaluating what patients may be communicating in difficult behavior.
▼ List types of nurses' responses that may impair awareness of the dynamics of patient problematic behavior.
▼ List resources available in most healthcare agencies for psychosocial support.

Nurses often see patients behaving at their worst because they are stressed and overwhelmed by their illness or hospitalization. And, often, these nurse-patient relationships change as the patient's healthcare needs change, requiring different types of involvement. Optimally, each nurse responds positively to every patient, but human nature makes that all but impossible. The next best strategy then is to learn the most effective ways to deal with those patients who are "difficult."

"Difficult patients" are usually defined by the amount of trouble and distress that the staff has in managing them. These patients often exhibit problem behaviors such as anger, regression, and out-of-control and/or manipulative behaviors (Fincannon, 1995). Nursing interventions may make the problem worse if the staff is unable to differentiate their responses to the behavior from their response to the person. If you think of these patients as having "difficult-to-care-for behaviors" rather than as "difficult patients," you may find that the staff's frustration decreases and more effective care strategies are identified. Sometimes these objectionable behaviors are used by the patient, with or without his or her awareness, to regain personal equilibrium and to reduce anxiety and fears and maintain control. Thus, while these behaviors may be causing stress for the staff, they are working just fine for the patient. Also, some patients are totally unaware that they are negatively affecting the staff. Once effective skills are learned to deal with these problem behaviors, the nurse may experience a sense of enhanced competence, and improved patient outcomes will follow.

Nurse-Patient Interactions

The nurse-patient interaction is based on the continuous flow of communication between the nurse and patient with input from both. The nurse's therapeutic use of self is the basic tool that enhances the interaction. Communication skills, an awareness of how personal responses can influence the patient, and a good knowledge base combine to enhance a positive nurse-patient interaction.

Difficult patient behaviors can negatively influence the nurse-patient interaction and, possibly, the quality of nursing care. Whenever a relationship is disrupted, the nurse needs to identify the source of the problem. Does it originate in the patient, in the nurse, in both? For example, a demanding patient who constantly rings the call bell may be communicating that she is afraid she will not recover and is seeking reassurance that someone will respond if she needs it. If the nurse interprets this to mean that the patient is communicating that she is doing her job poorly, she may become frustrated and angry. The nurse needs to objectively assess the situation to determine if the patient is truly looking for reassurance or if, because of the workload, the nurse is just not as tolerant as normal. Responding without assessing the situation could inhibit favorable nurse-patient interactions and negatively affect the patient's outcome.

To be effective, the nurse needs to treat the behaviors as symptoms and assess their cause. The nurse needs to explore her or his own attitudes and reactions that may be unwittingly initiating or perpetuating the undesired behavior. Better understanding can lead to a greater acceptance of both the patient's and nurse's feelings to create a more positive cycle of nurse-patient interactions. Compare in Table 4–1 how assessment and appropriate interventions can significantly alter patient outcomes.

Sometimes the only effective way to change a patient's behavior is for the nurse to change her or his response. If there is still no resolution of the situation, the nurse should seek the advice or interventions of other available resources to help understand the patient's behavior and the nurse's response to it and then select more effective interventions. If the patient continues manifesting difficult behaviors despite all efforts, the nurse should focus on self-awareness to remain objective.

Role Expectations

Clarifying the nurse's intertwining role expectations of patients in the sick role and oneself as the helper can provide a useful perspective. Keep in mind that nurses have chosen their roles as helpers but most patients have not deliberately chosen to become patients. A nurse may have chosen this profession for the personal satisfaction and

TABLE 4–1. **The Nursing Process With Difficult Patient Behaviors**

Assessment Step	Positive Cycle	Negative Cycle
Assessment	Nurse assesses patient's and her own understanding of what is happening. Nurse evaluates if she is stereotyping or reacting personally. Nurse gets assistance and support.	Patient does not explore issues. Patient responds only to surface level of communication. Patient reacts personally. Nurse complains to staff about patient.
Intervention	Nurse responds accurately and with empathy to patient.	Nurse avoids or rejects patient. Nurse is unable to control patient's behavior.
Patient outcome	Patient feels heard, accepted, and understood, resulting in less anxiety. Difficult behavior decreases. Patient can participate more fully in health care.	Patient feels alienated with escalation of undesirable behaviors. Potential exists for negative health outcome.

self-esteem resulting from attaining a high level of expertise. The patient, on the other hand, may feel that his or her self-esteem is threatened by entering the healthcare system. The patient is expected to accommodate the routines and expectations of the others. Some patients cannot accept this new role and may revert to using dysfunctional behaviors.

Optimally, the "good" patient is consistently cooperative; complies with the nurse's instructions and agency rules; is pleasant, polite, and respectful; shows improvement; and appreciates the nurse's help. These perfect patients ensure that the nurse meets his or her own role expectations; that is, the nurse feels helpful, effective, and accepted and valued by both patients and colleagues. "Difficult" patients produce the opposite effect. The nurse can experience frustration, anxiety, incompetence, lowered self-esteem, and a sense of being out of control.

Nurses need to objectively evaluate some common myths about these role expectations. A prevalent one is that nurses can control their patients' behavior to conform to expectations. They cannot. They can encourage, suggest, negotiate, and set limits, but only in very rare situations—such as when a patient poses a threat of imminent danger to himself or herself or to the staff—can the nurse force a patient into expected behaviors. A nurse who believes that he or she can control a patient's behavior is creating a set-up for failure.

Many nurses believe that only certain feelings toward patients are acceptable. Since nurses are human, they respond with a whole range of human emotions, including empathy, sympathy, disgust, love, hate, and, possibly, even sexual feelings. Experiencing all feelings is acceptable. Displaying these feelings to patients may not be. The nurse must use professional judgment in determining which feelings would be helpful to display to the patient and which would not. Responding genuinely to the patient with realistic concern is usually appropriate. If the nurse determines it would not be appropriate to display other feelings, he or she may want to find suitable ways to express them. Often just acknowledging the feelings to a trusted colleague can be beneficial.

Once the nurse has learned to accept and tolerate a broader range of human responses within oneself, he or she will develop more tolerance for formerly forbidden feelings displayed by patients. The nurse will be less likely to blame or avoid patients who stir up disturbing feelings. Often, before engaging with patients to work on problems, the nurse needs to work with ways to accept and assimilate personal experiences. Throughout this book, common nurses' reactions are listed as a way to help the reader identify them.

The following recommendations are listed to assist nurses in maintaining professional distance yet remaining available to patients:

- Listen to hear what the patient is really asking. People have a need to be heard. When a patient tells a nurse about his or her concerns and problems, this person needs someone to listen and understand the feelings and suffering to feel less alone. The nurse may erroneously believe that he or she has to do something or give advice.

- Assess the patient's ability to use comments or receive information about more negative emotions like anger before sharing this with the patient. There is a risk of alienating the patient.
- At times it may be therapeutic to share even very negative feelings. This should be done in a calm, matter-of-fact tone without accusation. For example, when working with a very provocative patient, point out that this behavior elicits angry responses and pushes others away. The patient may not be aware of the cause and effect. Bringing it to his or her attention may lead to a fruitful discussion of the patient's true fears underlying the behavior as well as to developing a realization of why others often react negatively.
- If a nurse determines that, even with the advice of specialists, he or she would not be able to work with the patient without bias, then alternate arrangements for patient care need to be made.

Patient Issues

COVERT COMMUNICATION

Consciously or unconsciously, patients often communicate their real needs and wishes indirectly, possibly because they may not even be aware of their fears. When their communication is not analyzed, the nurse may select ineffective interventions because he or she is dealing only with what the patient said, not what is really meant. Once the real concerns are identified, more effective interventions can be used. For example, the noncompliant patient may be indirectly expressing fear, the need for more reassurance, or the need for more help. If fear is the underlying issue, then interventions directed to reassure the patient will be the most successful.

TRANSFERENCE

This is a common issue with difficult-to-care-for patients. Sometimes even without being aware of it, the patient transfers early childhood perceptions, feelings, and experiences onto people with whom he or she is currently interacting. The patient may take positive or negative experiences with parents, teachers, siblings, or other significant people in his or her life and connect them to the nurse if there are superficial or substantial similarities between them. This usually occurs on an unconscious level, but the patient then feels, expects, and responds as if the nurse were that other person. For example, if the patient sees the nurse as his loving but somewhat controlling mother, he may respond with dependence tinged with resentment along with magical expectations of the nurse's effectiveness, reflecting earlier responses to his mother. If the nurse is viewed as a hostile, attacking parent, the patient may be hostile and defensive as a self-protection.

Other examples of patient behaviors suggesting transference include a preoccupation with a particular nurse, a desire to be the nurse's only patient, jealousy if the nurse spends time with other patients, and recurrent attempts to provoke a specific emotion from the nurse. A common warning sign of transference is when a patient displays a strong reaction to a single staff member.

If you suspect that the patient is using transference, use the following guideline:

- Find out if the patient is responding in similar ways to other staff.
- Determine, if possible, whether the patient acts in similar ways to other individuals in his or her personal life.
- Ask other staff members to provide support for the patient and a more balanced viewpoint.
- Avoid increasing the patient's dependency on you.
- Consult with a supervisor or specialist to determine appropriateness of gently confronting the patient with these issues.
- Set limits on the patient's behavior. Do not allow the patient to obtain special privileges.
- Do not personalize any hostility.

Nursing Issues

Usually, not every nurse will have the same amount of difficulty dealing with a patient who displays problematic behaviors. Each nurse will respond to the behavior based on individual expectations of correct and proper patient behavior, prior experience with working with a particular type of patient behavior, and the degree of success he or she may have had in dealing with a similar situation. Personal value systems, coping mechanisms, styles of communication, conflicts, and "pet peeves" will also play a role. The following issues may contribute to a deteriorating nurse-patient relationship.

IDENTIFICATION

The nurse may identify with a patient because of similarities such as age, sex, and social interests and then superimpose his or her own conflicts, values, and expectations onto the patient. So when the nurse seems to be responding to the patient, he or she is actually responding to oneself. A classic example of identification is a young female nurse who is caring for a critically ill woman her own age. The nurse sees herself in the patient and begins feeling intense sadness for all the things she (the nurse) has not yet accomplished in life. The nurse may do things for the patient that she would want for herself regardless of the significance for this patient.

COUNTERTRANSFERENCE

Countertransference occurs when the nurse transfers significant positive or negative early childhood figures and conflicts onto the patient. This may present problems if the nurse does not recognize what is happening and, therefore, chooses interventions based on faulty assessment findings. For example, the nurse whose father physically abused her may find herself reacting with fear or rage toward a particular male patient and initially may not understand why. If she does not recognize what is triggering her response, she may conclude that the problem is with the patient's behavior rather than her response to the patient.

For both countertransference and identification, the nurse must identify both personal feelings and the patient's behavior, speech, or attitudes that contribute to the discomfort; the nurse must then discriminate whether the difficulty lies with the patient's behavior or stems from his or her distorted or exaggerated response to it. It is always important for the nurse to compare his or her own reaction to one's usual way of responding and question other nurses to determine whether they have a similar reaction to the patient. If other staff have not had the same reaction to the patient, the nurse may want to examine their own personal feelings more closely. The following behaviors may suggest that the nurse is using countertransference (Lewis and Levy, 1982):

- Repeatedly experiences affectionate feelings toward certain patients
- Experiences depressed or uneasy feelings during or after interactions with certain patients
- Permits or even encourages resistance in the form of acting out
- Persistently attempts to impress a patient
- Cultivates a patient's continued dependence on nurse
- Is sadistic or unnecessarily sharp with a particular patient
- Experiences a strong need to care for patient
- Experiences conscious satisfaction from patient's praise, appreciation, and evidence of affection
- Constantly argues with the patient
- Experiences sudden increase or decrease in interest in patient
- Instantly likes or dislikes patient
- Does not trust anyone else to care for patient
- Feels intimidated by or is angry with the patient

JUDGMENTAL ATTITUDE

Judging another's behavior by personal values can significantly influence the nurse-patient relationship. Patients can usually sense these attitudes and may withhold important information for fear of being judged. The nurse may be unable or even unwilling to refrain from judging immediately but needs to be aware of these attitudes to diminish their impact on the patient.

RESCUE FEELINGS

The nurse may believe that he or she is the only person who really understands the patient and will be the one to save or cure a patient. This usually involves some internal needs of the nurse that are often reinforced by the patient. Secrets and secret alliances may result. Keep in mind, however, that becoming a rescuer undermines the patient's responsibility for his or her own health care.

LOSING CREDIBILITY

Stating facts such as "85 percent of patients have no complications with this type of surgery" is very different from telling a patient that he or she will not have any problems with upcoming surgery. In this example, if problems do occur after the nurse has stated that they would not, he or she will lose credibility, and the patient may stop sharing further concerns because the patient no longer feels confident in the nurse's opinions or information. Reassurance should be based on proper information and facts. Being evasive or dishonest destroys credibility.

LABELING

Labeling or referring to the patient by his or her diagnosis, problem ("he's just a junkie"), or even room number diminishes the value of the person. Almost without realizing it, once a label is used, nurses will begin to focus on the label and place less value on the patient's underlying needs and feelings. Optimal patient care requires that those needs and feelings be recognized and honored.

Strategies for Survival

Some overall recommendations can help nurses to cope better with difficult patient behaviors. Table 4–2 offers some general guidelines for selecting effective interventions.

Personal survival strategies also need to include strategies to maintain objectivity and prevent burnout. These can include using relaxation and stress management techniques and assertiveness training, as well as developing a professional support group to share concerns and help with problem solving. Developing a sense of team cooperation also lessens the chances of a single nurse's being called upon to meet everyone's needs. Attending classes

TABLE 4–2. **Staff Responses to Difficult-to-Care-for Patients**

Staff Responses	Intervention
Feeling inadequate to respond effectively to patient's symptoms	Lower emotional reactivity.
Feeling angry when patient gets angry	Maintain objectivity.
Fear of the patient who exhibits bizarre or unpredictable behavior or the patient who is confused, psychotic, or exhibits other psychiatric symptoms	Provide staff education on identifying and handling patients.
Identifying with patients who are the same age or race or who share similar life experience	Use empathy rather than sympathy to protect self and yet not harm patient.
Frustrated because there is not enough time or energy to work with patient	Share workload evenly.
Concern over being manipulated by patient's demands	Schedule consistent staffing.
Labeling patients rather than their behavior in an attempt to achieve an emotional distance	Foster staff value system that precludes patient labeling.
Uncomfortable with certain personal topics related to family dynamics or personal history	Support staff through discussion and education.

Source: Reproduced with permission of Fincannon, JL: Analysis of Psychiatric Referrals and Interventions in an Oncology Population. Oncology Nursing Forum 22(1):87, 1995.

and reading about managing commonly seen difficult patient behaviors gives the nurse more effective tools as well.

Maintaining a satisfying personal life is also very important. Nurses tend give of themselves as much in their personal life as they do at work. To prevent becoming burned out, one needs to create a balance in life. Developing supportive relationships and participating in enjoyable activities can decrease the pressure to have patients behave in ways that meet personal needs. Adequate rest and exercise and good nutrition are also extremely important.

Identifying Psychosocial Resource Personnel

In addition to the nurse's own personal strategies, many times outside assistance is needed. A first step is to identify the sources of help that are available in one's agency. Depending on the institution, any or all the following may be available:

- Social workers
- Clinical nurse specialists, nurse managers, educators
- Psychiatric liaison staff
- Psychiatrists or psychologists, including those specializing in chemical dependency, rehabilitation, or pain
- Chaplains
- Psychotherapists or staff members from other agencies who are familiar with the patient and his or her problem and previous treatment

Mental Health Consultation

At times agencies request outside consultation from mental health professionals for staff support and education, management of a crisis such as patient suicide, problem solving for difficult patient behaviors, or improving workplace communications. The consultant may be a mental health clinical nurse specialist, psychologist, psychiatrist, or social worker with consultation experience. This specialist needs to have experience and skill in providing consultation as well as some understanding of the type of problems the staff is encountering. The consultant may be from within or outside the agency. Staff attitudes can significantly influence whether this option can be used. Facilitative attitudes encourage use of these resources. These include:

- Feeling comfortable identifying problem areas and learning needs

- Recognizing that requesting assistance for areas outside personal knowledge or expertise is a sign of strength, not of weakness, and is necessary for professional development
- Approaching use of consultant as a resource and role model
- Anticipating the opportunity to gain insight

Hindering attitudes discourage or prevent use of resources. These include:

- Fearing exposure of inadequacies or embarrassment about not having all the answers
- Underestimating the specialized skill or knowledge needed to work with patients' problems
- Viewing patients' difficult-to-manage behaviors as deliberate or willful
- Calling the consultant too late and then challenging him or her to "fix" everything
- Harboring a prejudice against or fear of psychiatry
- Not maintaining confidentiality of group process

If the staff is meeting with the consultant as a group, the group leader will usually establish the ground rules for staff participation at the first meeting. If multiple sessions are planned, it will be necessary for all involved staff members to make a commitment to attend all the sessions. The administration needs to ensure adequate resources for coverage to ensure patient safety and reduce the level of staff discomfort about leaving their patients to attend the meetings. All members need to be aware of the objectives of these meetings. Hidden agendas, such as finding out who the troublemaker is, must be avoided.

Even though today's healthcare environment is facing tremendous economic pressures, mental health consultation has been recognized as providing a cost-effective way to enhance problem solving, reduce workplace stress, and, potentially, increase productivity. For example, staff anger that has been expressed by chronic lateness or increased sick time can be explored through consultation. This resource should therefore not be overlooked.

5 CRISIS INTERVENTION

LEARNING OBJECTIVES

▼ *Identify variables that influence response to a crisis.*
▼ *List interventions the nurse can use to reduce the impact of a crisis for a patient.*
▼ *Describe key questions to ask a patient experiencing a crisis.*

All people experience crises. Crisis is a state of disequilibrium resulting from a stressful event or perceived threat to self when usual coping mechanisms are ineffective and lead to the individual's experiencing increased anxiety. Nurses face patients and families in a crisis state as part of their daily routine.

It is impossible to predict what events will trigger a crisis in an individual. A diagnosis of serious illness, a breakup of a relationship, or a minor car accident may cause a crisis situation for one person but not another. Certain events, such as the death of a spouse, trigger a crisis in everyone.

Many factors influence how an individual responds to a specific situation and whether or not a crisis will ensue. Unresolved losses, coping with other stressful events at the same time, or being excessively tired or in pain, which may reduce one's ability to cope, increases the risk of viewing the situation as a crisis. Personal issues, such as low self-esteem, difficulty with anger, or need to control, may also cause an event to become a crisis in a vulnerable individual.

With or without intervention, a crisis will usually resolve in 4 to 6 weeks because it is much too difficult for the individual to maintain the high level of tension and distress. The person either develops some types of coping mechanisms to get through the situation, changes the goal, or redefines the problem.

A crisis represents both danger and opportunity. A person is at risk for emotional breakdown, but the period of vulnerability can also stimulate personal growth and strength. Crisis intervention is short-term active support that focuses on immediate problem solving and reestablishing emotional equilibrium can facilitate a positive and adaptive resolution.

Nurses' Reactions to a Patient Crisis

The way a nurse responds to a patient in crisis is about as varied as the way the individual will respond. Those factors that influence the patient's response will also influence the nurse's. Some common responses may be:

Feeling anxious or unsure about how to proceed

Becoming overinvolved and attempting to take over for the patient, possibly causing the patient to become dependent on the nurse

Viewing the patient's crisis as insignificant

Taking on some of the patient's anxiety

Setting unrealistic expectations or goals

Assessment

Aguilera (1994) identified three factors to determine the development of a crisis. They include:

Perception of the event: Successful resolution is more likely if the stressor is seen in a realistic, rather than in a distorted, way. For example, two students may get a C grade on an examination. One student may see this as an indication of the need to study harder and may realize that it is only a part of the final picture for the school year. The other student may view the grade as a personal failure, reflecting his low self-esteem and feelings of worthlessness.

Situational support: Lack of available resources or personal support systems added to the specific situation could be the factor that exacerbates a situation into a crisis. In contrast, having someone to turn to to vent grief or frustration can increase one's ability to cope.

Adequate coping mechanisms: Having proven mechanisms to deal with anxiety can prevent the situation's escalating into a crisis. If the individual has never used effective coping mechanisms or the mechanisms are not currently available, the situation could escalate into a crisis. For example, an individual who uses smoking or running as a mechanism to reduce stress may have a crisis response to being hospitalized in an intensive care unit because he will not be able to smoke or run.

To effectively assess the patient's response, follow these guidelines for conducting a crisis interview:

- Identify the precipitating event and determine its meaning.
  - What has happened in the past few days or hours?
  - If the patient describes an ongoing problem, what is

different today than yesterday about the problem? Be specific.
- What does the event mean to the patient?
- What is the patient most worried about in relation to the event?
- What are some of the consequences of the event?
- Does the patient see this event as influencing his or her future?
- Evaluate the patient's support system.
  - With whom does the patient have a close relationship?
  - To whom does the patient talk to when he or she has a problem?
  - Are these people available now?
  - Have these resources helped in the past?
  - Whom does the patient trust?
  - Are any other resources available in the patient's life such as a clergy member or a counselor?
- Evaluate previously used effective coping mechanisms.
  - What does the patient normally do to cope with stress?
  - What has he or she done now to cope with this situation?
  - If this hasn't helped, does the patient have any idea why not?
  - What has helped in the past in similar situations?

INTERVENTIONS

Crisis intervention is short-term problem-oriented support that ideally allows the individual to advance to a higher level of functioning as he or she develops new insights, strengths, and coping mechanisms. At the minimum the individual will return to the precrisis level of functioning. The crisis is considered unresolved if the person functions at a lower level after the crisis, for example, by his or her abusing substances, communicating ineffectively with family or loved ones, or exhibiting signs of depression or psychosis.

When facing a crisis situation, consider the following interventions:

- Make an accurate assessment of the precipitating event, the patient's perception of the event, and the available support systems and coping mechanisms. Also assess the patient's safety.
- Provide only small amounts of information at a time, and be prepared to repeat the information several times. Focus on concrete actions rather than vague ones.
- Communicate in a supportive, nonjudgmental way. Use gentle physical contact, as appropriate. Calming hand gestures, a calm voice, and an unhurried manner will help.
- Assist the patient to confront the reality of the event. This should be done slowly at first, such as gently bringing the patient back to a discussion of the car accident. More concrete, specific wording may be needed. This process may need to be repeated.
- Help the patient focus on one "here-and-now" problem at a time rather than jumping from one possible problem to another. For example, a patient who is frantic about his continuing pain may begin thinking about what will happen if the pain never stops. This will only escalate his anxiety. Rather, help him stay focused on dealing with the pain he is having now.
- In some situations, you may need to direct the person as to what to do next. His or her ability to make even the smallest decision may be compromised due to the overwhelming anxiety the crisis is producing.
- Encourage the patient to express his or her emotions in a socially acceptable manner.
- Assist with problem solving. This may include brainstorming all possible options and helping the patient narrow these down to the ones that can be used now. Focus on one or two possible options to give the patient a sense of control without overwhelming him or her with multiple options.
- Encourage the people in the patient's support system to become involved. Be sure to obtain the patient's permission before notifying family and friends to ensure that the patient maintains control of the situation. Be creative in identifying sources of support.

- Reinforce the patient's self-esteem by acknowledging how difficult the situation is and saying that you understand he or she is doing as best as possible to cope with it. Provide positive feedback.
- Reinforce effective coping mechanism such as deep breathing, exercising, or making prioritized lists.
- Identify other resources in the agency that could provide assistance. Avoid being the only staff member assisting this patient.
- Assess the need for medications to reduce anxiety.

Occasionally, a patient's response to a crisis requires more intense intervention including psychiatric treatment and/or hospitalization. The nurse needs to recognize signs of patient decompensation that go beyond the usual symptoms of a crisis. For example, suicidal behavior, evidence of psychotic thinking, or violent behavior that could endanger others needs to be identified and resources for intervention obtained. If these signs occur, be sure to obtain a consultation for specialized assistance.

LEGAL AND ETHICAL ISSUES

LEARNING OBJECTIVES

▼ *Describe the nurse's role in ensuring patient's rights.*
▼ *Discuss the impact of the Patient Self-Determination Act on patient care.*
▼ *Differentiate between the principle of double effect and euthanasia.*
▼ *List the steps in resolving an ethical dilemma.*

It is a nursing responsibility to safeguard the well-being of people entrusted to his or her care. Both legal mandates and ethical principles guide the nurse to determine the best way to meet this responsibility. Laws provide the mandates of acceptable social action and generally reflect the personal and professional values of society. Ethics provides a set of values that determines how to best conduct ourselves. Ethical principles that help guide our thinking and decision making include:

- *Autonomy:* The ability to choose for one's self and the freedom to act on that choice. To make an autonomous decision, the following components must be in place: adequate information, comprehension of risks and benefits of action, capacity to make a decision, and voluntariness.
- *Beneficence:* The responsibility to do good for the benefit of others.
- *Nonmaleficence:* The responsibility to never intentionally harm an individual and to protect those unable to protect themselves.
- *Justice:* Treating individuals equally and fairly.
- *Principle of double effect:* Using interventions that may indirectly, unintentionally, or unknowingly produce harmful effects such as administering needed pain medications to a dying patient, which will actually shorten his or her life.

Each individual brings personal ethical values, developed through individual life experiences, to every situation. Because there is no right or wrong when it comes to ethics, the nurse will be confronted with patients and colleagues who have conflicting values. The nurse can easily become confused or distressed unless one has formulated a foundation of personal beliefs and can maintain an open attitude toward others' beliefs.

Since state legal systems vary, it is important to know the laws of the state in which you practice. It is not uncommon to experience confusion between the law and one's personal ethical beliefs, so it is important to be aware of the difference. Sometimes, the nurse may feel bound to act on ethical grounds that could conflict with the law, but remember that one must comply with the law regardless of personal ethical beliefs. The nurse then has the right to work within the confines of the legal system to attempt to make changes to laws preceived as unjust or harmful to patients.

Patients' Rights

Nowhere do legal and ethical issues collide more than in the area of patients' rights. When the patient's expressed wishes contradict laws or what the nurse or other health team members view as the best treatment for the patient, dilemmas are created.

In 1972, the American Hospital Association adopted basic rights for patients in acute care hospitals. These are posted in most hospitals and healthcare agencies and provide guidelines for what patients can expect. The Joint Commission on Accreditation for Healthcare Organizations (JCAHO) also establishes general standards on patient rights. Any healthcare agency that seeks accreditation has minimum requirements for patients' rights they must meet. The 1995 JCAHO standards placed patients' rights in the first chapter, reflecting their perception of the importance of patient rights. The healthcare agency needs to respect the rights of patients, recognize that each patient is an individual with unique healthcare needs, and because of the importance of respecting each patient's personal dignity, provide considerate, respectful care focused on the patient's individual needs.

Federal and state laws guarantee the right of citizens to receive treatment by the least restrictive means, the right to prompt medical care and treatment, the right to be free of hazardous procedures, and the right to dignity, privacy, and humane care.

Patients with mental illness are guaranteed these same rights. Every state has enacted laws for the care and treatment of the mentally ill. Trends have been for greater emphasis on humane care and respect for individual civil rights. Most states have at least two types of in-patient psychiatric admissions including:

Voluntary: This is a patient in need of psychiatric treatment who is able and willing to consent for treatment.

In addition, the voluntary patient must be released on his or her request.

Involuntary: When a patient is a danger to himself or herself or to others or is completely unable to provide self-care, this person can be admitted to a psychiatric facility against his or her will.

Some variation of this policy exists in all states. Most states describe how long the patient can be held against his or her will. Even though someone is being held involuntarily, he or she still retains basic rights to dignity, privacy, and humane care. Mental illness is not equivalent to incompetence. The right to informed consent is also retained unless the person has been declared legally incompetent through a formal legal proceeding. If declared incompetent, then a court-appointed guardian gives consent.

INFORMED CONSENT

Informed consent is a freely made decision made by the patient or his or her legally authorized representative after full knowledge and understanding of risks, benefits, and available options about various treatment alternatives are obtained. Informed consent is based on the individual's right of self-determination. For any consent to be legal, it must be informed. It is required for any intentional touching of another. Without this consent or authorization, the person who touches can be charged with battery. Many procedures the nurse performs on a patient incorporate implied consent rather than a formal, written one. For example, when the nurse approaches a patient to take a blood pressure and the patient extends his or her arm, it is implied that he or she consents to the procedure. It is prudent to obtain a patient's consent before initiating any medical procedure. To ensure that the patient is able to give informed consent, he or she should be told the nature of the procedure, the burdens and benefits of the procedure, whether any alternative options exist, the probability that the proposed procedure will be successful, and the risks of not having the procedure.

When the patient is admitted to the hospital, he or she signs a general consent agreeing to receive routine care, services, and procedures. Any procedure beyond routine care for which there is more risk requires an additional signed informed consent. It is the physician's responsibility to provide the necessary information to the patient. Though the nurse can witness the patient's signature for consent and verify his or her understanding, the nurse cannot be the one to give the information. The patient has the right at any time to revoke consent either verbally or in writing.

If a patient is unable to give consent because of impaired cognition, consent is usually obtained from the patient's immediate family. Although this may not be legally binding, the physician generally finds this a prudent action. The physician may also seek out another physician to document why the procedure is needed. Only if the family member or significant other is the legal surrogate decision maker as identified by the durable power of attorney for healthcare can others give legal consent for the adult patient.

In an emergency where the patient is in a life-threatening situation, consent to treat is implied. Healthcare professionals are obligated to treat in an emergency.

COMPETENCY

Competency is a legal determination that a person is capable of sound decision making and management of his or her own life circumstances. This can only be done by a court of law. Mental capacity is the ability to reason without any signs of mental illness that could cloud the patient's judgment. This can be determined by a psychiatrist. Because competency is defined by law, psychiatrists or other physicians do not have the authority to determine it.

CONFIDENTIALITY

The right to privacy is a basic civil right that has implications for healthcare workers. All patients have the right to expect that information about them and their condition be shared only with appropriate people involved in the patients' care. Nurses have a legal duty to control indiscreet conversations in which privileged information could be overheard by others. The nurse has a legal duty to not disclose information about the patient without his or her consent to anyone who is not involved in the patient's care. Documentation needs to be protected in the same way.

USE OF RESTRAINTS

The decision to use restraints must be made with great care because restraints restrict the patient's rights and have in the past occasionally led to the neglect or abuse of patients. When a patient is in danger of imminently harming himself or herself or others, the least restrictive measures must be used first, and only if these fail are more restrictive measures considered. State laws and JCAHO have established standards for applying restraints and monitoring patients on whom they are used. Every healthcare organization will have specific policies on the nurse's responsibility, and these policies must be closely followed. See Chapter 8, specifically the section on aggressive and violent behavior, for more information on restraint use. When restraints are being considered, an ethical dilemma arises—violate the patient's rights (autonomy) or ensure the patient's safety (beneficence).

PATIENT SELF-DETERMINATION

The Patient Self-Determination Act (PSDA) went into effect in 1991 to ensure that patients in all healthcare agencies receiving Medicare and Medicaid funding are given adequate information on their right to accept or refuse medical treatment. In addition, the patient must be asked if he or she has an advance directive. If not, the patient must be provided with information on how to obtain one if he or she so wishes.

ADVANCE DIRECTIVES

An advance directive is a legal document that allows a person to state wishes about the direction of future medical care or designate another person to make medical decisions. It can include living wills, durable power of attorney, or similar documents. Though the format varies in each state, all 50 states have passed laws implementing some form of advance directive. Most often advance directives are used to determine care when decisions about resuscitation and aggressiveness of treatment in a critically or terminally ill individual must be made when the patient is no longer able to speak for himself or herself.

All healthcare professionals have an obligation to ensure that the patient's wishes are being honored. The nurse needs to intervene on the patient's behalf whenever there is doubt. Discussing the issues with the patient, patient's family, attending physician, and agency resources on resolving ethical dilemmas must be instituted if it is felt that the patient's wishes are not being followed.

END-OF-LIFE DECISIONS

Because the nurse is often the closest professional to the patient, he or she has an important role in participating in decisions regarding aggressiveness of care in critically ill and terminally ill patients. Issues that must be faced may include decisions to discontinue life support or other life-sustaining therapies such as hydration, artificial nutrition, and antibiotics. The nurse as patient advocate needs to be aware of the patient's wishes. This can be obtained directly from the patient or his or her advance directive, if available. If the patient is unable to communicate his or her wishes and has no advance directive, then the family member closest to the patient must be involved in determining what the patient would want. A surrogate decision maker, an individual designated by the patient to make decisions for him or her in the event of his or her being no longer able to do so, can also make these decisions. If no one is available to speak for the patient, the physician needs to determine what is appropriate medical care. In addition, agency policies and state laws will provide guidance on potential actions. Recent legal precedents (including Cruzan, 1990) have affirmed the right of competent adults to refuse treatments that will prolong their life, including artificial nutrition and hydration.

In addition to decisions to withdraw treatment, the nurse may be faced with decisions on administering adequate analgesics to a dying patient in pain even if administering these could hasten death. This practice differs from euthanasia, which is the deliberate action by an individual to end a patient's life at the patient's request. Administering analgesics or sedatives to the dying is generally justified under the ethical principle of double effect as long as the nurse's motivation is relief of symptoms rather than hastening death (see Table 6–1, What Does Not Constitute Euthanasia). If the nurse does not understand this difference, she may allow symptoms to go undertreated, and patients may suffer unnecessarily. The American Nurses' Association (1992) has established position statements to provide guidance for nurses on end-of-life decisions. Nurses can obtain copies of these statements by calling the American Nurses Association. These statements provide support for nurses by clarifying their roles in caring of these patients. If the nurse remains unsure or uncomfortable with decisions being made, he or she needs to seek out support from colleagues, supervisors, and clinical nurse specialists, as well as other representatives from the agency ethics resources. If the nurse remains uncomfortable, he or she needs to continue providing care to the patient until other staff can be identified to take over the patient's care. This will ensure that the patient's wishes will be carried out.

Nursing may also be faced with a patient who is suffering and verbalizes the wish to commit suicide to end the suffering. This nurse may be in sympathy with the patient but must follow the legal mandate to prevent suicide. This can create a dilemma for some nurses.

TABLE 6–1. **What Does Not Constitute Euthanasia**

- Giving a patient who is dying, hyposensitive, and in pain sufficient opioid to control pain (Principle of Double Effect)
- Giving a patient who is dying and dyspenic sufficient morphine to control symptoms (Principle of Double Effect)
- Sedating a patient who is symptomatic or distressed at his or her request (Principle of Autonomy)
- Withholding nutrition or hydration at the request of the patient who is dying (Principle of Autonomy)

Source: From Coyle, N: The euthanasia and physician-assisted suicide debate: Issues for nursing. Oncol Nurs Forum (Suppl) 19(7):41, 1992.

Ethical Dilemmas

All healthcare organizations must have policies in place to address and resolve ethical dilemmas. Many agencies will have formal ethics committees; however, such committees are not required. JCAHO requires all healthcare agencies to have a mechanism to address ethical issues, and nursing staff need to have access to this process. Nurses need to be aware of ethics-related policies and use the resources available to them. Steps in resolving ethical dilemmas include the following:

1. Determine what ethical principles are in conflict. Consider the burdens and benefits of each and possible courses of action.
2. Identify who the participants are, the appropriate history and background of their association with and knowledge of the patient, and their values.
3. Identify your feelings and personal values.
4. Identify applicable policies and laws.
5. Inform supervisors of dilemma, and seek their input to identify agency resources that may be of help. Such resources may include members of the agency ethics committee or consultants such as clergy, clinical nurse specialists, and social workers.
6. Coordinate a case conference with other team members and attending physician to discuss pertinent issues.
7. Arrange a formal ethics consultation with members of the healthcare team, the patient's family, and the patient if possible. Generally ethics committees and consultants provide guidance and support rather than definitive or binding decisions. Ethics consultation provides a supportive environment in which to share concerns and identify possible courses of action. Ethics committees often establish agency ethics policies as well.
8. Share the resolution with colleagues, and be aware of any feelings in you that may have been stirred up by the situation.

7 PROBLEMS WITH ANXIETY

The Anxious Patient

LEARNING OBJECTIVES

▼ *Differentiate among the cognitive, affective, behavioral, and physical symptoms of patients with anxiety.*

▼ *Use the different manifestations of anxiety to assess a patient experiencing anxiety.*

▼ *Select the most appropriate interventions for dealing with the patient with anxiety.*

▼ *Identify possible nurses' reactions to an anxious patient.*

Anxiety is the primary emotion from which most other emotions, such as anger, guilt, shame, and grief, are generated. The term *anxiety* conjures up images of people

Glossary

Anxiety—An unpleasant feeling of tension, apprehension, and uneasiness or a diffuse feeling of dread or unexplained discomfort; accompanied by physiologic, psychologic, and behavioral symptoms; serves as an early warning that alerts one to an impending real or symbolic threat to self, significant others, or way of life and motivates the individual to take corrective action to relieve the unpleasant feelings. The source of the anxiety is often nonspecific or unknown to the individual.

Panic—An attack of acute, intense, and overwhelming anxiety accompanied by a considerable degree of personality disorganization, such as being unable to think clearly or solve problems.

Panic attack—A sudden, unpredictable, intense episode of severe anxiety characterized by personality disorganization, a fear of losing one's mind, going crazy, being unable to control one's behavior; a sense of impending doom, helplessness, and being trapped.

Posttraumatic stress disorder—Anxiety and stress symptoms that occur after a massive traumatic event; often includes the feeling that the event is recurring.

Posttraumatic stress response—A persistent, disorganizing, and distressing reaction to a catastrophic event that affects the person's emotional, cognitive, and behavioral dimensions and relationships; extends beyond the time of the immediate crisis.

State anxiety—A transitory experience that varies in intensity, fluctuates over time, and tends to occur in relation to a specific situation anticipated in the future or currently happening.

Trait anxiety—A stable personality characteristic that predisposes some people to more frequent and intense anxiety in relation to stressful events.

pacing and wringing their hands with a pounding heart and rapid breathing when they are taking an important test in school or waiting to hear from their doctor about a biopsy. Words such as *worry, concern, fear*, and *uncertainty* are often associated with the term *anxiety*.

Anxiety can also have positive meaning, implying eagerness and readiness to face a challenge or perform some skill. Being mildly anxious can enhance experiences such as performing a piano recital or completing a term paper. Anxiety is a healthy response to novel and unique experiences. In fact, being mildly anxious helps you to perform at your best, as perceptual, emotional, and physiologic arousal can enhance learning, problem solving, satisfaction, and pleasure during and after an event. Just as pain serves as a cue and a response to potential or actual physical danger, anxiety can serve as a cue and response to emotional, social, or spiritual danger.

Anxiety is a universal experience. People vary significantly in their ability to manage feelings of anxiety and in their styles and patterns of coping with anxiety-producing situations. Knowing the meaning to the person of the subjective experience is essential in understanding how to intervene with a particular patient. For nursing treatment purposes, anxiety is categorized into four levels: mild, moderate, severe, and panic (see Table 7–1, Characteristics of Anxiety Levels).

Mild or moderate anxiety usually speeds up physiologic functions, whereas severe anxiety may slow them down. Prolonged panic can result in complete paralysis of functioning, in the extreme resulting in death. Anxiety can also be classified as normal or abnormal. Both are characterized by the same feelings and behaviors (uncertainties, helplessness, an intense sense of personal discomfort), and the level of anxiety may be equally intense.

Normal anxiety results from a realistic perception of danger and prepares the person for defense or change in face of the threat. Normal anxiety can be motivating and useful. Abnormal anxiety arises when the perception of danger is distorted, unrealistic, and out of proportion, resulting in maladaptive, defensive coping and inappropriate behavior.

TABLE 7–1. **Characteristics of Anxiety Levels**

Level	Characteristics
Mild	• Enhanced ability to deal with stressor • Heightened awareness, problem-solving abilities, increased attention to details • Increased curiosity, asks questions • Alert, confident • Logical thinking intact
Moderate	• Hesitation and procrastination • Narrowing of perceptual field • Selective inattention • Change in voice pitch; speech rate accelerates • Frequent change of topics • Repetitive questioning; joking • Increased respiratory rate, heart rate, palpitations • Muscle tension • Dry mouth • Changing body positions frequently; restlessness • Purposeless activity (wringing hands, pacing)
Severe	• Highly distorted perceptual and cognitive function • Fear of losing control • Inability to learn • Focus on small or scattered detail; inability to see connections between events • Selective inattention; inability to concentrate • Difficult and inappropriate verbalizations • Sense of impending doom • Sweating • Hyperventilation, tachycardia • Urinary frequency and urgency • Nausea • Headache, dizziness • Gross motor tremors, trembling, shaking • Purposeless activity (pacing, hand-wringing) • Numbness or tingling sensations • Dilated pupils
Panic	• Dyspnea; choking feeling; chest pain • Extreme discomfort; emotional pain • Unrealistic, distorted perception of situation • Disruption of visual field; distortion and enlargement of detail • Inability to speak; unintelligible communication; incoherent speech • Vomiting; incontinence • Feeling of personality disintegration • Fear of going crazy; fear of dying

Etiology

Theoretical approaches to anxiety are wide ranging. In the *biologic* perspective, anxiety is the uneasy feeling aroused by a threat or danger and is accompanied by a physiologic response. This response prepares the person for "fight or flight." The fight response (sympathetic stimulation) causes changes primarily in the cardiovascular and neuroendocrine systems. During the flight response (parasympathetic stimulation), as occurs in acute fear states, an effort is made to conserve body resources. Other evidence suggests a biologic basis for anxiety. For example, researchers have found that the metabolism of monamines and the function of the limbic system are central to the expression of emotions such as anxiety. Researchers have also discovered that benzodiazepines can reduce chronic anxiety and that sodium lactate can lessen the frequency and strength of panic attacks.

In Freudian *psychoanalytical theory*, anxiety represents a person's struggle with the demands and prohibitions in his or her environment, including the internal struggle among the person's instinctual drives (id), the realistic assessment of the possibility for need fulfillment (ego), and the conscience (superego). Anxiety is a signal from the ego that an unacceptable drive is pressing for conscious discharge. A conflict results between the drive, usually of a sexual or aggressive nature, and fear of punishment or disapproval. Phobias are fears that are disproportionate to the situation and cannot be explained or reasoned away. The significance and meaning of anxiety depend on the nature of the underlying conflict.

Interpersonal theorists believe that anxiety arises from experiences in relationships with significant others throughout a person's development. If a child is treated malevolently, the foundation is laid for the child to become insecure and to feel inferior and anxious in future situations. The child is forced to use coping strategies to allay anxiety; these then become part of the personality of the adult.

Learning-behavioral theorists explain anxiety as the result of a conditioning process in which a neutral stimulus has come to represent punishment, pain, or fear. The individual learns to reduce anxiety by avoiding a negative stimulus or by approaching a positive reinforcer. Extinction of behavior is a process of reducing response strength by nonreinforcement.

An eclectic understanding of anxiety, incorporating components of all these theories, is most helpful. Thus anxiety can be understood as experienced at conscious, unconscious, or preconscious levels. Sources of anxiety fall into two major categories:

Threats to biologic integrity: Actual or impending interference with basic human needs such as food, drink, shelter, warmth, safety, and health

Threats to self-security or self-esteem:
- Unmet expectations important to self-integrity
- Unmet needs for status and prestige
- Anticipated disapproval by significant others
- Inability to gain or reinforce self-respect or to gain recognition from others
- A severe, sudden, unexpected threat to sense of security, self-esteem, well-being
- Guilt or discrepancies between self-perception and actual behavior

Experiences with anxiety in early life lead to the development of coping behaviors, personality traits, and defense mechanisms intended to reduce anxiety and increase a sense of security. Over time, the person develops characteristic patterns of relief behaviors intended to provide comfort and protection in the face of anxiety. When these behaviors, traits, or mechanisms fail to relieve anxiety, the patient experiences intense emotional or physical discomfort.

Behavioral responses to anxiety can be constructive (problem solving, task oriented) or destructive (defensive, aggressive, violent). When anxiety levels exceed a person's adaptive coping abilities, maladaptive behaviors may develop. Disturbed coping mechanisms are characterized by the inability to make choices, conflict, repetition and rigidity, and alienation. Frustration and anxiety can lead to anger, hostility, and violence.

Anxiety often increases when a person expects one thing and is suddenly confronted with something very different. The same stressor may not always lead to anxiety or the same level of anxiety in everyone or in the same person at different times. Generally, the patient experiences anxiety as very painful and unbearable for any length of time. Behavior patterns used to cope with anxiety include:

Acting out: Converting anxiety into anger, which is either directly or indirectly expressed

Paralysis or retreating: Withdrawing or being immobilized by anxiety

Somatizing: Converting anxiety into physical symptoms, such as stomachache, headache

Avoidance: Evasive behaviors performed unconsciously to ward off or relieve anxiety before it is directly experienced (consuming alcoholic beverages, sleeping, keeping busy)

Constructive action: Using anxiety to learn and problem solve (set goals, learn new skills, seek information)

Syndromes of abnormal anxiety include:

Panic attacks (panic disorder): Acute, intense attacks of anxiety associated with extreme changes in physical and emotional behavior that can last from minutes to hours. Panic disorder is severely debilitating and characterized by sudden, intense, and discrete periods of anxiety and fear that may occur without warning in previously calm and untroubled individuals. Recent research points to physical and/or organic causes for some patients.

Posttraumatic stress syndrome (PTSD): The patient reexperiences the trauma of a prior traumatic event (rape, assault, military combat, floods, earthquakes, major car accidents, airplane crashes, bombings, torture). The syndrome is usually more severe and lasts longer when the cause is an artificial, rather than a natural, disaster. Three subtypes of PTSD are recognized:

○ *Acute:* Symptoms begin within 6 months of event and do not last longer than 6 months

○ *Chronic:* Symptoms last for 6 months or more

○ *Delayed:* Symptoms begin after a latency period of 6 months or more

Reexperiencing the trauma may include recurrent and intrusive recollections of the event, recurrent dreams or nightmares of the event, or sudden acting or feeling as if the event were recurring because of an association with an environmental or mental stimulus. Other behaviors and affect associated with the syndrome include decreased interest in usually significant activities, feelings of detachment or estrangement from others. Symptoms not present before the trauma include hyperalertness or exaggerated startle response, sleep disturbance, guilt about surviving while others died or about behavior required for survival, memory impairment, difficulty concentrating, avoidance of activities that arouse recollection of the event, or intensification of symptoms by exposure to events that symbolize or resemble the traumatic event.

Phobia (phobic state): A phobic reaction is an intense irrational fear response to an external object or situation. Unlike an anxiety reaction, where the anxiety is free-floating and the person cannot identify the cause or source, a phobia is a persistent fear of specific places, things, or situations. The major dynamic mechanism of phobic behavior is the displacement of the original anxiety from its real source and the symbolization of the stressor in the phobia (fear of sex becomes a fear of snakes).

The hallmark of phobias is that they are irrational and persist even though the person recognizes that they are irrational. The unconscious operations involved in the phobia help the person to control anxiety by providing a specific object to which to attach it. The phobic person can then control the intensity of the anxiety by avoiding the object and/or situation to which the anxiety has become attached. Some of the more common phobias include *claustrophobia* (fear of closed places), *agoraphobia* (fear of leaving home and/or fear of open spaces), *acrophobia* (fear of heights), *xenophobia* (fear of strangers), and *zoophobia* (fear of animals).

Related Clinical Concerns

Anxiety is perhaps the most common complaint in medical practice. Anxiety presents in many ways and with great variation in intensity and duration; therefore, treatment must be individualized and monitored very closely. Anxiety may be caused by or a consequence of many other medical and psychiatric problems such as cardiac and vascular disorders, sleep disorders, hyperthyroidism, depression with agitation, dementia, and delirium, hypochondriasis, schizophrenia, mania, and personality disorders such as obsessive compulsiveness. Some medications, caffeine intoxication, and withdrawal from alcohol or sedatives may cause anxiety. Physical illness or underlying major psychiatric syndromes must be considered and ruled out before treatment for anxiety is undertaken.

Lifespan Issues

CHILDHOOD

The anxiety most frequently experienced by children is separation anxiety. When separation from those to whom the child is attached occurs, excessive anxiety to the point of panic may occur. Onset may be as early as preschool age. The child may refuse to go to sleep or go to school. Physical symptoms, such as headache, stomachache, nausea, and vomiting are also common.

ELDERLY

Anxiety in the aged has not been systematically investigated. It is the consensus of clinical gerontologists that anxiety is a common response to the stresses of late life, including fear of dependency, illness and dying, and multiple losses of friends, home, or lifestyle. A long-standing disposition to excessive anxiety can persist into late life and usually does not diminish the ability to function in the patient who has adapted to it. Anxiety in the elderly may be the presenting symptom of a new illness, especially depression with agitation, or of early dementia or of a low-grade or chronic toxic state due to the consumption of drugs or alcohol.

Possible Nurses' Reactions

• May be apprehensive and even fearful about caring for patients experiencing severe anxiety or a panic attack. Such intense anxiety can be very contagious not only with staff but also with other patients.

- May try to determine the cause of the patient's anxiety and do what is possible to reassure and assist the patient to decrease it, then become frustrated when the patient's anxiety continues.
- May find the patient too strenuous to work with for more than a day at a time if anxiety does not subside as the nurse anticipates it should.
- May interpret the anxiety as a weakness in the patient who is seen as unable or unwilling to control it or may judge the anxiety to be part of a more serious psychologic problem and thus feel very uncomfortable caring for the patient.
- May prefer to keep the patient sedated.
- May feel resentment and even hostility toward anxious patients who require more attention and time than their physical conditions alone warrant.
- May want to avoid family or significant others who are also quite anxious and make unreasonable requests in a demanding or complaining manner. Most of these behaviors may be caused by the families' own frustration or apprehension in dealing with the patients' anxiety, and they are frequently unaware that their behavior is affecting the staff.

Assessment

Behavior and/or Appearance

See Table 7-1, Characteristics of Anxiety Levels.

Mood and/or Emotions

- Dread, fear, apprehension
- Lack of control or self-confidence
- Guilt
- Anger
- Grief
- Sense of imminent catastrophe

Thoughts, Beliefs, and Perceptions

- Narrowed focus of attention
- Inability to focus on reality

- Inability to learn or remember; forgetfulness
- Inability to reason or solve problems
- Difficulty concentrating; lack of awareness of environment
- Distorted perceptions

Relationships and Interactions

- Withdrawal and isolation; avoidance behaviors
- Demanding, complaining, quarreling; attention-seeking behavior
- Defensive; uses denial
- Tense, strained relationships; others frustrated over dealing with patient's anxiety and maladaptive coping

Physical Responses

See Table 7–1, Characteristics of Anxiety Levels.

Pertinent History

- Medical conditions that present with anxiety as a symptom such as thyroid, pituitary, and adrenocortical disorders, hypoglycemia, and an impending heart attack
- Amphetamine usage
- Synergistic or idiosyncratic drug reactions
- Alcohol or sedative withdrawal
- Cerebral vascular disorders
- Pancreatic disorder
- Sequelae to head injury
- Chronic anxiety
- Recent loss of loved one or significant object; work; finances; or self-esteem
- Phobic behavior
- Recent reexposure to anxiety-causing situation

Collaborative Management

Pharmacologic

Benzodiazepines are the medications most commonly prescribed for treating most types of anxiety, including short-term (situational) anxiety, long-term (trait) anxiety, and especially panic attacks. Unfortunately, because they are so efficacious and safe, these medications are often prescribed without full appreciation of their potential problems (see Chapter 20, Pharmacology).

Psychologic Treatments

Anxiety may be treated by therapeutic modalities such as guided imagery and muscle relaxation, exercise and rest programs, and music and art therapy as adjuncts to medication or alone. All mental health disciplines, psychiatric mental health nurses, psychiatric social workers, psychologists, and psychiatrists may use these interventions.

Nursing Management

ANXIETY MANIFESTED BY TENSION, DISTRESS, UNCERTAINTY RELATED TO THREAT TO HEALTH, SELF-CONCEPT AND LIFESTYLE.

Patient Outcomes

- Demonstrates decreased level of anxiety
- Reports feeling less anxious after using coping strategies
- Uses coping strategies effectively when anxiety is recognized
- Demonstrates increased ability to prevent episodes of anxiety by problem solving

Interventions

- Speak in a calm, quiet voice; convey a sense of confidence and control and a tolerant, understanding attitude.
- Place patient in quiet environment; reduce distracting stimuli such as noise, activity, and light.
- Use discretion in conversation with patient and near patient's room.
- Reduce demands placed on patient until anxiety is reduced. Provide rest periods between tests, activities, and visitors.
- Provide diversional activity and exercise. Monitor changes in level of activity.
- Allow others who provide support for the patient, such as clergy, social workers, or volunteers, to visit patient.

As appropriate, explain tests and equipment to them so they can in turn be more relaxed around patient. Be careful to ensure patient privacy.

- Provide realistic feedback about patient's situation. Do not give false reassurances. Help patient understand the anxiety by having him or her name the feeling.
- Encourage patient to express feelings. Remember that sometimes crying and being angry are appropriate.
- Have patient identify what happened just before the anxiety started, and try to identify the causative event. Discuss the possible connection between the precipitating event and the meaning it has for the patient.
- Determine patient's usual coping mechanism in similar situations.
- Encourage the patient to recall and think through similar instances of anxiety. What alternative behaviors could be used to cope more adaptively.
- Attempt to discuss what patient understands as cause of anxiety or panic once the anxiety level is reduced.
- Stay with patient, but do not require explanations for the distress. Individuals experiencing severe or panic-level anxiety may become more agitated by attempts to communicate with them.
- Provide physical measures to relieve anxiety, as appropriate, such as a warm bath, back rub, or walk. Discuss other techniques for reducing anxiety when patient is calmer and more rested, for example, relaxation exercises and stress-reduction techniques. Encourage slow, deep breathing if patient is hyperventilating. Breathing with patient to the set pattern may be helpful.
- Assist the patient in learning and problem solving when anxiety is diminished enough to allow concentration.
- Evaluate the need for antianxiety medications. Antianxiety medications can be very effective in relieving panic. If none are ordered, consult with physician for appropriate pharmacologic therapy.
- Assess for potential injury or violence to self or others.
- Provide feedback about patient's current coping ability, and reinforce any attempts to cope adaptively.
- Refer the patient with recurrent anxiety and maladaptive coping mechanisms for further psychiatric or psychologic evaluation and treatment.

- For patients with panic-level anxiety:
  - Take patient to a quiet area with minimal stimuli.
  - Administer ordered antianxiety medications as needed. Ask what medications patient has used in past.
  - Remain with patient through the attack.
  - Give patient clear, honest feedback: "You are having a panic attack; I will stay with you."

INEFFECTIVE INDIVIDUAL COPING EVIDENCED BY ANXIETY, FEAR, AVOIDANCE OF OBJECTS OR EVENTS, IRRATIONAL THOUGHTS RELATED TO PHOBIAS, EXTREME GUILT.

Patient Outcomes

- Demonstrate increased ability to think rationally and without undue guilt.
- Identify thoughts and/or situations that evoke anxiety.
- Show decreased anxiety related to improved thought processes and problem solving.
- Demonstrate appropriate coping strategy for reducing anxiety related to phobia.

Interventions

- Realize that phobic reactions are irrational and are not changed by rational, logical explanations. Adapt your care to avoid anxiety-producing events. For instance, do not require a claustrophobic patient to use an elevator.
- Promote communication that reinforces rational thinking and decreases guilt.
- Verify your interpretation of what patient is experiencing. For instance, you might say, "I understand that you are afraid to go to the radiology department."
- Use words familiar to patient when describing new events or expectations.
- Assist patient to clarify thoughts and avoid misinterpretation by asking the meaning of anything he or she says that you do not understand.
- Do not talk around or whisper near patient. Include the patient in conversation, and check that he or she heard what you actually said by asking him or her to repeat it.
- Set limits on discussing irrational material. Focus on topics based in reality that you can verify.
- Avoid belittling patient who misinterprets stimuli or is irrational.

- Assist patient to set limits on own behavior; suggest alternative ways to cope with anxiety. For instance, you might suggest that he or she take a walk instead of crying.
- Be aware of the potential for violence. Observe for changes in behavior indicating increased anxiety, irrational thoughts, or any destructive behavior that requires attention.
- Anticipate difficulties in adjusting to return or transfer to home or other facility. Discuss any concerns with the family.
- Allow the patient to have some control in anxiety-provoking situation. Do not force the patient to do anything that seems to be extremely frightening to him or her.
- Provide the time to discuss anxieties and fears while continuing supportive verbal and behavioral interventions.
- If anxiety is not managed by preceding interventions, refer the patient with phobias to a psychiatrist, psychologist, psychiatric mental health nurse, or social worker for more specific treatment, such as desensitization or behavioral modification.

ALTERNATE NURSING DIAGNOSES

Altered comfort
Altered thought processes
Altered role performance
Fear
Noncompliance
Posttrauma response
Self-esteem disturbance
Sleep deprivation
Social isolation
Spiritual distress

WHEN TO CALL FOR HELP

✔ Increased anxiety leading to refusal of treatment or noncompliance
✔ Onset of paranoid psychotic thinking
✔ Onset of panic attack
✔ Staff conflict over management of patient behavior
✔ Increased staff anxiety over caring for patient

Patient and Family Education

- Teach patient and family anxiety-reducing exercises and/or activities such as muscle relaxation and guided imagery, or listening to music.
- Discuss with patient and family the causes and treatment of patient's anxiety.
- If patient is using antianxiety medications, review the need to monitor their use and potential problems when overused or discontinued without weaning.
- Provide written instruction where possible as patient may have limited retention.

Charting Tips

- Use objective assessment and nonjudgmental terms to describe behavior.
- Use patient's own words to describe amount and type of anxiety experienced.
- Note which interventions are most helpful in decreasing patient's anxiety and specific treatments that patient successfully learned to control own anxiety.
- Document family and/or significant others' responses to education about anxiety-reducing methods.
- Document use of antianxiety medications and patient's response to them.

Discharge Planning

- Discharge can be a particularly anxiety-provoking time for many patients. Begin discharge planning early and include all caretakers in planning for home care.
- Allow enough time to discuss alternatives, and provide as much emotional support as possible during the transition time.
- Discuss available community resources, their functions, services, and capabilities as well as their limitations.
- If transferring patient to another facility or agency for follow-up care, provide information about patient's progress and successful interventions for dealing with anxiety.
- Refer to a psychiatrist if patient has frequent panic attacks or chronic, moderate to severe anxiety.

- To ensure consistency, record and communicate to family responsible for patient after discharge those interventions that worked well.

Nursing Outcomes

- Staff caring for patient tolerates patient's anxiety and responds with support and understanding. Staff assists patient in understanding cause and reactions to anxiety.
- Staff assists patient in learning appropriate strategies for reducing anxiety.
- Treatment and care plan are carried out consistently.

Suggested Learning Activities

- Role-play managing a patient experiencing a panic attack.
- Share past experiences dealing with patient anxiety and "spread" of anxiety to other patients.
- Learn how to do muscle relaxation or guided imagery exercises to reduce and/or control your own anxiety.
- Attend support groups for patients with panic disorders or other phobias.
- Participate in a critical incident stress debriefing in which mental health professionals work with staff to work through feelings after a disaster like a plane crash or an earthquake.

8

PROBLEMS WITH ANGER

The Angry Patient

LEARNING OBJECTIVES

▼ *Identify three positive functions of anger.*
▼ *Identify possible nurses' reactions to an angry patient.*
▼ *Differentiate among assertive, passive, and hostile expressions of anger.*
▼ *Select the most appropriate interventions for dealing with an angry patient.*

Anger, a normal response to frustration, rejection, and fear, can cause difficulty in our lives, especially when we have been taught that it is unacceptable to feel angry, have learned to display our anger inappropriately, or have developed a sense of fear that the anger can lead to abandonment. However, learning to deal with anger is an ongoing process, and when we learn how to deal with our anger and others' anger appropriately, we can gain a positive feeling of control, a sense of power and energy, and increased self-esteem.

Anger can be viewed along a continuum. At one extreme is passive-aggressive behavior in which a person avoids direct, open expression of anger but finds hidden ways to express it. At the other extreme is aggressive expression in which a person inflicts pain on others when

---

Glossary

Anger—A state of emotional excitement and tension induced by intense displeasure, frustration, and/or anxiety in response to a perceived threat.

Rational anger—Anger expressed in a direct, socially acceptable manner.

Assertiveness—Behavior directed toward claiming one's rights without denying the rights of others.

Assertiveness training—Learning behavioral techniques that allow an individual to stand up for his or her own rights without infringing on the rights of others.

Frustration—Feelings generated from the inability to meet a goal.

Passive-aggressive—Behavior characterized by angry, hostile feelings that are expressed indirectly, leading to impaired communication and inappropriate expression. This behavior masks anger in such a way as to obstruct honesty in relationships. It may also be associated with obsessive-compulsive personality, borderline personality, and depression.

Hostility—Feelings of anger and resentment that are destructive.

he or she expresses anger. Rational anger falls in the middle. When anger is rational, feelings are expressed in a direct, socially acceptable manner that allows the person to gain some control over the threat without causing harm to others.

Etiology

No single theory can explain the complex emotion of anger. Most likely, an intertwining of biological, psychologic, and sociocultural factors create each individual's unique response.

Biologic theories of anger look at the physiologic tensions created by hormones, such as testosterone and estrogen, and neural transmitters, such as dopamine and serotonin, and other sources and the need to discharge these tensions in order to be healthy.

Psychologic theories look at the various dynamics and learned responses that cause anger. Children often use inappropriate anger responses, such as temper tantrums, to deal with frustration. Positive reinforcement for this behavior can cause inappropriate anger responses to continue into adulthood. When the child's caregivers are demanding, hypercritical, and punitive, the child may develop coping mechanisms aimed at avoiding directly expressing anger for fear of displeasing the caregiver and risking emotional abandonment or retaliation. These coping mechanisms often lead to a passive-aggressive anger response and resentment, which eventually erupt into inappropriate or destructive behavior. Anger can sometimes be a normal response to fear and help the person gain control of a perceived threat, or it can be part of the adaptive process in adjusting to a loss.

Sociocultural factors also play an important role in the way an individual expresses anger. Social groups, including families, often display common patterns in the degree of acceptance of expressed anger. For example, in some families yelling and aggressive confrontation are acceptable means of dealing with anger and conflict, while in others, any overt display of anger is not tolerated. While both of these styles may work within the individual families, they may not be the healthiest ways of dealing with anger.

Women are often socialized to deal with anger differently from men. They may tend to displace or suppress angry feelings and attempt to give in and compromise rather than deal with the conflict directly. This behavior can lead to passive-aggressive responses or resentment that may eventually become destructive. Such repression can also be detrimental and lead to misunderstanding when dealing with male colleagues.

Clinical Concerns

Medical conditions, such as chronic illness or loss of body function, may strain one's coping abilities and lead to an uncharacteristic display of anger.

Abuse of mind-altering substances may reduce inhibitions and negatively influence the anger response.

Lifespan Issues

CHILDHOOD

Children normally respond with anger when faced with frustration. When raised in an environment where intense anger and violence are accepted, they can develop overly aggressive anger response including cruelty to others and intolerance for frustration. Conversely, children who are taught that anger is unacceptable may tend to suppress or deny angry feelings and can develop extreme distress and guilt when faced with conflict. Children who learn appropriate ways to relieve tensions are more able to express anger rationally. Because children are vulnerable, they may be at increased risk of injury caused by inappropriate expressions of anger by caregivers.

ADULTS

Adults who must deal with difficult life experiences, such as a chronic illness or the onset of an acute illness compounding stressful life events, can become very angry. This anger can further complicate the disease by depleting coping skills and interfering with the recommended medical treatment.

ELDERLY

Uncharacteristic displays of anger in the elderly may be due to frustration caused by a variety of physical, mental, and lifestyle changes such as dementia, altered sensory function, altered mobility, changes in sleep-rest patterns, effects of medications, loss of loved ones, and fear of dying. Inappropriate behavior may cause the elderly to be alienated, further increasing their sense of fear, frustration, and possible confusion. Additionally, the vulnerable elderly are at risk of being victims of another's anger.

Possible Nurses' Reactions

- May take patient's anger personally, causing an unhealthy emotional response.
- May respond defensively by using an aggressive response or avoidance. This can accelerate the anger cycle.
- May attribute the patient's anger to a specific event, such as the quality of care provided, and respond by feeling unappreciated and resentful.
- May feel uncomfortable or fearful and respond by suppressing or denying the anger.
- May avoid confronting the patient for fear of emotional or physical pain.

Assessment

Behavior and/or Appearance

- Loud voice, change in pitch, or very soft voice, forcing other to strain to hear (see Table 8–1)
- Intense eye contact or avoidance of eye contact
- Rapid, pacing movement
- Ruminating about an issue
- Passive-aggressive behavior, possibly including sarcastic humor; chronic complaining; socially annoying habits; pseudocompliance (agreeing to do something but not doing it)
- Possible physical violence

TABLE 8–1. **Comparing Behavioral Responses to Anger**

Traits	Passive	Assertive	Aggressive
Speech content	Negative: "Can I, Should I" Puts self down	Positive: "I can, I will" "I" messages	Hostile: "You never . . . You always . . ." Derogatory
Voice	Whispers Whiny, weak	Firm, clear	Loud
Posture	Drooping	Erect, relaxed	Tense
Eye contact	Looks down	Appropriate	Invasive
Gestures	Fidgets	Appropriate	Threatening

Mood and/or Emotions

- Annoyance, discomfort, frustration, continuous state of tension
- May be quick to anger, then let it go or take time to "stew" before expressing anger
- Guilt
- Powerlessness
- Passive-aggressive emotional response possibly including being sullen, yet denying any concerns, or inappropriate cheerfulness for the situation.

Thoughts, Beliefs, and Perceptions

- May believe anger is normal and can be expressed without hurting others
- May take responsibility appropriately without blaming others
- May be angry at others but still care for them
- May lack ability to express true feelings
- May fear loss of love if anger is expressed directly
- May fear emotional or physical abandonment if anger is expressed
- May feel a sense of power when angry

Relationships and Interactions

- May communicate concerns clearly to avoid additional misunderstanding
- May avoid hostile or angry persons
- May be catered to by others who fear patient's anger

Physical Responses

- Fight-or-flight response during confrontations, possibly including rapid pulse, increased blood pressure, rapid breathing, muscle tension, sweating, or intense feelings of wanting to attack or run
- Episodes of headaches, depression, sleep alterations, pain, or gastrointestinal symptoms associated with repressed anger

Collaborative Management

Pharmacologic

Antianxiety medications, including benzodiazepines, are sometimes used for short-term relief of feelings of tension and anger, However, these should not be used as a substitute for acknowledging and dealing with anger, and they should not interfere with pharmocologic actions of medications being taken for the underlying medical condition.

Nursing Management

ANXIETY EVIDENCED BY TENSION, DISTRESS, UNCERTAINTY, RESTLESSNESS, OR DISPLEASURE RELATED TO THREAT TO SELF-CONCEPT, FRUSTRATION, OR UNCONSCIOUS CONFLICT.

Patient Outcomes

- Verbalizes concerns and frustrations directly at an appropriate time
- Demonstrates reduced tension including lowered voice and more appropriate anger response

- Demonstrates problem-solving skills when faced with frustration
- Demonstrates behaviors to calm self when faced with frustration

Interventions

- Use therapeutic communication techniques including open-ended questions, appropriate eye contact, and supportive gestures to encourage patient to vent feelings and concerns. Avoid providing solutions before the patient has a chance to relieve tensions.
- Listen with concern without being patronizing or condescending. Phrases such as "Tell me what happened next" or "That really sounds frustrating" allow the patient to feel accepted and understood. Avoid phrases that escalate feelings of powerlessness, such as "Calm down" or "It can't be that bad."
- If needed, direct the patient to a more private setting to express his or her feelings. Having others view the demonstration of anger can make it more difficult to back down and contribute to escalation of hostility or aggression.
- When the tension of the situation is reduced, focus on identifying and validating the problem, and explore options on how to deal with the problems more constructively. Ask the patient which methods he or she has used successfully in the past when dealing with frustration. Teach problem-solving skills. Assist the patient to identify and use more effective coping mechanisms.
- Teach tension-reducing techniques, such as deep-breathing, counting to 10, walking away, and talking to self about remaining in control.
- Encourage the patient to express angry feelings toward the appropriate person. Role playing before the confrontation may help the patient choose effective strategies.
- Recognize that an angry outburst may result from an accumulation of multiple stressors and cause the patient to overreact.
- If the patient is justifiably angry because of something you have done or not done, accept appropriate respon-

sibility. Work with the patient or colleagues to resolve the problem. Accepting and validating the patient's feelings sends the message that you value his or her viewpoint.
- Encourage children to vent frustration by redirecting their activity, such as hitting a pillow and engaging in exercise.

INEFFECTIVE INDIVIDUAL COPING EVIDENCED BY INAPPROPRIATE EXPRESSION OF ANGER, DISTRESS, DESTRUCTIVE BEHAVIOR TO SELF OR OTHERS, AND RELATED TO THREAT TO SELF-ESTEEM OR UNCONSCIOUS CONFLICT.

PATIENT OUTCOMES

- Able to identify personal strength that may help to reduce stress
- Accepts personal limits in dealing with inappropriate demands
- Demonstrates effective skills for dealing with frustration

Interventions

- Identify ways to increase the person's self-esteem as part of expressing anger by treating him or her respectfully and acknowledging his or her skills or attributes. For example, when dealing with an angry child's confrontation about his or her parent's care, state, "Your father is lucky to have you as his advocate." Avoid a defensive response or ignoring complaints.
- Convey a sense of trust in the patient's ability to respond appropriately to the stressor.
- Focus on the patient's strengths to deal with frustration. Help him or her identify which coping skills have been successful in the past.
- Teach the patient that anger is a normal response to loss. Some individuals are unable to accept this anger as normal and experience unneeded guilt.
- Encourage the patient to clearly state the cause of the problem to avoid erroneous assumptions.
- If the patient rejects or finds fault with all of your suggestions, place the responsibility for choosing the appropriate response on the patient. You might say, "We've

discussed many options. Now it is up to you to consider which one is best for you."
- Set clear limits on the patient's expressions of anger toward the staff. Refuse to listen to extensive complaining if the patient is not willing to participate in determining an acceptable solution.
- Be assertive when explaining which types of behavior are not appropriate.
- Be consistent with the demands the patient can set on the staff.
- Be a role model for expressing negative emotions in a positive manner. Use "I messages," such as "I feel angry" rather than accusing the other person, which makes them defensive. speak firmly without yelling, and avoid threatening gestures when confronting issues.

ALTERNATE NURSING DIAGNOSES

Impaired social interactions
Noncompliance
Violence, high risk for
Self-concept disturbance

WHEN TO CALL FOR HELP

✔ Increased aggressiveness; violent behavior, including damaging property; increasing use of abusive language, threats made to patients or staff
✔ Onset of paranoid thinking or psychotic behavior
✔ Onset of extreme obsessive-compulsive behavior
✔ Increased staff conflict over management of patient behavior
✔ Increased staff anxiety over caring for patient

Patient and Family Education

- Teach assertiveness skills by role modeling appropriate responses and helping the patient practice these skills.
- Review with the patient frequently encountered frustrations, and explain that giving up control of the outcome may be the most effective strategy for dealing with them.

- Review potential negative health effects of inappropriate anger expression.
- If the patient is using antianxiety medications, review the need to monitor their use, and avoid using them in place of trying to resolve the cause of anger.

Charting Tips

- Use objective, nonjudgmental terms to describe behavior.
- Document patient's response to frustration.
- Document limits set on care plan or treatment plan for consistency.
- Document use of antianxiety medications and patient's response to them.

Discharge Planning

- Communicate plan of care to all involved in discharge planning.
- Inform any appropriate agencies of patient behaviors to avoid miscommunication.
- Refer patient to counseling services or assertiveness training, if needed.
- Encourage patient's active participation in treatment plan.

Nursing Outcomes

- Staff caring for patient selects interventions that allow the patient to express rational anger.
- Treatment and care plan are carried out consistently.
- Staff responds to patient's demands with support and understanding.

Suggested Learning Activities

- Attend assertiveness training class.
- Role play assertive communication with colleagues.
- Share past experiences of dealing with anger.
- Attend class on conflict resolution.

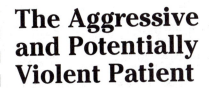

The Aggressive and Potentially Violent Patient

LEARNING OBJECTIVES

▼ *Identify factors that precipitate aggressive behavior.*
▼ *Describe effective techniques for verbal deescalation of aggressive behavior.*
▼ *List possible nursing staff reactions to violent behavior in patients.*
▼ *List interventions a nurse could use in working with a violent patient.*

It has been estimated that over half of healthcare professionals will be assaulted by a patient sometime in their career, probably reflecting the increase in aggression and violence in society (Blair and New, 1992). Nurses are especially at risk because they are often the ones working with patients most closely. Historically, nurses working with psychiatric patients have been taught to be alert to and manage violent, assaultive behavior; however, now nurses working in emergency departments, general hospitals, clinics, and nursing homes must be prepared to deal with it. Healthcare facilities must institute security measures to ensure the safety of staff and patients and to reduce the fear of impending violence among staff and visitors. Consistently being confronted with aggressive and potentially violent patients can cause excessive fear, stress, job dissatisfaction, lost work time, reduced staff morale, and possible injury.

Though studies linking violence and mental illness are inconsistent (Blair and New, 1991), previous violent behavior and a history of psychiatric illness, particularly

---

Glossary

Aggression—Any verbal or nonverbal, actual or attempted, forceful abuse of the self or another person or object.

Assaultive behavior—An intentional act that is designed to make another person fearful and produces harm.

Hostility—Anger that is destructive in nature and purpose as opposed to rational anger that is appropriate to the situation and is not destructive in intent.

Intimidation—The use of threats to frighten and control.

Rage—Engulfing emotional experience of extreme anger.

Violent behavior—Exertion of extreme force or destructive acts with intent to hurt another and which cause injury.

schizophrenia, paranoia, borderline personality disorder, personality disorders, and posttraumatic stress disorder remain the most frequent risk factors associated with predicting an aggressive outburst. Other major risk factors include drug and alcohol use. Studies show that young males are by far the most frequent perpetrators of violent acts.

The causes of the increased violence in our society and, consequently, in health care are varied and complex. Some of these causes include:

- Attitudinal changes in society with increased acceptance of violent response to authority figures
- Increased use of mind-altering alcohol and drugs
- Court decisions that give psychiatric patients the right to refuse treatment and/or medication
- Patients more likely to be treated as outpatients rather than inpatients
- Healthcare staff inadequately prepared to respond to aggression or who deny the risk of violence
- Increasing frustrations in healthcare settings including inadequate staffing and long waits
- Impersonal care, which may stress already frustrated patients
- Easy availability of firearms
- Media coverage of violence which triggers additional crimes

Using restraints to manage potentially violent patients can create ethical dilemmas for the nurse concerning patient autonomy, human dignity, and informed consent. In 1993, the Joint Commission on Accreditation of Health Care Organizations (JCAHO) created standards for physical restraints, requiring each agency to provide clear policies and education on appropriate restraint use. The aim is to reduce the incidence of injuries that can result from restraint use, such as loss of mobility, skin breakdown, and, possibly, death from strangulation. Before applying restraints, the patient must be carefully assessed and alternative measures must be exhausted. This is especially important in the elderly since they are particularly vulnerable to injury, increasing confusion, and paranoia.

Etiology

Aggressive, violent behavior has many causes. Most studies on the causes of aggression have been done on subjects with mental illness and/or prison populations, which may skew the results.

Biologic theories include genetics, which links chromosomal abnormalities to aggressive behavior, hormone imbalances, particularly testosterone, and neurotransmitter irregularities, specifically the abnormal secretions of dopamine and serotonin.

Psychologic theories on aggression are related to a person's view of the world as a source of anxiety. Individuals prone to violence often have low self-esteem and need to maintain control in order to enhance their own feelings of power and self-worth. Aggressive behavior temporarily reduces the anxiety and creates a temporary sense of power. In addition, individuals with poor impulse control or a personality disorder may use violence to intimidate others. Aggressive individuals may have limited ability to tolerate frustration and demand to have their needs met immediately. Individuals who have experienced emotional deprivation in childhood may be particularly vulnerable to responding with violent outbursts when they sense an attack on their self-esteem.

Social learning theory views aggression as a learned behavior. Individuals with a tendency toward aggressive, violent behavior may be more likely to respond to stressors such as illness, school or work pressures, or relationship problems with anger and hostility because they have learned that such behavior temporarily reduces their anxiety.

Sociocultural theories look at an aggressive individual's poor interpersonal skills. Exposure to aggression and violence as part of family life may also be a significantly influential factor. Children who are treated with violence may view violence as a normal way to deal with others. The cycle of family violence continues when children learn to use violence as their only coping mechanism instead of more socially acceptable ones. Poverty, deprivation, and hopelessness can also increase the risk of violent behavior.

Related Clinical Concerns

A wide variety of organic disorders may be associated with aggressive and violent behavior. These include:

INTRACRANIAL DISORDERS
Brain tumors
Head injury
Seizure disorders
Cerebrovascular accident
Dementia and/or organic brain syndrome

SYSTEMIC DISORDERS
Endocrine disorders such as thyroid storm, Cushing's syndrome
Electrolyte imbalance
Oxygen deficiency
Hypoperfusion
Septicemia
Hepatic encephalopathy

EXPOSURE TO SUBSTANCES
Acute alcohol intoxication, withdrawal, and delirium tremens
Use of mind-altering substances such as PCP and amphetamines
Withdrawal from barbiturates and sedatives
Use of aromatic hydrocarbons (glue, paint)
Use of medications such as steroids, central nervous system stimulants, and anti-Parkinson agents
Exposure to toxic chemicals, pesticides, lead

Lifespan Issues

CHILDHOOD

Consistent exposure to violence in childhood is a major factor contributing to the cycle of child abuse and family violence. Children who learn to use violent behavior to cope with frustrations and problems are likely to carry these behaviors into adulthood and may need to learn effective coping skills. Early signs of problems may include cruelty to animals and other children as well as difficulty controlling responses to frustration. The alarming presence of violence in schools and neighborhoods and in the media has increased the number of children who are exposed to seeing aggressive behavior and weapons used to resolve frustration in what may appear to them to be socially acceptable, normal behavior. Aggressive and violent behavior in children may also be caused by autism, mental retardation, learning disabilities, and attention deficit disorders.

ADOLESCENCE

Adolescents may act out aggressive feelings by participating in self-destructive behavior such as drug and/or alcohol use, smoking, or crime. Using mind-altering substances increases the risk of violent behavior.

ADULTS

Aggressive behavior in adults often reflects the learned life-long patterns. For instance, persons who abuse their spouse often have experienced abuse in their parents' relationship or been abused themselves as children.

ELDERLY

As with anger, violent behavior can be a life-long pattern or be caused by organic conditions or adverse reactions to medications. Aggressive behavior may also be a self-protective response related to confusion, fear, or sensory loss. Most frequently, aggressive behavior in the elderly is associated with Alzheimer's disease, senile dementia, cerebrovascular accidents, metabolic disorders, and hypoxia.

Possible Nurses' Reactions

- May fear being hurt by the violent or aggressive patient, which is the most common reaction. This fear can cause the nurse to use poor judgment or totally deny feeling fearful. Other common fear responses include avoiding the patient or bending the rules in an attempt to appease the patient. All of these responses can affect continuity of patient care.

- May feel abused and unappreciated, leading to defensive responses such as attempting to punish the patient. Defensive responses can escalate anger.
- May feel guilty for not being able to control the behavior or feel uncomfortable for participating in applying restraints.
- May feel offended or frustrated because the patient does not respond to care positively.

Assessment

Behavior and/or Appearance

- Pacing, restless
- Tense facial expression and body language
- Unpredictable behavior
- Loud voice, shouting, use of obscenities, argumentative
- Overreacting to stimuli such as noise
- Exhibiting poor impulse control evidenced by acting quickly before considering consequences of actions
- Grasping potential weapons and attempting to use them

Mood and/or Emotions

- Anger, resentment, rage
- Anxiety; fear of loss of control leading to panic
- Inappropriate affect for situation

Thoughts, Beliefs, and Perceptions

- Low self-esteem
- Low frustration tolerance
- Thoughts and/or plans to harm someone
- Inability to trust others to follow through without strong intimidation and suspiciousness
- Hallucinations, paranoid delusions
- Views others as out to hurt them
- Sense of being out of control

Relationships and Interactions

- Difficulty with close relationships; lack of trust, which causes person to fear closeness
- Others fearful of and avoid aggressive person, believing that they might be hurt or manipulated
- Family and friends have learned to meet person's demands to avoid aggressive response or exhibiting passive-aggressive behaviors in response to the person's demands

Physical Responses

- Increased muscle tension
- Increased heart rate and blood pressure
- Altered level of consciousness, confusion, lethargy
- Possible abnormal laboratory values including blood sugar, blood alcohol, drug screening
- Increased use of medications

Pertinent History

- History of violent behavior, particularly assault
- Psychiatric diagnosis
- Substance and/or alcohol abuse
- Physical, emotional, or sexual abuse in childhood

Collaborative Management

Pharmacologic

Use appropriate medications in adequate doses as an alternative or adjunct to physical restraints to manage aggressive behavior.

Pharmacologic management of acute aggressive and/or violent behavior may require rapid neuroleptization (also known as *rapid tranquilization*), which involves regular, frequent administration of antipsychotic medications such as haloperidol (Haldol). Parenteral administration may be required if oral route is not feasible. If the patient is in physical restraints, parenteral administration reduces the risk of aspiration. Haloperidol, 5 mg, may be administered every 30 to 60 minutes until symptoms are under control.

TABLE 8–2. **Encouraging an Uncooperative Patient to Take Medication**

- Have the nurse with the best relationship with patient offer the medication. Avoid power struggles and confrontations, which would most likely escalate the situation.
- Have the medication in hand so that it can be given quickly when the patient gives consent. The patient may change his or her mind suddenly.
- Be prepared for the patient to spit out the medication. This is especially common in the elderly aggressive patient.
- Use liquid oral medication if available. It is absorbed more quickly and is less likely to be "cheeked." If medication needs to be given by injection, work quickly. Have adequate staff available in case violence erupts.
- Review with the patient the benefits of medication, and help him or her gain control of his or her feelings.

Dosage should be reduced in the elderly. When using this drug, monitor the patient closely for hypotension and signs of extrapyramidal symptoms including akathesias and dystonia (see Chapter 20).

Antianxiety medications and sedatives may also be useful. Anticonvulsants, such as carbamazepine (Tegretol), have been used with some success. Lithium and beta-blockers, such as propranolol, are other alternatives. When using these drugs, evaluate how they may interfere with the medications ordered to treat the patient's underlying medical condition.

Convincing an aggressive, agitated patient to accept medication can be difficult and may lead the nurse to face an ethical dilemma of giving medication against a patient's will. Be aware of hospital and/or agency policies and state laws regarding patient rights (see Table 8–2).

Nursing Management

RISK FOR VIOLENCE, DIRECTED TO OTHERS EVIDENCED BY OVERT HOSTILITY AND/OR AGGRESSION TO OTHERS, THREATENING OTHERS, POSSESSION OF POTENTIAL WEAPON, ASSAULTING OTHERS RELATED TO IMPAIRED JUDGMENT, FEELINGS OF POWERLESSNESS, IM-

PULSIVE BEHAVIOR, INABILITY TO EVALUATE REALITY SECONDARY TO NEUROLOGIC PROBLEMS, PSYCHOTIC THOUGHTS, AND/OR DRUG/ALCOHOL USE.

Patient Outcomes

- Demonstrates increased self-control while in nurses' care
- Does not harm others or self while in nurses' care
- Demonstrates alternative coping mechanisms to reduce tension while in nurses' care
- Behavior does not escalate while in nurses' care

Interventions

- Help patient to verbalize angry feelings by reflecting and by clarifying your understanding of these feelings. Communicate your interest by appropriate eye contact, restating what patient has said, and asking questions. Help patient identify source of anger. Recognize that response to illness may make the person feel helpless with the need to strike out to gain a sense of control.
- If needed, allow patient to release tension physically on inanimate objects such as pillows and prescribed exercise, as appropriate.
- Do not take patient's behavior personally. For example, if a patient calls you derogatory names, refrain from reacting emotionally. Rather, remind yourself that you represent an authority figure to the patient and he or she is reacting to you in that way. Remember that patient may use derogatory remarks as a way to bolster his or her own self-esteem and seem to zero in on your sensitive, vulnerable points, such as weight or speech patterns. Avoid responding with sarcasm or ridicule.
- Do not ignore aggressive behavior in hopes that it will go away. It needs to be addressed. Minimization of behavior and ineffective limit setting are the most frequent factors contributing to escalation to violence.
- Set clear, consistent limits in a timely manner on what will and will not be tolerated. Clarify any specific consequences of patient behavior. For example, "If you attempt to hurt anyone, we will be compelled to control your behavior, which may mean using restraints" (see Table 8–3).

TABLE 8–3. **Setting Limits**

1. Explain exactly which behavior is inappropriate. Don't assume the individual knows which behavior is inappropriate.
2. Explain why the behavior is inappropriate. Don't assume the individual knows why the behavior is inappropriate.
3. Give the individual reasonable choices or consequences. Present them as choices, and always present the positive first.
4. Allow time—if you don't allow time to comply, it may be perceived as an ultimatum.
5. Enforce consequences—limits don't work unless you follow through with the consequences.

Source: Reprinted from the Art of Setting Limits Participant Manual, p. 8, with permission of the National Crisis Prevention Institute, Inc., © 1991.

- Identify one or two staff members who are comfortable with the patient to handle most of the care if possible to help provide in consistent interventions. Evaluate whether a male or female staff member has a more calming influence. Sometimes a male's presence is too threatening and powerful. Other times it is reassuring to the patient that a male staff member is available. A male patient may be less likely to hurt a woman and may see her as nurturing and supportive. Conversely the male patient may view the female staff as less able to provide control or have other conflicted feelings toward women (see Table 8–4).
- Free patient's environment of extra stimulation, such as noise or an agitated roommate. Extra stimulation may reduce impulse control. Remove objects around patients that could be used as potential weapons such as portable IV poles or food tray and/or utensils. Consider providing plastic food dishes and utensils. Avoid startling patient. Call patient by name before walking into room. Avoid sudden movements that the patient may interpret as threatening.
- Remain calm, and communicate that you are in control and can handle the situation. Use a moderate, firm voice and calming hand gestures. Avoid touching patient.
- Place yourself between door and patient. Always have a

TABLE 8–4. **Summary of Staff Interventions**

Patient	Staff
Anxiety	Verbal intervention: • Assess. • Use verbal calming techniques. • Attempt to calm patient. • Do not invade patient's personal space; avoid antagonizing.
Threatening	Set Limits: • Continue verbal calming techniques • Set clear and definite limits. • Be directive and matter of fact. • Be prepared to enforce limits.
Acting out aggression	Physical management: • Recognize mounting tension. • Have a plan. • Designate team leader. • Use only after other measures fail.
Tension reduction	Emotional support: • Allow patient to express feelings. • Listen nonjudgmentally. • Show concern for patient, not anger. • Discuss events with colleagues. • Avoid blaming.

Source: Adapted from Haven and Piscitello, 1989, and Lewis, 1993.

quick exit available. Never turn your back on the patient. Keep door of room open. Let other staff know you are going in patient's room. Protect other patients who may get in the way of the violent individual. For patients at home, always be aware of your surroundings and be alert to possible exits. Consider going to a home with colleagues when there is a known risk of aggressive behavior. Leave the home immediately if there is any sign of out-of-control behavior.

• Never force an agitated patient to have a test or treatment. Power struggles will escalate aggression. Rather, prioritize care that must be given, and focus only on that. Explain all procedures, and ask patient's permission before beginning. Give patient choices as often as possible.

• If the patient is psychotic, he or she may be hearing

voices. If so, ask what the voices are telling him to do. This gives you more information on what to expect. Hallucinations that command the patient to initiate aggression can an extremely powerful force for the patient to overcome.
- A nurse who has been assaulted in the past and is now faced with a potentially violent patient may bring fears from this past experience, which could inhibit his or her response. Sharing these fears with colleagues may provide much needed support.
- If a patient makes threats to harm specific people, the nurse needs to notify his or her supervisor and follow protocol for notifying potential victims.
- A visitor who becomes aggressive or violent needs to be reported to the agency security staff immediately and removed from the patient care area.

RISK FOR INJURY EVIDENCED BY FALLS, PAIN, TRAUMA, SKIN BREAKDOWN RELATED TO RESTRAINING PATIENT TO CONTROL VIOLENT BEHAVIOR.

Patient Outcomes

- Remains free of injury and complications during restraint application
- Demonstrates control of behavior once restraints are removed

Interventions

- Never attempt to restrain a patient by yourself. Have adequate staff available, usually three to five persons, and a plan of action before attempting to physically control a patient. Recruit reliable help from all possible sources, such as security. Assess their experience in managing a violent patient and review the plan. Decide in advance who will grab which arm or leg if patient must be restrained. The presence of a number of staff (show of force) alone may subdue a patient.
- Designate one person to talk with the patient and another to direct the other staff. Only one staff member should talk with patient, preferably someone who knows the patient. It is important to communicate in a firm manner,

speaking slowly. Lack of leadership can cause confusing and contradictory messages and result in someone's being hurt or the patient's escaping.

- Maintain a firm base of support for balance if you are suddenly pushed. Remove name badge, eyeglasses, jewelry, and so on to avoid injury.
- If patient is resisting, he or she may need to be distracted. Each staff member should grab one of the patient's limbs when given the command by the coordinating person and take patient down to the floor or bed quickly. Attempt to cradle patient's head to prevent injury.
- The decision to use restraints should be made only after other efforts to reduce tension have been tried and proven ineffective. A physician's order must be obtained. If there is no time to obtain an order, it must be obtained immediately after the event.
- Once decision is made to restrain patient, act quickly and decisively. Determine what appropriate type of restraint is to be applied before approaching patient. Restraints include cloth chest and limb restraints or leather (hard), locked restraints. (*Note*: When using hard restraints, make sure you have the key, and double-check that they are locked after applying them to patient.) Have equipment ready before approaching patient.
- Once restraints are applied to bed frame, take the time to talk with the patient in a calm, concerned manner to try to humanize situation. Call patient by his or her name.
- Make sure patient has no potential weapons within reach. Patient needs to be searched for sharp objects, matches, and so on.
- Administer medications as ordered.
- Be aware of agency policy regarding application of restraints. Requirements for monitoring patients while in restraints, reasons for restraints, doctor's orders, and the length of time each order remains valid should be clearly spelled out in agency policies. If you are not sure about using restraints on someone, discuss with your supervisor to weigh your obligations to protect the patient versus going against the patient's wishes.
- Monitor patient closely, and document findings according to agency policy including vital signs, circulation extremities, and input/output.

- Remove restraints, and observe patient closely when the situation is under control. Consider removing one limb at a time so that patient has time to adjust. For the high-risk patient, keep one arm and one leg in restraints at all times until it is clear that patient can be released. Inform other staff that patient has been released. Establish clear criteria for reapplying restraints with patient and staff. Prepare family for patient's condition, as appropriate.
- Once the patient has regained control, discuss with him or her why that intervention was used, and allow opportunity to express feelings. This increases his or her sense of control and decreases dehumanization.
- If patient has a gun or other weapon, never attempt to disarm him or her. Contact security and/or law enforcement agency as soon as possible. Focus on getting assistance and protecting patients and staff. Patients and staff should remain in a safe area until help arrives.
- Consider taking a specialized class on use of defensive techniques such as management of assaultive behavior. Proper training is essential to prevent injury to patients and staff. Staff members can practice with each other how they would handle a violent patient.

ALTERNATE NURSING DIAGNOSIS

Altered thought processes
Ineffective individual coping
Noncompliance
Risk for injury

WHEN TO CALL FOR HELP

✔ Escalation of behavior from aggressive to violent
✔ Patient in possession of a weapon
✔ Inadequate staff available to control behavior
✔ Increased staff anxiety over caring for the patient

Patient and Family Education

- Review early warning signs of escalation of aggressive behavior with patient and his or her family.

- Instruct patient on role of alcohol and drugs in contributing to aggressive behavior.
- Instruct on use of prescribed medications to control tension. Instruct on when to ask for PRN medications.
- If patient is in restraints, review with him or her criteria for removal and reinstatement.

Charting Tips

- Document all actions taken to prevent violent behavior.
- Document application of restraints including type, length of time in restraints, reasons for application, patient response, release of limbs, and care given while in restraints. (Document per agency policy.) Document vital sign monitoring.
- Document need for and response to medication given.
- Document any threats patient makes.
- Document all interventions and responses to them.

Discharge Planning

- Provide information to patient's family and/or caregivers about emergency psychiatric services, if needed. Discuss potential for violence with family to share possible strategies from nursing care plan.
- Provide information on shelters and/or domestic violence services, if appropriate.
- If patient is being transferred to another facility, share concerns about patient's behavior and interventions.
- Provide information to family and caregivers on what to do if behavior is out of control. Encourage them to call for help immediately.
- Provide information on drug treatment if appropriate.

Nursing Outcomes

- Staff creates a safe environment (see Table 8–5).
- Staff is free from injury.
- Staff demonstrates appropriate interventions to control aggressive behavior.
- Documentation reflects appropriate assessment and monitoring of patient in restraints.

TABLE 8–5. **Steps to Ensure Patient and Workplace Safety**

- Be particularly vigilant during change of shifts and on nightshift. Most events occur between 8:30 p.m. and 10:30 a.m.
- Minimize stress factors such as long waits, crowded, confined spaces, and inflexible policies for patients where possible.
- Avoid wearing jewelry or neckties that can be grabbed or tugged.
- Immediately report all assaults to your supervisor and security.
- Be aware that many agency security staffs have minimal training.
- Receive education on local gangs and gang violence.
- Participate in agency safety committees to ensure that adequate security measures are in place.

- Medication given as ordered with appropriate monitoring.
- Staff takes opportunity to share feelings after managing a violent patient.
- Staff reports to supervisors any threats the patient makes to others.

Suggested Learning Activities

- Discuss security measures within your agency.
- Review agency policies and state laws on restraint application and administration of psychotropic medications.
- Take a course on managing assaultive behavior.
- With your colleagues, share experiences and feelings when working with violent patients or personal experiences with violence.

9

PROBLEMS WITH AFFECT AND MOOD

The Depressed Patient

LEARNING OBJECTIVES

▼ *Differentiate feeling depressed from a depressive disorder.*
▼ *Describe common physical symptoms seen in depressive disorders.*
▼ *Describe interventions for the patient with low self-esteem.*
▼ *Describe possible nurses' reactions to the depressed patient.*

Feeling down, discouraged, and depressed is something all people experience at some time in their life. Periods of emotional highs and lows are normal. Feeling depressed, however, is very different from depressive illness or clinical depression. Depression is a psychiatric illness characterized by a cluster of symptoms including prolonged depressed mood, lowered self-esteem, pessimistic thoughts, and loss of pleasure or interest in former activities. It is a painful, debilitating illness. It needs to be differentiated from short-term depressed moods or grief reactions, which are normal. Although grief displays many of the signs and symptoms of depression, it is a time-limited condition in response to an obvious loss and does not cause lowered self-esteem.

Glossary

Depression—Primary psychiatric illness manifested by characteristic symptom clusters such as depressed mood, lowered self-esteem, pessimistic thoughts, and loss of pleasure or interest in former activities.

Masked depression—Concealed depression where patient is not aware of depressed mood or does not display obvious sadness. The depression is expressed through other means as physical complaints and/or diverse psychiatric symptoms such as phobias or compulsions.

Melancholia—Severe form of major depression with somatic symptoms including hypochondriasis, insomnia, anorexia, and somatic delusions.

Dysthymic disorder—Mild to moderate chronic depression that lasts at least 2 years. Previously called a "neurotic depression."

Anhedonia—Loss of pleasure in activities or interests that were previously enjoyed.

Psychomotor agitation—Classic symptom cluster of depression including restlessness with rapid, agitated, purposeless movements like pacing or wringing hands.

Psychomotor retardation—Classic symptom cluster of depression including slow movements and speech.

Depression is the most common reason for seeking out mental health professionals. Because the symptoms of depression can be hidden, vague, or atypical, and may present as physical symptoms instead of a mood disturbance, primary care physicians may be the first to see this patient. Surveys consistently show that 6 to 8 percent of all outpatients in the primary care setting have major depressive disorders (DHHS, 1993). However, the symptoms of depression can often go unrecognized and are often misdiagnosed. Undiagnosed and untreated depression is considered a major national health concern contributing to poor work performance, family disruption, substance abuse, and premature death due to suicide or lack of self-care. Women are twice as likely to suffer from depression than men. It crosses all ethnic lines. In addition, depression can be part of a bipolar disorder (manic depression), psychosis, eating disorder, or dementia. Depression can also be a secondary problem to a primary problem such as substance abuse or schizophrenia.

Once a person experiences a depressive episode, he or she is at a higher risk for recurrence. After one depressive episode, an individual has a 50 percent chance of another; after two episodes, there is a 70 to 80 percent risk of another; and after three episodes, the individual is at very high risk for chronic disability from depression (Kupfer, 1991).

Etiology

No single theory of depression is accepted by all theorists and clinicians. Different theories may apply to the divergent pathways that patients travel to arrive at the various types of depression.

Biological theories have focused on an insufficiency of neurotransmitters, especially norepinephrine and serotonin. These insufficiencies may be the result of inherited or environmental factors. The effectiveness of antidepressants may result from enhancing levels of these neurotransmitters. The most severe depressions are predominantly biologically determined.

Genetics may be a factor in more severe depressions. Relatives of people with depression have a higher incidence of this illness than those in the general population.

Psychologic theories about a predisposition to depression have focused on a personal history of deprivation, trauma, or significant loss during childhood. These patients may be more susceptible to depression as current losses revive memories of former losses.

Depression can be viewed as forbidden anger that has been turned inward. Classic psychoanalytic theory identified depression as the reaction to the loss of a significant person who has been both hated and loved. The patient handles this ambivalence by turning the hatred inward, resulting in depression and low self-esteem, while the memory of the departed person remains beloved and idealized.

Certain predominant symptoms such as low self-esteem, helplessness, and disturbed thoughts seen in the past as end products of depression are now being evaluated as possible causes of or contributors to depression in the *cause-versus-effect theory*. For instance, low self-esteem may be based on the faulty development of an adequate, competent sense of self during childhood. As a child, the person received attention and approval only when meeting parental needs and expectations. As an adult, the absence of external support and praise and especially the loss of a supportive person may make the patient vulnerable to collapse of self-esteem, which triggers depression.

Learned helplessness is displayed by a lack of adequate effort based on the belief that a person cannot be effective in getting needs met nor making an impact. This person grows up in an environment that did not respond to any actions or initiative taken (Seligman, 1975).

Distorted thinking can generate a depression. Typically, there are negative expectations about the self, world, and the future. If a patient consistently overgeneralizes any mistake into the conclusion "I can't do anything right" and judges self as deficient, those negative beliefs can build toward depression. Negative expectations of the world such as receiving no help from others or expecting only criticism reinforce helplessness and lead to hopelessness (Beck, 1979).

Related Clinical Concerns

Clinically significant depressive symptoms are detectable in about 12 to 36 percent of the medically ill population (DHHS, 1993). The patient's response to a medical illness could cause depression, and in some cases physiologic problems could contribute to depression. In some medical disorders, depression is a symptom. Those disorders include:

- Stroke

TABLE 9–1. **Drugs That Cause Depression**

General Drug Categories	
Anticonvulsants	
Barbituates	
Benzodiazepines	
Beta-blockers	
Contraceptives, oral	
Corticosteroids	
Digitalis	
Opioids	
Procaine derivatives	
Sedative/hypnotics	
Sulfonamides	
Thiazides	
Thyroid hormones	
Specific Drugs	**Trade Name**
Acyclovir	Zovirax
Clonodine	Catapres
Disulfiram	Antabuse
Isoniazid	INH
Isosorbide dinitrate	Isordil
Levadopa	L-Dopa
Methyldopa	Aldomet
Metoclopramide	Reglan
Nifidepine	Procardia
Reserpine	Serpasil
Tamoxifen	Nolvadex
Trimethoprimsulfamethoxazole	Bactrim

Source: Drugs that cause psychiatric symptoms, with permission Medical Letter 35(65), July 23, 1993.

- Myocardial infarction
- Adrenal disorders
- Dementia
- Diabetes
- Some cancers (especially advanced cancers)
- Hypothyroidism
- Some brain tumors

In addition, medications could trigger depression (see Table 9–1).

Lifespan Issues

CHILDHOOD

Experts do not agree on the prevalence of depression in children; however, there is consensus that it does occur even in young children. Depression could be the aftermath of emotional deprivation, abuse, or separation. Because the child may be unable to express feelings or worries, other signs need to be analyzed including acting-out behaviors, conduct disorders, inappropriate aggression, not meeting developmental tasks, sleep disorders, inability to experience joy (anhedonia), and self-destructive behaviors. There is a higher risk of depression in children when one or both parents suffer from major depression. Depression can also be a secondary reaction to other problems such as learning disorders and substance abuse. Children have been treated successfully with antidepressants in conjunction with psychotherapeutic interventions.

ADOLESCENCE

Adolescents often do not verbally express feelings of depression as they may fear exhibiting feelings of vulnerability and dependency. Rather, their feelings of depression come out in self-destructive and/or antisocial behaviors including sexual promiscuity, school truancy, threats, or petty crime. Some experts believe that substance abuse and eating disorders in adolescence may be masking or related to depression. A depression-prone adolescent with low self-esteem will have greater difficulty achieving a positive sense of self as an adult. Adolescent victims of abuse are particularly vulnerable to depression.

POSTPARTUM

Debate continues as to whether the etiology of postpartum depression is solely hormonal or represents an intermingling of psychologic and physiologic stressors. Though postpartum "blues" (a few days of labile mood after the birth of a baby) is extremely common, more severe reactions are relatively rare. Postpartum depression can include psychotic symptoms of delusions that often concern the newborn infant. Bonding with the infant is disrupted. Women with a psychiatric history including bipolar disorder are at higher risk. Once a woman experiences a major postpartum depression with psychotic features, the risk of recurrence is between 30 and 50 percent in subsequent deliveries (DSM-IV, 1994).

ELDERLY

Depression is the most common emotional disorder of old age. The elderly are at higher risk because they experience more multiple losses and medical illnesses than the rest of the population. Depression can be superimposed on dementia or confused with pseudodementia, since common depressive symptoms in the elderly include confusion, distractibility, and memory loss. In addition, some of the physical symptoms of depression like fatigue, anorexia, constipation, and psychomotor retardation can be confused with physical illness, medication interactions, substance abuse, or "signs of old age." Treatment with antidepressants must be very closely supervised due to the possibility of severe side effects.

Possible Nurses' Reactions

- May feel depressed when working with these patients. A patient's despair and unhappiness can be very painful to be around and could lead to the nurse's avoiding the patient.
- May reject the patient due to the nurse's perception of the patient's dependency. Or may become overinvolved because of patient's needs and inadvertently create more dependency.

- May resent patient because of the longer time it takes to provide care.
- May feel angry or frustrated with depressed patient who isn't "helping himself" or can't just "snap out of it."
- May feel inadequate when unable to make a quick impact on a patient's depression. Nurse may create unrealistic expectations of patient's recovery.
- Staff may have inaccurate beliefs about the cause of depression, which may lead to their minimizing the degree of the patient's suffering.
- Because of the high prevalence of depression in our society, the nurse may have personally experienced it or may have witnessed a family member's struggle with depression. This can cause the nurse to identify with the depressed patient and reexperience these feelings.
- Reaction may depend on whether the nurse believes that the expression of sadness is an acceptable behavior; for example, the nurse may believe sadness is acceptable in women but not in men.

Assessment

Behavior and/or Appearance

- Persistently sad, anguished, or apathetic facial expression
- Dejected appearance: Head down, poor eye contact, posture slumped as if bearing a heavy weight
- Psychomotor agitation and/or retardation
- Decreased interest in grooming and self-care
- Decreased sexual interest
- Makes statements like "I don't care anymore"
- May have difficulty with even simple tasks
- Anhedonia

Mood and/or Emotions

- Dysphoric mood: Verbalizes feelings of sadness and depression
- Inability to enjoy activities that were enjoyed previously
- Low self-esteem with feelings of worthlessness and inadequacy

- Feeling ineffective, powerless, and helpless
- Pessimistic: May appear brooding and express feelings of futility and despair
- Feelings of great heaviness
- Mild to high levels of anxiety possibly including panic attacks and irritability
- Unexpressed anger, turned inward against self
- May express generalized anger
- Ambivalence; may feel two opposing ways at the same time

Thoughts, Beliefs, and Perceptions

- Thoughts slowed
- Poor concentration with possible temporary impairment of recent memory
- Self-doubt with relentless rumination and obsessions
- Lack of self-worth: Believes self undeserving of good experiences
- Indecisiveness
- Preoccupation with body changes
- Loss of perspective: May reject positive comments from others; gives self no credit for achievements
- Excessive guilt: Condemns self; feels deserving of punishment
- Narrowing of interest to self
- Possible suicidal thoughts
- Confusion
- In severe depression: Delusions; hallucinations that express feelings of worthlessness; guilt
- Believes life has no meaning and that there is no future

Relationships and Interactions

- Withdrawal from social interactions
- Deterioration of relationships because of preoccupation with self, anger, and anxiety
- Increasing dependence on others due to inability to make decisions or care for self

Physical Responses

- Slowed physiologic functioning evidenced by:

- ◦ Lethargy and fatigue especially in the mornings
- ◦ Constipation
- ◦ Decreased appetite with weight loss or increased appetite with weight gain
- ◦ Sleep problems including early morning awakening, frequent awakenings, waking up feeling tired, sleeping all the time
- ◦ Body aches; pains such as headaches; indigestion; dizziness
- • Thyroid function tests may be ordered to rule out hypothyroidism

Pertinent History

- • Past history of depression, bipolar disorder, panic attacks, suicide attempts
- • Family history of depression
- • History of substance abuse
- • History of stroke or myocardial infarction (particularly high rate of depression)

Collaborative Management

Pharmacologic

Antidepressants can be a very effective treatment for a moderate to severe major depressive disorder. Since there are so many on the market, the specific medication choice is based on side effects, patient profile, history of prior response, type of depression, concurrent medical or psychiatric illnesses, and other medications the patient is taking. See Chapter 20 for a detailed discussion of antidepressants, their side effects, and nursing implications. Most antidepressants require at least 3 to 4 weeks of use before full benefits are obtained. Often, relief of other symptoms occurs prior to a change in the patient's subjective sense of feeling better. Side effects must be monitored closely. The patient may need to remain on a maintenance dose of antidepressant for many years.

If the patient is experiencing anxiety, panic attacks, hallucinations, or delusions, other medications may need to be added.

Psychotherapy

Psychotherapy is recommended for mild to moderate major depression and in conjunction with antidepressants in more severe depressions. The federal guidelines on depression (DHHS, 1993) recommend a short-term trial of 6 to 12 weeks of psychotherapy to determine symptom response. If there is no significant improvement after 12 weeks, antidepressants should be added or changed. One short-term psychotherapy approach is cognitive therapy. This method is brief, structured, directive treatment designed to alter the negative thoughts so common in depression. Group therapy can also be helpful to enhance the patient's socialization.

Electroconvulsive Therapy

Electroconvulsive therapy (ECT) is a first-line treatment option only for patients with more severe or psychotic forms of depression. It may also be used for those who have failed to respond to other therapies or those with medical conditions that preclude the use of antidepressants.

Nursing Management

SELF-CARE DEFICIT EVIDENCED BY DECREASED ABILITY TO MANAGE OWN HYGIENE, GROOMING, FEEDING, AND DAILY ACTIVITIES RELATED TO LOSS OF ENERGY, INHIBITION OF MOTIVATION, ANXIETY, AND/OR DEPENDENCY.

Patient Outcomes

* Increased participation in self-care, daily activities
* Improved grooming and hygiene

Interventions

* Determine patient's level of self-care prior to onset of depressive symptoms to set realistic goals.
* Assess whether the patient is expressing certain psychologic needs such as dependency or rebellion by not performing self-care. Observe whether patient acts more independently when unaware of being watched.

- Encourage as much independence as possible. Take the time to allow patient to do things for himself or herself. Assign care to staff member who may have more time or is especially patient. Make sure all staff members reinforce patient's participation. Encourage patient's participation in decisions about timing sequence, and approaches to self-care.
- Create a positive attitude that patient can learn and progress with practice. Avoid taking over for the patient if he or she has trouble.
- Break down tasks into small steps so patient can experience some success. For instance, have the patient focus on washing his or her face rather than completing the whole bath.
- Create an environment to ease patient's participation, such as having proper utensils available at mealtime or having the walker available in room if patient is ambulating to bathroom.
- Provide reassurance and encouragement. Avoid minimizing patient's problems or infantilizing him or her.
- At times, a nurse may need to make all decisions for a very depressed patient such as when to eat. Then, as the patient begins to improve, limited options can be presented. With further improvement, the patient should take on increasing decision-making.

SELF-ESTEEM DISTURBANCE EVIDENCED BY STATEMENTS OF LOW SELF-ESTEEM, MISINTERPRETING POSITIVE OR PLEASURABLE EXPERIENCES, EXPRESSIONS OF SHAME AND GUILT RELATED TO FEELINGS, THOUGHTS OF WORTHLESSNESS, FAILURES, AND NEGATIVE REINFORCEMENT.

Patient Outcomes

- Identifies positive aspects of self
- Modifies unrealistic expectations for self
- Demonstrates reduced symptoms of depression

Interventions

- Provide emotional nurturing through empathetic listening and supportive encouragement. By treating the patient as a valued individual, self-esteem will be enhanced.

- Avoid blanket reassurances like "things will get better soon." These tend to alienate the patient who may feel that you don't understand his or her pain.
- Encourage patient to share feelings, especially negative ones. If this is too difficult, consider alternative means of expression such as writing about feelings or drawing.
- Point out any specific improvement, no matter how small. Depressed people often do not see improvement because they are so focused on the negative. Consider keeping a progress chart at the bedside to record concrete accomplishments such as the number of times the patient ambulates or the percentage of food he or she eats.
- Encourage patient to speak up if he or she disagrees or feels his or her rights are being violated. Reinforce assertive response.
- Recognize and point out manifestations of self-destructive or self-undermining thinking or behavior:
  - Requiring self to be perfect or setting unattainable goals
  - Assuming responsibility for and feeling guilt about failures and events that are outside the patient's control
  - Basing entire feeling of self-worth on one achievement or attribute, a single relationship, or obtaining approval from others
  - Projecting own feelings of self-hate onto family, staff, or friends, such as "All the nurses hate me." "My family blames me for my illness"
  - Expressing self-hate directly via suicidal thoughts and behavior
  - Expressing self-hate indirectly with repeated accidents, noncompliance, provoking or being antagonistic to others, thereby unwittingly creating rejection
  - Covering poor self-esteem with anger, blaming, or other maneuvers that displace responsibility onto others
- Suggest the patient identify a few achievements from the past.
- Discuss and practice with patient alternate ways to respond to stress and to ask for what he or she wants.

POWERLESSNESS Evidenced by lack of initiative, non-achievement of realistic goals, passivity; nonparticipation in decision making related to decreased motivation, decreased energy, hopelessness, perfectionistic expectations or sadness.

Patient Outcomes

- Identifies factors that he or she can control
- Participates in decisions about his or her care

Interventions

- Encourage the patient to describe feelings or the experience of powerlessness. Let the patient know you are interested and you understand his or her pain. For instance, you may state, "You believe there is no hope for you to ever feel better."
- Once the patient indicates that he or she feels understood, suggest alternate viewpoints. Work with patient to identify times in life when he or she felt better or felt more in control.
- Work with the patient to identify realistic goals to work toward. Encourage having patience and accepted current limitations. Break down goals into small steps, and recognize progress as each is achieved.
- Allow the patient to maintain reasonable control over some of the daily routine if able.
- Have the patient list specific situations in which he or she felt powerless. Correct distorted assumptions, discuss alternative ways to handle situations, and identify helpful resources.
- Direct the patient to other topics if he or she obsesses on unrealistic goals or things that cannot be changed.

ALTERNATE NURSING DIAGNOSES

Altered nutrition
Anxiety
Dysfunctional grieving
Hopelessness
Impaired social interaction

Impaired thought processes
Ineffective individual coping
Risk for injury
Sleep pattern disturbance
Social isolation

WHEN TO CALL FOR HELP

✔ Extreme self-care deficit to point of not being able to care for basic needs
✔ Suicidal thoughts, threats, or attempts
✔ Hallucinations or delusions
✔ Severe side effects from antidepressants including severe urinary retention, dramatic fluctuations in blood pressure, cardiac complications, seizures

Patient and Family Education

- Teach the patient that depression can generate feelings of helplessness, powerlessness, and pessimism. Encourage the patient to delay major decisions and actions based on those feelings, and reinforce that the severe symptoms will lift with treatment and time.
- For patients on antidepressants, review potential side effects and importance of taking the medication even when they start feeling better. Patient should know which side effects to report to physician.
- Inform the patient that other medications are available if the side effects from the current one are too uncomfortable.
- Encourage the patient to maintain a schedule of activity.
- Explain to the family the symptoms of depression, medication management, and interventions and what they can do to assist and encourage patient.
- Teach the patient and family to report signs of increasing depression or suicidal thoughts.
- Teach the patient that long-term, enduring self-esteem comes from beliefs about self as a valuable human being and is expressed through achievements, relationships, and healthful living.

- Inform the patient that the negative assumptions about himself or herself are not necessarily true.

Charting Tips

- Document patient activity, intake, sleep patterns, bowel patterns.
- Document any expressed suicide thoughts, plans, or attempts.
- Document side effects of medication.
- Document patient response to encouragement or support.

Discharge Planning

- Strongly encourage patient to seek out counseling. Give appropriate referrals.
- If patient is unable to care for himself or herself or is potentially suicidal, work with other members of the team as well as family to determine discharge options. Patient may need psychiatric hospitalization or temporary placement in a board and care or convalescent facility.
- Refer patient for home health care for follow-up on medication compliance and self-care activities.
- Encourage patient to maintain follow-up with physician.

Nursing Outcomes

- Staff demonstrates interventions that promote patient's self-worth.
- Staff demonstrates appropriate, nonjudgmental, objective care.
- Staff remains involved and motivated to provide care to patient.
- Antidepressants are administered as ordered, and side effects monitored.

Suggested Learning Activities

- Arrange for an inservice from a mental health professional who works with depressed patients, a specialist in

geriatric psychiatry, and/or pharmacist on medication management.
- Attend support programs or group therapy for depressed individuals if possible.
- Share experiences with colleagues on working with depressed patients.

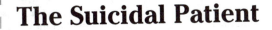

The Suicidal Patient

LEARNING OBJECTIVES

▼ *Identify risk factors for suicide.*
▼ *Differentiate between a suicide attempt and suicide gesture.*
▼ *Describe effective interventions to protect the high-risk patient in the hospital.*
▼ *Describe common nurses' reactions to the suicidal patient.*

Some nurses mistakenly believe suicidal patients are found only in psychiatric settings. However, patients with suicidal tendencies are not always easily identified, and they can be the same patients you care for in an intensive care unit, medical unit, nursing home, or at home.

Many people have experienced momentary self-destructive thoughts. But obsessive preoccupation with these thoughts and acting on them is another matter. Thinking about suicide does not mean the individual will act on those thoughts; however, anyone who talks about, threatens, or attempts suicide must be taken seriously. In approximately 70 percent of suicides, the individual has one or more active or chronic medical illnesses at the time of death (DHHS, 1993). See Table 9–2, Suicide: Intensity of Risk, for key risk factors.

There are approximately seven suicide attempts for every completed suicide. Women make more attempts than men, but men are more likely to complete suicide because they tend to use more lethal methods, particu-

---

Glossary

Suicide—A broad range of behaviors in which a person causes his or her own death.

Suicide attempt—Any act intended to end in suicide.

Suicidal ideation—Thoughts about harming oneself.

Suicide gesture—Any action that appears to be a suicide attempt but that is actually contrived or manipulative and that results in only minimal harm, such as superficial cuts on the wrist or a small overdose of sleeping pills.

Suicide threat—Verbal threat to commit suicide.

Completed suicide—Suicide attempt resulting in death.

Lethality—The level of risk in suicide method chosen to cause death. The more lethal methods include guns, jumping, and hanging. Lower lethality methods include superficially slashing wrists, inhaling house gas, and ingesting pills since death is not immediate and there is more of a chance of being found and treated.

TABLE 9–2. **Suicide: Intensity of Risk**

Behaviors or Symptoms	Intensity of Risk		
	Low	Moderate	High
Anxiety	Mild	Moderate	High, or panic state
Depression	Mild	Moderate	Severe
Isolation or withdrawal	Some feelings of isolation; no withdrawal	Some feelings of helplessness, hopelessness, or withdrawal	Hopeless, Helpless, withdrawn, self-deprecating
Daily functioning	Fairly good in most activities	Moderately good in some activities	Not good in any activities
Resources	Several	Some	Few or none
Coping strategies or devices being used	Generally constructive	Some that are constructive	Predominantly constructive
Significant others	Several available	Few or only one available	Only one or none available
Previous psychiatric help	None, or positive attitude toward	Yes, and moderately satisfied with	Negative view of help received
Lifestyle	Stable	Moderately stable	Unstable
Alcohol or drug use	Infrequently to excess	Frequently to excess	Continual use
Previous suicide attempts	None or low lethality	One or more of moderate lethality	Multiple attempts of high lethality
Disorientation or disorganization	None	Some	Marked

TABLE 9–2. **Suicide: Intensity of Risk** (*Continued*)

Behaviors or Symptoms	Intensity of Risk		
	Low	Moderate	High
Hostility Suicide plan	Little or none Vague fleeting thoughts but no plan	Some Frequent thoughts; occasional ideas about a plan	Marked Frequent or constant thought with a specific plan

Source: Adapted with permission from Suicide: Assessment and Interventions, by Hatton, C, and Valente S, Appleton-Century-Crofts, Norwalk, CT, 1984.

larly guns. Generally, the risk for suicide is greater when the plan is more detailed and the method more lethal and accessible.

Statistics show that suicide is the tenth leading cause of death in this country. However, it may be higher because hidden suicides such as "accidental" overdoses, auto accidents, noncompliance with medical regimens, or not seeking medical care for symptoms are not reported as suicides.

Because suicide is basically not accepted by our culture, it generates anxiety that has lead to a number of myths. See Table 9–3, Clearing Up the Myths About Suicide.

Surviving family and friends of the suicide victim often experience complicated grief reactions that may affect them for the rest of their lives. They are faced with the stigma of this form of death as well as many unresolved feelings of anger and guilt. Unfortunately, they may receive less support from others because of the discomfort around the cause of death. In addition, many life insurance policies do not cover self-inflicted death, so the surviving family may be economically devastated.

Etiology

Suicide is not a disease in itself but a symptom of some underlying problem. *Biologic and genetic* theories are

TABLE 9–3. **Clearing Up the Myths About Suicide**

Myth	Truth
Asking people about their suicide thoughts will make them more likely to act on them.	Most patients are not afraid to talk about their thoughts of committing suicide and are usually grateful that someone is available and cares. Talking can reduce the sense of isolation.
All people who attempt suicide have a psychiatric disorder.	People can become overwhelmed with life circumstances without having a psychiatric disorder.
A person who talks about suicide won't do it.	Approximately 80 percent of individuals who attempt or complete suicide give some definite verbal or indirect clues. As many as 50 percent have seen their physician within the previous month, often with vague somatic complaints.
A person who attempts suicide won't try again.	Almost 75 percent of those individuals who complete suicide have attempted it at least once before.
People who attempt suicide are always determined to die.	Many individuals are ambivalent and are using the suicide as a cry for help.
People who attempt suicide just want attention.	Even if the suicide attempt is manipulative, the individual may go on to complete the suicide.
As the person becomes less depressed the risk of suicide decreases.	As the depression lifts, the individual's energy level can increase before feelings of hopelessness are relieved. Once the individual makes the decision that suicide is an effective solution to the problems, his or her mood may even elevate.

closely tied to those causing depression. It is believed that low levels of the neurotransmitters, serotonin and norepinephrine, are a factor in the decision to commit suicide. There is also a strong link to alcohol and substance abuse. Suicide behavior also runs in families. This may be related to genetics or to psychological factors in which suicide is viewed as an acceptable way to cope. Family members of individuals who have committed suicide have a 15 times greater risk of suicide.

Psychologic theory focuses on a number of motivating forces. Suicide can be a way to escape deep psychologic pain or atone for past sins. Intense feelings of hopelessness and helplessness are key factors. It can also be related to unacceptable feelings of aggression, which the individual turns inward. The individual could also have a belief of being reunited with a loved one. Another motivating force could be the wish to instill guilt in a significant person who is perceived as abandoning or rejecting the suicidal person. Individuals with limited coping reserves who become overwhelmed with stress may have a tendency to seek self-destructive acts as a way to escape these overwhelming feelings. Because the suicidal person may be severely depressed, the theories on etiology of depression and substance abuse may also relate to suicide. Alcohol plays a significant role in many suicides.

Suicidal behavior can also be a symptom of psychosis as the person acts out hallucinations or delusions. Command hallucinations, where voices tell the patient to kill himself or herself, create a very high risk. This individual may experience severe anxiety and distress as well as lack judgment and/or reality testing. Suicide may be viewed as a way to escape overwhelming distress or disturbed thoughts.

Suicidal gestures with nonlethal self-mutilation may occur in individuals who have poor impulse control or who go to these extremes to get attention or control others. An individual with a history of multiple threats and gestures may have a personality disorder such as a borderline personality disorder.

Sociologic views look at a person who may feel alienated from others. A susceptible individual who no longer feels part of his or her culture or social group could be at an increased risk if cultural or religious taboos against suicide are not very strong. In some individuals, suicide is a way of expressing political beliefs. Economic losses or unemployment could also play a role as a person feels trapped and powerless to change. Suicide is an increasing problem in minority and economically deprived groups.

Related Clinical Concerns

Physical illness is a frequent contributor to suicidal behavior. Illnesses associated with suffering and dependency, such as advanced cancer and AIDS, are associated with higher suicide rates. Uncontrolled pain and delirium are the key variables with these illnesses. Controversy over the terminal patient's "right" to commit suicide has recently received much attention. Right to die groups have supported initiatives in several states seeking physician-assisted suicide for terminal patients. In these initiatives, a terminally ill patient could request his or her doctor to administer a lethal dose of medication or give him or her a prescription for a lethal dose of sleeping pills at a time of the patient's choosing. The patient's ability to remain in control until death is a key motivation for this action. Other illnesses, such as multiple sclerosis and Huntington's disease, that may not be terminal but are chronic and debilitating may also be associated with increased suicide risk. Suicidal patients with physical illnesses should be carefully evaluated and treated for depression. In addition every effort to identify and control any uncomfortable symptoms will enhance quality of life.

Medications that contribute to depressive or psychotic symptoms could also precipitate a suicide attempt. See Tables 9–1 and 11–3 for lists of medications that contribute to these symptoms. Patients with suicidal tendencies who are taking prescribed analgesics, tranquilizers, or sleeping pills may be at risk for saving up medications to use later for a possible suicide attempt. Some patients may prefer to suffer with pain or anxiety because they are more focused on accumulating medications for possible future use.

Lifespan Issues

CHILDHOOD

Though the rate of suicide in children is low, any time it occurs is cause for great concern and analysis. Recently it has received increased attention because the rates have increased. Young children have tried to kill themselves by jumping out of windows, hanging themselves, or running in front of moving cars. These actions are generally impulsive and in response to intense emotion. A suicidal act may be an attempt to gain power, punish a parent, or escape stressful situations. It could also be a response to parental neglect, rejection, or abuse. A young child who does not understand the finality of death may not understand the consequences of his or her action. In addition, children could also be imitating parental behaviors. Suicidal behavior can also be related to substance abuse and school problems.

ADOLESCENCE

Suicidal behavior in adolescents is considered a serious health problem. It is the second leading cause of death in teens following accidents. And some accidents could be concealed suicide attempts. Teens who are depressed, socially isolated, or using drugs and alcohol are at highest risk. Low self-esteem, history of abuse, not fitting in with peers, and school pressures may be other risk factors. As with adults, girls make more attempts, and boys are more likely to use more lethal methods, such as firearms. The availability of firearms in our society is believed to contribute to the increase in teenage suicides. Carbon monoxide poisoning and ingestion of pills are other common methods used by adolescents. High-risk behaviors like drug use, drag racing, and gang activity could be masking suicidal thoughts.

"Cluster" suicide, in which adolescents copy an episode of suicide of an acquaintance or celebrity, is a recent and alarming trend. To some teens the suicide of an idol can be romanticized.

ELDERLY

The elderly commit suicide more often than any other age group in the United States. Elderly men over age 80 are at highest risk. Guns remain the most frequent method. Suicide statistics in the elderly are probably even higher due to the prevalence of passive suicides. Elderly are more likely to use noncompliance with medical regimen or refusal to eat as a way to hasten their death. Risk factors include living alone, widowhood, lack of financial resources, poor health, and social isolation. In addition, misuse of alcohol and antianxiety medications may contribute.

Possible Nurses' Reactions

- Because of personal religious or moral beliefs, a nurse may identify a suicidal patient as weak or bad.
- May experience feelings of anxiety with patients, which may prevent the nurse from recognizing warning signs.
- May lack adequate training to work with suicidal patients and avoid dealing with them for fear of saying the wrong thing or contributing to their suicide.
- May have beliefs of rescuing patient and then experience intense guilt if patient does attempt or complete suicide. May take patient's behavior as a personal rejection.
- May feel angry with these patients for creating so much chaos, especially if the nurse perceives that the patient seems to have so much to live for, such as children and a good job. The nurse can feel in conflict because he or she is devoted to promoting health and saving lives.
- May deny or minimize suicidal behavior as a defense against anxiety and helplessness.
- Patient's behavior could stir up personal feelings of depression.

Assessment

Behavior and/or Appearance

- Direct verbal statements ("I wish I were dead")
- Indirect verbal statements ("You won't see me when you come back to work" or asking about specific suicide methods)
- Giving away possessions
- Agitation
- Sudden changes in eating, sleeping, or usual activities
- Neglecting appearance or hygiene
- Drawing up a will
- Refusing medications

Mood and/or Emotions

- Depression or despair
- Sudden lifting of depression, sudden elevation in mood
- Apathy
- Hopelessness
- Helplessness
- Anxiety
- Bitter anger

Thoughts, Beliefs, and Perceptions

- Disorganized, chaotic, irrational thinking
- Tunnel vision—unable to see options other than death
- Poor judgment
- Persecutory delusions and hallucinations, especially commands
- Excessive guilt or self-blame
- Low self-esteem

Relationships and Interactions

- Social isolation; withdrawn; feels alone and abandoned
- Recent loss of significant person through death or separation
- Recent tumultuous termination or interruptions of psychiatric treatment

Physical Responses

- Chronic debilitating illness
- Unrelieved pain
- Terminal illness
- Recent, catastrophic loss of physical abilities

Pertinent History

- History of suicide attempts
- Self-destructive behavior, such as drug abuse, reckless acts, or self-mutilation
- Family history of suicide attempts or depression
- Psychiatric illness
- Recent significant loss

Collaborative Interventions

Pharmacologic

Suicidal patients may benefit from taking antianxiety medication, such as lorezepam, to reduce feelings of intense anxiety or distress. In addition, antipsychotic and antimanic medication may be prescribed as needed. If antidepressants are being started, it is important to remember that it will take a number of weeks to lift depression, so other interventions must be used in the interim to prevent suicide. Antidepressants could actually increase suicide risk if the patient gets a sudden burst of energy to act out the plan before the depression lifts. In addition overdosing on antidepressants are an increasingly frequent method of suicide.

Adequate symptom management for pain and other distressing symptoms must be provided to the patient with a serious or terminal illness. A patient's belief that his or her symptoms cannot be controlled could be a contributing factor in suicide.

Patients at high risk for suicide may need to have medications administered in liquid form or parenterally to avoid "cheeking" pills that could be hoarded and used in an overdose attempt later. Outpatients should be given only a few days' supply of any medication that could potentially be used in a suicide attempt.

Nursing Management

HOPELESSNESS EVIDENCED BY EXPECTATIONS THAT THERE WILL BE NO IMPROVEMENT IN SITUATION RELATED TO DEPRESSION; OVERWHELMED BY LIFE CIRCUMSTANCES.

Patient Outcomes

- Verbalizes more optimistic expectations for the future
- Initiates realistic plans for the immediate future
- Demonstrates initiative in decision making

Interventions

- Recognize that extreme hopelessness is a strong indicator of suicide and should be thoroughly assessed.
- Listen to patient's concerns and issues with which he or she is struggling. Convey empathy to promote verbalizing about doubts and fears. Reflect back patient's despair without agreeing with it. For instance, you might say "You describe a world that seems empty."
- Encourage patient to discuss recent events or stresses that have contributed to the hopeless view. Offer alternative analysis viewing the event without arguing or minimizing patient's concerns. Minimizing or joking about the patient's feelings will increase the patient's sense of isolation and lack of trust.
- Emphasize the patient's strengths and problem-solving abilities. Describe a recent situation in which you observed the patient being successful. Have him or her describe a past success. Patients who are overwhelmed often have difficulty thinking clearly about future goals or viewing themselves objectively. Point out obstacles or negative thinking that get in the way of effective problem solving.
- Provide a balanced point of view to counteract patient's tendency to judge himself or herself so harshly. Point out unrealistic, perfectionistic thinking. Offer more constructive interpretations to open real options for the future.
- Acknowledge that you understand the patient feels that everything is useless and nothing will help but also that you believe something helpful can be done.

RISK FOR SELF-HARM EVIDENCED BY SUICIDE ATTEMPTS, SELF-MUTILATION, SUICIDE PLAN RELATED TO SUICIDE IDEATION, POOR IMPULSE CONTROL, DEPRESSION.

Patient Outcomes

- Remains free from injury
- Verbalizes intent not to harm self
- Expresses more optimistic view of future

Interventions

- Make a thorough assessment of patient's suicidal risk. Be aware that research is being conducted to develop assessment rating scales to better predict suicide potential.
- Determine if patient has a plan and how potentially lethal and available that plan is. See Table 9–4, Assessing Suicide Lethality. A patient in the hospital who talks about using a gun to kill himself or herself, would be at lower risk as long as he or she does not have a gun available to him or her. A patient who has a stash of medication would be at higher risk. Seek input from other professionals to participate in this assessment. If your agency has mental health professionals on staff, it is essential to involve them in the assessment.
- Talk openly with patient about your concern that he or she is suicidal. Let them know you are concerned and

TABLE 9–4. **Assessing Suicide Lethality**

1. Do you think about hurting or killing yourself? *If yes:*
2. Do you have a plan? How have you considered doing it? *If yes:*
3. Do you think you may or will do something to act on your thoughts? *If yes:* Where and when? Do you feel you have control over your own behavior?
4. Do you have the means available (such as, rope [could be a rolled-up sheet], gun, saved-up pills)?
5. Have you ever tried to harm yourself in the past? *If yes:* How? Did you expect to survive?
6. Are you willing to contract or notify staff whenever you feel you may act on these thoughts?

Our side of the contract is to be available and actively help you during these times.

If patient denies having a suicide plan, ask about other plans for the future and support systems.

1. What do you see yourself doing in a week, in a month, and in one year from now?
2. Do you feel optimistic or pessimistic about the future?
3. Do you have family members or friends with whom you can freely discuss your problems?

available to help. However, do not promise confidentiality about information he or she shares with you. Let the patient know that optimal care is possible only when the entire health team knows the facts.

- If the patient has attempted suicide, see Table 9–5, Assessing After a Suicide Attempt. Patient may or may not still be suicidal.
- Talk to patient about making a no-suicide contract with you. This involves asking him or her to wait or postpone action so that you and other professionals have time to help. Point out that depression is not permanent and that with time, medication, and therapy there is hope for a change but that death is permanent and cuts off other options.
- Make sure all members of the health-care team are aware of the patient's risk for suicide. Staff must be supportive and empathetic and familiar with treatment plan.
- For patients assessed to be at high risk for suicide:
  - Follow agency policy for need for continuous supervision. Discourage use of family for this purpose.
  - If in the hospital, place the patient in room close to nurses' station or in an ICU where closer monitoring is possible.

TABLE 9–5. **Assessing After a Suicide Attempt**

1. Did the patient expect to die? (yes, no, uncertain) Did the patient think his or her chance for dying was high, medium, or low?
2. Did suicide attempt appear to be highly lethal in intent?
3. How does the patient now feel about surviving? (relieved, sorry, angry) If the patient regrets surviving, question him or her about any current plan to attempt suicide.
4. If the patient's objective in suicide attempt or gesture was to manipulate a significant other to behave differently, have the sought-after changes occurred? Does the patient have alternative, more adaptive methods for coping?
5. Is support system present? (helpful, unhelpful)
6. Does the patient have any hope for future? How optimistic or pessimistic is he or she?
7. Is the patient willing to make a no-suicide contract?

- ○ Avoid checking on patient at predictable intervals.
- ○ Check more frequently during danger times, such as changes of shift, when patient may think staff will be preoccupied
- ○ Remove any objects in the room that could be used to inflict self-harm such as glasses, razors, belts, or lighters. Be aware of agency policy regarding need to search personal belongings or do a body search.
- ○ Make sure windows cannot be opened.
- ○ Physical restraints may need to be used for brief periods to prevent self-harm if all other interventions have been ineffective.
- Make sure family and friends are not bringing in potentially dangerous items such as medications, alcohol, or razors.
- Arrangements should be made to transfer the suicidal patient to a psychiatric unit as soon as medically stable.
- For patient who is not in the hospital, make sure family and friends are aware of the possible suicide risk. This patient probably should not be left alone. Give him or her resources to contact such as hotlines or therapists' phone numbers. Make sure patient has a list of phone numbers for support people he or she can call.

INEFFECTIVE INDIVIDUAL COPING EVIDENCED BY REPEATED SUICIDE THREATS AND GESTURES RELATED TO STUNTED AREAS OF PERSONALITY DEVELOPMENT WITH INTERMITTENT SELF-DESTRUCTIVE IMPULSES.

Patient Outcomes

- Decrease in self-destructive behaviors
- Demonstrates more adaptive means of communicating thoughts, feelings, and needs

Interventions

- Determine if self-destructive behavior is a pattern.
- Remain calm, treat patient's suicide threats and gestures in matter-of-fact manner, and demonstrate a neutral approach. Treat any physical injury without excessive emotion. Avoid creating a sense of alarm about the patient's

behavior. *Caution*: Do not dismiss any threat or gesture as manipulative or not serious. Any self-destructive threat or gesture should be taken seriously and not ignored.

- Ask the patient to identify any disturbing thoughts or feelings that occurred just before the threat or action. Encourage him or her to put thoughts and feelings into words rather than acting them out impulsively and destructively. Teach that sometimes anger hides more painful feelings such as sadness and rejection.
- Confront the patient who wants revenge and retaliation. These patients may state "They'll be sorry when I'm dead." Remind patient this is not a solution as he or she won't be there to see the results.
- Encourage the patient to alert staff if feeling out of control or when having thoughts of self-harm. Consider discussing a no-suicide contract to provide guidelines for behavior.
- Establish limits with patient on amount of time staff will spend listening to patient's concerns. Set limits on the patient's use of verbal abuse and demands.
- Review with the patient possible causes for self-destructive behavior that could include an attempt to get others to assume responsibility for patient's life. This patient needs to be encouraged to take more self responsibility. See Chapter 12, The Manipulative Patient, for additional interventions.
- Keep in mind that this patient is usually not aware of the manipulative appearance of his or her behavior. Diplomatically provide feedback about effects of this behavior on others, such as alienating supportive people.

ALTERNATE NURSING DIAGNOSES

Altered thought processes
Anxiety
Grieving
Risk for self-mutilation
Self-concept disturbance
Spiritual distress

WHEN TO CALL FOR HELP

✔ Self-mutilation
✔ Suicide threats or attempts
✔ Access to highly lethal methods such as firearms, car in an enclosed space, or sleeping pills in a high-risk patient
✔ Hallucinations or delusions
✔ Lack of staff available to manage suicidal patient
✔ Increasing staff anxiety and fear over patient's behavior

Patient and Family Education

- Teach patient that his or her view of options available becomes narrowed when depressed and/or suicidal. Review alternative ways of thinking or viewing his or her problems.
- Review with the patient that he or she needs to reach out to others for support and assistance.
- Teach the patient to reach out immediately when feeling urge to harm self.
- Encourage the patient to report and seek out adequate treatment for uncomfortable symptoms of physical illness, possibly including analgesics, to reduce any suffering.
- Teach alternative outlets for anger rather than self-destructive ones.
- Make sure patient and family understand the purpose of close observation by staff if actively suicidal.
- Make sure the family is aware of signs of increasing suicide risk and are aware of what they should do.
- In the event that a patient does commit suicide, prepare family for the complex grief reaction that may follow. See Table 9–6, Information for Survivors of Suicide.

Charting Tips

- Document all behaviors that could be considered a suicide thought, threat, or action.
- Note patient's response to suicide assessment.

TABLE 9–6. **Information for Survivors of Suicide**

- Recognize that their grief may have an added burden of guilt, shame, and anger.
- Sharing their grief with others about the cause of death will put the tragedy out in the open and provide added support.
- Recognize that factors contributing to the suicide may be out of the family's control.
- Provide information on dynamics of suicide.
- Encourage attendance at bereavement support groups specific for survivors of suicide.

- Document all measures in place to prevent suicide.
- Document patient's response to a no-suicide contract.
- Document any information from others on availability of potential methods for suicide available to the patient.

Discharge Planning

- Make sure the patient and family have information on referrals for follow-up counseling. They should also have emergency numbers such as suicide hotlines.
- Determine if psychiatric evaluation needs to be made before the patient is discharged or leaves the agency.
- Determine the appropriate quantities of prescribed medications to send home with the patient.
- Refer for home health follow-up, and make sure the agency is aware of the patient's suicide risk. Refer for psychiatric home care, if available.
- For high suicide risk, the patient may need to be transferred to a psychiatric hospital.

Nursing Outcomes

- Staff provides safe, appropriate, nonjudgmental care.
- Staff recognizes suicidal behavior and acts appropriately.
- Staff communicates effectively while caring for patient.

Suggested Learning Activities

- Arrange for inservice education from mental health professional on managing the suicidal patient.

- Discuss agency policies with supervisors and colleagues on managing the high-risk patient.
- Visit local suicide prevention center.
- Attend bereavement group for survivors of suicide.
- Discuss attitudes toward euthanasia and physician-assisted suicide with colleagues.
- Contact the American Association of Suicidology for statistics on suicide and information for survivors.

The Grieving Patient

LEARNING OBJECTIVES

▼ *Describe the variables that contribute to the intensity of the grief response.*
▼ *Describe some common behavioral responses to grief in children.*
▼ *Identify dysfunctional grief reactions.*
▼ *Describe effective nursing interventions to assist the grieving family.*
▼ *Describe common nursing staff reactions to the grieving patient.*

Experiencing loss, such as friends' moving away, losing functional abilities or physical health, and the death of loved ones, is a normal part of life. Grief is the normal human response that usually follows these experiences. As things change in our lives, we must adapt. This process of adaptation is called *grieving*. The purpose of grief is to begin to face the loss, work through the emotions, and eventually let go of it with renewed energy to focus on new relationships and goals. Because all individuals respond to a loss differently, the process of adapting varies widely and can take days, months, or even years. Variables that can influence the sense of loss include:

- The meaning of the lost object to the person (Generally the more important the loss is to the person, the more intense the reaction.)
- Degree of preparation and past unresolved losses
- Physical health
- The degree of ambivalence in the relationship (Often the more mixed the feelings are, such as in a love/hate relationship, the more difficult the grieving process may become.)
- Support system available

Glossary

Anticipatory grief—Grief response prior to and in preparation for a significant actual or potential loss.

Loss—Situation, real or potential, in which a valued object is rendered inaccessible or is altered in such a way that it no longer has the valued qualities.

Grief—Subjective, emotional response to a loss.

Mourning—The process by which grief is resolved.

Dysfunctional grief—Grief reaction that does not follow the usual pattern and may include delayed, distorted grief.

Delayed grief—The absence of grief behavior when it would be normally expected.

Distorted grief—Abnormal extension or overelaboration of grief behavior.

Bereavement—State of having suffered a loss.

• Concurrent stressors

Culture also influences the way an individual responds to loss. Most cultures have specific rituals and traditions that provide support and reassurance during the grieving process.

Grief caused by a death can be influenced by the cause of death. Unexpected deaths can leave the grieving person unprepared. Death resulting from a cause with a social stigma, such as suicide or AIDS, can be particularly difficult. With suicide, death is unexpected, violent, and possibly preventable. Survivors may experience intense anger, guilt, and self-blame. Those who lose a loved one from AIDS may have had time to prepare for the death, but many complicated feelings may still need to be resolved before grieving can be accomplished. Reactions from society to deaths caused by problems such as these, may affect the type of support the mourners receive.

Etiology

There is no one comprehensive theory that explains normal grief. Research has shown that grief occurs in a sequence of phases or stages with predictable symptoms that change over time and that these stages do not necessarily progress in an orderly, set fashion.

Acute grief symptoms were first described in Lindemann's classic study of 1944 following the Coconut Grove Fire in Boston. Symptoms include sighing, sobbing, and hyperventilating as well as a sense of unreality and shock as the first reactions to facing a major loss. Elisabeth Kübler-Ross and George Engel both described behavioral stages through which individuals advance in their progression toward resolution (see Table 9–7). These stages give us guides for expected behaviors, but each individual goes through the process in his or her own way and pace.

During the initial period of shock, the mourner may experience denial as a protective mechanism from the overwhelming stress to block out the pain. As denial and shock fade, the mourner begins to face the sadness of the loss. In addition to depression, there may be periods of anger and guilt. Anger can be directed at the lost person for leaving, (the person responsible for the situation), or it can be dis-

TABLE 9–7. **Adapting to Loss**

Stage	Purpose	Behavior
Engel's Stages: Adapting to Loss of a Person or Object		
Shock and disbelief	• Protect self from the pain of reality • Reality too painful for the person to take into consciousness	• Numbness, dazed appearance; denial of event
Developing awareness	• Emotional response as person realizes loss has occured; emotional reactions also signal to others their need for support and caring	• Sad, emotional; pangs of grief; intense suffering; sobbing, hyperventilating
Resolution	• Work of grieving as true scope of loss becomes incorporated; integration and acceptance of loss into one's life	• Reliving past; anger, depression
Kübler-Ross's Stages: Adapting to a Loss of Self		
Denial	• Unconscious avoidance to protect self from painful reality	• "No, not me." • Lack of expected reaction; using unproved treatment methods; doctor shopping to avoid confronting diagnosis
Anger	• Attempt to take control when feeling out of control by attacking, blaming others	• "Why me?" • Irrational demands; criticizing staff; hostile behavior
Bargaining	• Attempting to change reality by making agreement, bargains for more time • Indicates beginning acceptance	• "It's me, but . . ." • "I want to live til my son's wedding, then I'll accept death." • Making bargains with God to change if can have more time, change reality

TABLE 9–7. **Adapting to Loss** (*Continued*)

Stage	Purpose	Behavior
Kübler-Ross's Stages: Adapting to a Loss of Self		
Depression	• Work of grief as realization hits • Involves despair, the pain of experiencing loss	• "It's me." • Sad, tearful, life review
Acceptance	• Resolution of feelings about death • Neither happy nor sad • Acceptance of reality, sense of peace and letting go	• Comforting others to accept impending death; remembering the past with fondness but without fighting to hang on to life

Source: Adapted from Engel, 1964, and Kübler-Ross, 1969.

placed onto others. Guilt feelings, possibly evidenced by self-reproach for real or imagined acts of negligence or omissions, can be especially painful. All of these behaviors force the individual to confront the pain over and over again. However, not all reactions cause the individual to feel discomfort. Some can provide comfort such as having a sense of being watched over by the lost person.

The ability to tolerate intense emotions, increasing periods of stability, taking on new roles and relationships, and having the energy to invest oneself in new endeavors may indicate that the individual is recovering. Remembering both the positives and negatives of the lost person can indicate successful completion of grieving. However, brief periods of intense feelings may still occur at significant times, such as anniversaries and holidays.

Because each individual is unique, the extent of a grief reaction can vary. People may grieve as deeply over a loss of a pet or a longed for goal as the death of a family member. Traditionally one year is the time frame for grieving a major loss but longer or shorter periods are also normal.

Related Clinical Concerns

The physical stress of grief can place the mourner at risk for health problems. Lack of sleep, poor eating, and changes in routine can predispose the individual to illness. Loss of spouse in the elderly is associated with higher morbidity and mortality rates. Two months after a death, the bereaved elderly report more illness, greater use of medications, and poor health ratings.

Lifespan Issues

CHILDHOOD

Often adults try to protect children by not including them in the crisis or expressions of grief of other family members. However, they need to be included in the process, based on their level of development, so that they do not feel abandoned and left to face their fear and loss alone. Children generally display grief differently than adults, and it is important not to misinterpret these behaviors to mean that they are not grieving or that they are unaware of what is happening. They often use symbolic or nonverbal language to communicate their awareness of loss and may even feel ashamed of their loss because they feel differently from their peers. Since they may also need more time to really assimilate what has happened, grief reactions may be delayed (see Table 9–8).

ELDERLY

The elderly face multiple changes often including loss of spouse, peers, job, financial status, health, and mobility. In spite of the extent of these losses, most elderly seem able to adapt probably because of their past experience. However, the death of a spouse or partner still remains one of the major losses in life. This loss requires multiple life changes that become more difficult with increasing age. Grief can be masked in symptoms of dementia, depression, suicidal ideation, and substance abuse.

Possible Nurses' Reactions

• May feel helpless and uncomfortable with a sense of not knowing what to say. This could lead to avoidance or inappropriate hopefulness.

TABLE 9–8. **Children's Understanding of Death**

Age	Understanding of Death	Common Behaviors in Response to Death
Infant/toddler	• Unable to comprehend death • Fears separation and abandonment	• Frightened, difficulty separating
3–5 years	• Views illness as punishment for real or imagined wrongdoings • May view death as sleep; cannot comprehend death • Magical thinking; may think they caused the event by their thoughts or actions	• Sadness • Clinging to parent • Nightmares, sleep disruption • Regression in toilet habits • Complaints of stomachache and headaches • Temper tantrums
School age	• Associates death with punishment, mutilation, violence • May feel responsible for event • By age 9, understands that death is final	• School phobia, diminished school performance • Aggressive behavior • Preoccupation with parent's health • Loss of appetite • Change in relationship with friends
Adolescence	• Understands own mortality • May seem to have adult view of death but not emotional view	• Acting out; substance abuse • Increased time with peers • Withdrawal from family • Depression

- May fear saying the wrong thing that will cause the patient or family to feel more pain.
- May become detached from the dying patient to avoid the pain of losing him or her.
- May fear losing control of emotions.
- May make judgments regarding the degree of intensity of

grief behavior such as a family that is "not upset enough."
- May become detached from the situation and attempt to minimize the loss to the patient with phrases like "this was for the best," or "at least you can have more children."
- May unrealistically expect an optimal dying situation for the patient with family at the bedside, everyone open with their feelings, and conflicts resolved. This may be the nurse's need, rather than patient's.
- May expect all people to experience the stages of grief in the same way.
- May relive past, and unresolved losses causing intense emotions.

Assessment

Behavior and/or Appearance

- Crying, agitation
- Extreme change from usual behavior patterns
- Unable to concentrate, distractible
- Taking on behavior traits of lost person
- No apparent reaction when one would be expected
- Unkempt, not caring for self

Mood and/or Emotions

- Shock, numbness
- Depression (See Table 9–9)
- Anxiety, panic
- Mood swings
- No obvious emotional reaction or it is inappropriate to situation
- Anger
- Guilt, remorse
- Feeling relief that ordeal is over

Thoughts, Beliefs, and Perceptions

- Self-blame
- Idealizing lost person

TABLE 9–9. **Differentiating Grief from Depression**

	Uncomplicated Grief	**Major Depression**
Reactions	• Labile • Heightened when thinking of loss	• Mood consistently low • Prolonged, severe symptoms lasting over 2 months
Behavior	• Variable, shifts from sharing pain to being alone • Variable restriction of pleasure	• Completely withdrawn or fear of being alone • Persistent restriction of pleasure
Sleep patterns	• Periodic episodes of inability to sleep	• Wakes early morning
Anger	• Often expressed	• Turned inward
Sadness	• Varying periods	• Consistently sad
Cognition	• Preoccupied with loss • Self-esteem not as affected	• Focused on self • Feels worthless; has negative self-image
History	• Generally no history of depression	• History of depression or other psychiatric illness
Responsiveness	• Responds to warmth and support	• Hopelessness • Limited response to support
Loss	• Recognizable, current	• Often not related to an identified loss

Source: Adapted with permission. Schneider, J M: Clinically significant differences between grief, pathological grief, and depression. Patient Counselling and Health Education, 4th quarter, p 276, 1980.

- Only remembering the positives
- Ruminating over events leading to the loss
- Obsession with the deceased
- Illusory phenomena where mourner thinks lost person is present
- Preoccupied with thoughts that can only bring pain
- Imagining the lost person is watching over mourner
- Difficulty making decisions

Relationships and Interactions

- Seeks support from others, may become more dependent
- Fears being alone
- Unable to participate in conversation because of preoccupation with loss
- Feeling that others do not understand the pain ("How can they have a good time when I hurt so much?")
- Projection of anger onto others

Physical Responses

- Initial symptoms may include hyperventilating, sighing, sobbing, muscle tension, chest pain, fainting
- Gastrointestinal distress
- Loss of appetite
- Change in bowel habits
- Insomnia, constant fatigue
- Dehydration

Pertinent History

- Unresolved and/or multiple past losses
- Ambivalent relationship with lost person
- History of psychiatric disorder, and/or substance abuse
- Tendency to isolate self

Collaborative Interventions

Pharmacologic

Sedatives and tranquilizers are often used in the early stages of grief to reduce the impact of the intense emotions and promote rest and sleep. However, these medications suppress the intense emotions and interfere with the purpose of the grief process. Antidepressants may be useful, along with psychotherapy, when depressive symptoms are prolonged.

Spiritual

As people face loss and grief, they may be more likely to reach out for spiritual support. They may question their beliefs, talk about an afterlife, and face past wrongdoings. Allow the patient to express feelings, and, as needed, seek out clergy available within the agency or ask the patient's or family's own clergy to assist. Churches may also offer special support programs. If the patient requests, provide information on important religious rituals such as the Sacrament of the Sick and prayer, and provide religious articles such as Bibles, prayer books, medals, rosary, candles, and special clothing. Clergy may also provide important support for staff who may be struggling with helping patient or family with spiritual issues.

Nursing Management

ANTICIPATORY GRIEVING EVIDENCED BY DISTRESS AT POTENTIAL LOSS, INCLUDING DEPRESSION, ANGER, AND GUILT RELATED TO TERMINAL ILLNESS.

Patient Outcomes

- Acknowledges potential loss
- Expresses concerns, feelings of grief
- Verbalizes feeling of being supported in the grieving process
- Identifies potential coping mechanisms, support systems

Interventions

- Accept grieving behavior. Recognize that responses to grief are highly individual.
- Use open-ended questions and reflection to give patient the opportunity to share feelings and concerns. Listen for patient readiness to discuss issues about facing dying. For example, a patient may say "I don't think I'll be around much longer." The nurse can respond by saying "Tell me what you're worried about."
- Recognize that your role may be a listener if patient has need to vent feelings. Providing an accepting environment to share these feelings is extremely important. Let the patient determine what issues he or she needs to

explore. The patient may feel more comfortable discussing his or her grief with a nurse because of not wanting to upset family and friends.

- Facilitate communication between family and patient, if appropriate. Ask patient if he or she would like you to share personal concerns with family if communication has been blocked. Prepare family for some of patient's concerns.
- Be aware of need to preserve hopefulness. Recognize that hope may take on many faces in the dying patient. It could move from hope for a miracle, to hope to have less pain, to hope to live until a grandchild's wedding. Be careful not to promote inappropriate hopefulness based on your own needs or discomforts.
- Recognize that behaviors, such as frequent demands, criticisms, frequent questioning, and family conflict, may indicate the family members' sense of loss of control in preparing to face the death of a loved one. Provide the family with some areas of control and decision making in patient's care. Acknowledge their important role as patient advocate and the difficult situation they are facing.
- Encourage family to express feelings of sadness and grief. Talk with them about what to expect. Assess need for privacy versus not wanting to be alone.
- Determine family readiness to talk about facing patient's death. Some important questions may include their understanding of the prognosis and treatment plan and the patient's care. Talk with family away from patient to determine readiness, and then determine if it is appropriate for all to talk together.
- Remember that family members still have other responsibilities such as childcare and job. Talk with them about how they are managing, and support their decisions about when to stay and leave. Assess if they are getting adequate sleep and food. They may be looking for permission to care for themselves.
- Speak with parents away from their children. Assist the parents on how to begin preparing their child for receiving the information about the situation. This may include encouraging children to talk about their feelings, drawing their feelings, being given a role in helping the dying per-

son, allowing them to maintain some normalcy in routine such as attending school and providing opportunities for play. Parents should let the children's teachers know what is happening.

- Support cultural and religious beliefs during the dying process. Recognize that mourners may have rituals that need to be carried out such as chanting, or lighting candles.

- Keep family informed on the patient's condition. Provide information on what to expect, what they can do for the patient, and what nurses are doing. Reinforce the need for a referral to hospice care, as needed.

- Once patient has died, inform family members in private. Give them the opportunity to have some private time with patient. Assist them in getting other family members to the bedside, if possible, to provide support. Provide information on procedures regarding mortuary arrangements, when appropriate. If appropriate, provide information on organ donations and autopsy.

DYSFUNCTIONAL GRIEVING EVIDENCED BY INHIBITION, SUPPRESSION, ABSENCE, PROLONGATION, OR DISTORTED GRIEF REACTIONS RELATED TO SIGNIFICANT LOSS, MULTIPLE LOSSES, UNRESOLVED GUILT, LACK OF SUPPORT SYSTEM, DIFFICULTY EXPRESSING FEELINGS.

Patient Outcomes

- Acknowledges the loss
- Demonstrates absence of abnormal, prolonged, excessive reactions to loss
- Resumes or develops social relationships.
- Expresses feelings expected with the loss

Interventions

- Recognize that the individual needs to confront the loss slowly and accept it into his or her reality at their own pace. Part of this process will include talking about the loss, reliving memories, talking about events leading to the loss, and expressing feelings.

- Use supportive phrases such as "It must be hard for you now" or "I'm so sorry to hear of your loss." These phrases acknowledge the loss and encourage the person to tell his or her story. Avoid phrases such as "At least you had him for 20 years." These statements diminish the loss to the mourner and can lead to feeling isolated and misunderstood.
- Monitor for signs of dysfunctional grieving including prolonged denial, lack of emotional response, living in the past, or self-destructive behavior. If the mourner exhibits these behaviors, monitor closely and talk with him or her about your concerns. If possible, refer to bereavement counseling.
- Encourage involvement in new activities and meeting new people. Help the person to set small goals to begin these activities very slowly, and identify realistic expectations.
- Assist the mourner to redefine the relationship with the lost person or object. This includes remembering the positives and negatives and acknowledging possible angry feelings.
- If the mourner does not acknowledge the loss, bring up the subject. You might say "I notice you never mention your deceased husband. How has it been for you?"
- Provide spiritual support as requested. Encourage involvement of clergy.

ALTERNATE NURSING DIAGNOSES

Anxiety
Body image disturbance
Ineffective family coping, compromised
Ineffective individual coping
Knowledge deficit
Powerlessness
Self-esteem disturbance
Sleep pattern disturbance
Social isolation
Spiritual distress

WHEN TO CALL FOR HELP

Professional consultation is important if the patient exhibits:

✔ Disturbing behavior including hallucinating, delusions, obsessions
✔ Evidence of intense prolonged preoccupation with lost person
✔ Long periods of depression possibly including suicidal thoughts and/or gestures
✔ Living in the past many months or years after loss occurred
✔ No emotional reaction to loss for a prolonged period of time

Or, if the staff exhibits:

✔ Intense emotional reaction to death of patient
✔ Difficulty in dealing with personal grief to the extent that it impacts on patient care

Patient and Family Education

- Prepare patient and family for the normal stages of grieving.
- Inform them that anticipatory grief does not necessarily reduce the emotional impact of the loss. Mourners still may expect an intense reaction.
- Provide information on advance directives. Encourage the patient to clarify his or her wishes on topics such as treatment options and resuscitation, and share these with the physicians and family.
- Tell the family the signs of dysfunctional grief and encourage them to seek help if they begin to experience them.
- Tell the patient that feelings of anger and guilt may be normal. Encourage seeking professional help if he or she is having difficulty resolving these feelings.
- Encourage mourner to be very patient through this process. Time is needed to slowly face the grief. Discourage making major decisions early on in grieving.
- Discourage use of tranquilizers as a way to avoid intense emotions.

- If appropriate, encourage dying patient to make a videotape or other form of legacy for the family, especially if there are young children.
- Provide information on organ donation and mortuary arrangements, if appropriate, for dying patient or family.
- Let the mourner know that his or her feelings may be intensified at key times such as holidays and anniversaries and that they may last for a few days.
- Encourage good nutrition and good health habits, especially for the elderly. Encourage seeking medical attention, as needed, during the bereavement period because he or she is at an increased risk of illness.
- Prepare mourner and family for delayed grief reaction when intense feelings may occur in response to future loss.

Charting Tips

- Document grieving behaviors.
- Document medication use such as tranquilizers and analgesics.
- Document patient and family awareness of prognosis and closeness of death.
- Avoid documenting judgments about patient behavior.

Discharge Planning

- Provide information on bereavement counseling and support groups. Provide the information in writing as mourners may be unable to concentrate.
- Inform referring agencies and home health agencies about potential grief reactions. Refer dying patients to a hospice program for additional support, as indicated.
- Identify opportunities for socialization. Encourage involvement in activities when appropriate.
- Encourage involvement of family and friends to expand mourner's support system.

Nursing Outcomes

- Accepts and supports grief responses of patient and family

- Demonstrates increased comfort in providing support for grieving patient and family.
- Seeks support from colleagues on facing grief of losing a patient.
- Demonstrates evidence of allowing mourner to grieve at own pace.

Suggested Learning Activities

- Arrange for inservice by hospice professionals to discuss caring for the dying patient and family.
- Invite local clergy to discuss rituals and/or traditions around the grieving process for variety of religions.
- Share past experiences with colleagues or own experiences with grief.
- Sit in on a bereavement support group, if possible.

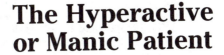

The Hyperactive
or Manic Patient

LEARNING OBJECTIVES

▼ *List the outstanding characteristics of mania.*
▼ *List possible contributing factors to manic episodes.*
▼ *Describe effective nursing interventions for a manic*
   episode.
▼ *Describe possible nurses' reactions to manic behavior.*

In the early phase of a manic episode an individual can become engaging, outgoing, and charming, presenting as one who is achieving and successful with excessive energy and optimism. During the hypomanic episode, people remain at this level. Unfortunately, mania can accelerate to a continuously frenzied, out-of-control pace, leading to seriously impaired decision making and potentially very hazardous activity. A patient in an escalated manic phase frequently denies the seriousness or even

Glossary

Manic episode—A distinct period during which there is an abnormally and persistently elated, expansive, or irritable mood possibly accompanied by inflated self-esteem or grandiosity, decreased need for sleep, pressured speech, flight of ideas, or subjective experience that thoughts are racing, distractibility, increased involvement in goal-directed activities or psychomotor agitation, and excessive involvement in pleasurable activities with a high potential for painful consequences. Psychotic features may arise.

Mixed episode—A period during which the criteria are met for both a manic episode and for a major depressive episode nearly every day.

Hypomanic episode—A distinct period that is similar to a manic episode but the symptoms are not as severe. There is no marked impairment in social or occupational functioning. Psychotic features are not present.

Rapid cycling—At least four episodes of a mood disturbance in the previous 12 months that meet criteria for a major expressive episode, manic, mixed, or hypomanic episode.

Cyclothymic disorder—A chronic mood disturbance of at least 2 years, which can be thought of as a muted version of bipolar disorder.

Schizoaffective disorder—An uninterrupted period of illness during which, at some time, there is a major depressive, manic, or mixed episode concurrent with the characteristic symptoms of schizophrenia.

the existence of illness, both medical and psychiatric. This individual could walk endless miles for days, expecting cars to clear a path for him or her, ignore the need for any food and sleep, and disregard any physical impairment.

An increasing manic episode, which usually occurs over a few days, can be viewed as a series of stages during which the symptoms become more intense and severe. For example, an initial overestimation of abilities ("I can earn more money than any other salesman in the United States") can balloon to grandiose delusions ("I am Jesus Christ") and hallucinations. What begins as pressured, rapid, but still organized speaking can escalate to constant loose flitting verbalizations from topic to topic with little or no connections, and eventually, incoherence. Irritability, especially when demands are not met, can escalate into belligerent explosiveness and combativeness. And restlessness can peak into a state of continuous motion. If the patient is not medicated, a manic episode can last months.

Interestingly, descriptions of manic episodes reflect a mirror image of depression. Depression is characterized by an insidious slowing down of movement, thought, self-esteem, and initiative, which is accompanied by dejected, constricting, pessimistic, and even despairing mood. Internally focused guilt (even when not deserved) abounds, and anger is self-directed. In mania, everything seems to speed up including thought, speech, decisions, and activity. Mood and self-esteem skyrockets upward with a belief that all desires and dreams can be fulfilled. Externally focused, anger is directed outward, guilt is noticeably absent, and blame is put on others. In the extreme forms of both depression and mania, there is a psychotic break with reality, including delusions and/or hallucinations.

Bipolar disorder, formerly called "manic depression," is best viewed as a recurrent illness in which there are symptom-free periods. More than 90 percent of patients who experience a first manic episode go on to have future episodes. The majority of individuals with bipolar disorders return to a fully functional level between episodes. Manic episodes (and hypomanic episodes) often precede or follow major depressive episodes in a characteristic

TABLE 9–10. **Comparing Episodes in Bipolar I and Bipolar II Disorders**

	Bipolar I Disorder	**Bipolar II Disorder**
Mania	• Manic or mixed episode(s) *must* occur. • Hypomanic episode(s) can occur.	• Hypomanic episode(s) *must* occur. • Manic or mixed episode(s) cannot occur.
Depression	• Major depressive episode(s) can occur.	• Major depressive episode(s) *must* occur.

Note: Mixed episodes have been listed under mania for organizational purposes although they are an almost daily intermingling of both manic and major depressive episodes.

pattern for a particular person. The frequency of manic episodes varies. Some have periodic episodes separated by years, and some have close repetition. Long-term, even lifelong, medication may be necessary. (Medication-free trials should be tried only under physician supervision.)

DSM-IV further defines two types of bipolar disorders: bipolar I and bipolar II (See Table 9–10):

Bipolar I disorder: Characterized by the occurrence of one or more manic episodes or mixed episodes. Often, but not always, individuals also have one or more major depressive episodes.

Bipolar II disorder: Characterized by the occurrence of one or more major depressive episodes with the presence (or history) of at least one hypomanic episode.

Etiology

Bipolar disorder is a complex phenomenon in which a variety of factors converge.

Biologic theory predominates. Studies indicate that this disorder is caused by an imbalance in neurotransmitters, particularly norepinephrine and serotonin. Increase is believed to be present in manic episodes and decreased in depressive ones. Impaired interrelationships of the hormonal and endocrine systems are currently being explored. Investigation of brain electrical activity is also being studied since valproate, carbamazepine, and other anticonvulsants have been successfully used with lithium-resistant manic episodes. Electroencephalographic changes have been also linked to mood disturbances. Disruptions in circadian rhythms and exposure to light, as in light therapy for depression with seasonal pattern, can contribute to manic episodes.

A *genetic* link has also been demonstrated through family studies. Bipolar patients have a significantly greater percentage of relatives with bipolar disorder and depressive disorder than the general population. Studies done on twins and adopted individuals provide strong evidence of a genetic influence for bipolar I disorder.

Sociologically, there are no reports of differential incidence of bipolar I disorder based on race or ethnicity. Bipolar I disorder is approximately equally common in men and women, although mania is more often the initial episode in males and depression in women. Bipolar II disorder may be somewhat more common in women.

Psychologic theory views mania as a defensive flight from an underlying extreme depression with its attendant painful feelings of hopelessness, worthlessness, and emptiness. It is suggested that the individual uses denial as a defense mechanism. Hypotheses requiring further investigation are that the patient uses manic symptoms to covertly get dependency needs met, the patient is highly dependent on approval from others to maintain self-esteem, and the patient uses manic symptoms to prevent others from setting limits and containing out-of-control behavior.

Related Clinical Concerns

Hyperactive symptoms caused by substance abuse, medication use, or a general medical condition are not considered to be a bipolar disease. Under these circumstances, the diagnoses would be substance-induced mood disorder or mood disorder due to a general medical condition (see Table 9–11).

TABLE 9–11. **Drug, Medical, and Traumatic Causes of Manic and Hypomanic Symptoms**

Drug-Related	*Metobolic Disturbance*
Isoniazid	Postoperative states
Procarbazine	Hemodialysis
Levodopa	Vitamin B_{12} deficiency
Bromide	Addison's disease
Decongestants	Cushing's disease
Bronchodilators	Postinfection states
Procyclidine	Dialysis
Calcium replacement	Hyperthyroidism
Phencyclidine	
Metoclopramine	*Neurologic Conditions*
Corticosteroids	Right temporal seizure focus
Hallucinogens	Multiple sclerosis
Sympathomimetic amines	Right cerebral hemisphere damage
Disulfiram	Epilepsy
Alcohol	Huntington's disease
Barbiturates	Postcerebrovascular accident
Anticholinergics	
Benzodiazepines	*Other Conditions*
Antidepressants	Neoplasms
Amphetamines	Postisolation syndrome
Cocaine	Right temporal lobotomy
Cyclosporine	Posttraumatic confusion
Zivovudine (AZT)	
Infection	
Influenza	
Q fever	
Neurosyphilis	
Post-St. Louis type A encephalitis	
"Benign" herpes simplex encephalitis	
AIDS (HIV)	

Source: Adapted from Goodwin and Jamison: Manic-Depressive Illness, Oxford University Press, New York, 1990, with permission.

Manic episodes can be induced by other somatic treatments for depression, such as electroconvulsive (ECT or "shock") therapy or light therapy for depression with seasonal pattern (exposure to increased amount of bright visible-spectrum light during seasons of the year with diminished daylight).

Sleep disturbance is both a symptom of manic episodes and an irritant that can exacerbate manic episodes and worsen the overall condition. In hospitalized patients who have a history of bipolar disease, it is essential to encourage the patient to maintain a normal sleep-wake cycle and to obtain adequate hours of sleep each night.

Lifespan Issues

CHILDHOOD

Studies indicate that 20 to 30 percent of bipolar disorders have onset before age 20. The true diagnosis may need to be clarified in observing the patterns and manifestations of future episodes. The possibility of manic episode(s) occurring in young children is controversial. Since the incidence of manic episodes in children before the age of 12 years is extremely rare, there is a danger of a child with this disorder being labeled a "problem child" or being misdiagnosed as attention-deficit disordered with hyperactivity.

ADOLESCENCE

Manic episodes in adolescents are more likely to include psychotic features and can be misdiagnosed as schizophrenia. Behavioral problems can lead to the misdiagnosis of conduct disorder. Approximately 10 to 15 percent of adolescents with recurrent major depressive episodes will go on to develop bipolar I disorder. Assessments should include a family history of mood disorders.

In adolescents, manic and hypomanic episodes may be associated with school truancy, antisocial behavior, school failure, or substance abuse. A significant minority of adolescents appear to have a history of long-standing behavior problems that precede the onset of a frank manic episode. It is unclear whether these problems represent a prolonged prodrome to bipolar disorder or an independent disorder.

Antimanic medications can be used in adjusted doses along with pychotherapeutic interventions.

ADULTHOOD

The majority of first manic episodes in bipolar disorder occur between the ages of 20 and 30 years with a preponderance in the early twenties. If the onset of a first manic episode occurs in a patient 40 years or older who has no prior psychiatric illness, then medical conditions and drug-inducing manic symptoms should be ruled out.

"Postpartum onset" is applied to manic, depressive, or mixed episodes that occur within 4 weeks after delivery of a child. The symptomology remains the same. If delusions are present, they often concern the newborn child. If a manic episode develops in the postpartum period, there may be an increased risk for recurrence in subsequent postpartum periods.

In the adult years, uncontrolled symptoms can result in job losses, marital and other relationship breakups, grave financial problems, or serious legal repercussions from violating laws. During manic episodes parents may be unable to care for and provide safety for a child. Child abuse, spousal abuse, or other violent behaviors may occur during severe manic episodes or during those with psychotic features.

ELDERLY

The intervals between episodes tend to decrease in bipolar I disorder and to increase in bipolar II disorder as an individual ages. Medical conditions and drug reactions as causative factors in manic episodes need to be carefully evaluated, particularly when initial episodes occur in the elderly. Managing patients with bipolar disorder in long-term care settings can create major challenges for the staff.

Possible Nurses' Reactions

- May be entertained or amused by the initial exuberance and acting out
- May become irritable, anxious, or angry when patient is noncompliant with healthcare regimen or hospital routine
- May become embarrassed or sense lowered self-esteem if the nurse believes that a "good" nurse should be able to control patients or prevent them from behaving strangely
- May feel verbally abused and unrecognized by the patient

- May feel manipulated, outsmarted, and defensive, needing to justify actions and motives
- May feel frightened if patient becomes violent

Assessment

Behavior and/or Appearance

- Very interactive and engaging with others
- Pressured speech (profuse, rapid, as if generated by an engine)
- Excessive in all areas: bizarre, garish, flamboyant, eccentric
- Poor personal grooming
- Noticeably excessive amount of makeup, provocative clothing
- Restlessness, hyperactivity with constant moving and pacing
- Flitting attempts to participate in multiple activities, few to completion, impulsive
- Poor judgment in decision making; undertakes risky or dangerous endeavors without awareness of consequences, such as buying sprees, foolish business investments, and reckless driving; hypersexuality
- Inappropriate behavior to situation
- Complaints, hostile comments, and angry tirades; may be violent

Mood and/or Emotions

- Elation; heightened sense of pleasure; unrealistic optimism
- Lack of shame or guilt
- Anger escalating to rage especially when wishes thwarted
- Labile mood swings including depression, irritability, and anger

Thoughts, Beliefs, and Perceptions

- Distracted; unable to concentrate on task at hand; overly attuned and responsive to stimulation from people and events

- Grandiose overestimation of own abilities, talents; exaggeration of past achievements; inflated self-esteem; impaired judgment
- Complicated plans to acquire unlimited fame, fortune, and/or power
- Poor insight; unaware of his or her distortion and negative effect on others
- Makes puns, plays on words, and jokes
- Flight of ideas (continuously jumps rapidly from one topic to another)
- Suspicious
- Delusions and/or hallucinations of grandiosity or persecution

Relationships and Interactions

- Excessively gregarious; can be charming
- Able to form superficial relationships quickly but becomes manipulative, demanding, intrusive, taunting
- Attempts to engage everyone into their plans and activities
- Lacks true concern for others
- Manipulates self-esteem of others by flattery
- Constantly demands attention
- Irresponsible; gives quick, deceptively plausible excuses for own actions; puts responsibility on others
- Intimidating

Physical Responses

- Initial overeating; weight gain, even food hoarding
- As mania escalates, inadequate nutritional intake leading to weight loss and even dehydration
- Physical exhaustion
- Insomnia
- May exhibit side effects of drug abuse and symptoms of general medical conditions that can cause mania

Pertinent History

- Earlier episodes or family history of depressive and/or manic episodes

- Dramatic changes in personality during manic phases (e.g., usually quiet person becomes flamboyant and blatantly seductive)
- Psychiatric outpatient treatment or hospitalization or psychiatric diagnosis of schizophrenia or schizoaffective disorder; differential diagnosis often confused since extremes of manic episodes have similar symptoms
- History of substance abuse

Collaborative Management

Pharmacologic

Patients may need to take antimanic medications for the rest of their lives; therefore, education and compliance are very important.

Lithium carbonate is the most common first-line medication used in typical manic episodes of bipolar disorder. Lower maintenance doses are often continued in the intervals between episodes. Blood levels and side effects need to be monitored since lithium can reach a toxic range possibly causing seizures, coma, and even death. Therapeutic lithium levels are between 0.5 and 1.5 mEq/L for most patients. Blood lithium levels can be elevated when there is significant lowering of body fluids such as limited fluid intake, profuse sweating, or chronic diarrhea. It is essential to constantly monitor for adverse drug reactions since some individuals can become toxic at blood levels considered normal for most people. Onset of sedation, nausea, and vomiting are early warning signs of lithium toxicity. As toxicity increases, tremors and muscle twitching may occur.

Lithium can take 7 to 10 days to reach desired effect. If psychotic symptoms are present, antipsychotics can be used on a regular or as-needed basis. The need should diminish as lithium or other antimanic medications reach therapeutic levels.

Antimanic drugs are available only in oral forms. If the patient is unable to take oral medications, other medications may be used, such as antipsychotics or antianxiety drugs, that can be given parenterally.

Anticonvulsants, such as carbamazepine, are also used. Carbamazepine can cause agranulocytosis with lethal implications. The incidence of this adverse effect is low; however, it is important to continually monitor the patient for changes in white blood cell and granulocyte count and any signs of infection. Agranulocytosis subsides promptly when the drug is removed.

Dietary

A patient in an escalated manic phase may be too restless to sit and eat foods. Patients may need "finger foods" that can be carried, such as sandwiches and milkshakes. A high-caloric diet should be provided if patient is in constant movement.

Psychotherapy

To gain the patient's acceptance of maintaining the medication regimen, the patient needs to accept the reality of having a bipolar disorder. This requires that the patient have the time to work through the denial and, later, anger over having an incurable condition. Medications can control the frequency and intensity of manic episodes, but exacerbations can still happen. The patient may need assistance in dealing with shame over behavior during manic episodes. He or she may also need to learn how to discriminate normal from abnormal moods and will probably need help in learning to tolerate more dysphoric feelings and moods.

As life becomes flatter and is less colorful without mania, the patient may need to grieve the losses associated with giving up mania, such as fantasies, highs and/or euphoric states, increased level of energy and sexuality, decreased need for sleep, and possibly, decreased degree of productivity and creativity.

Developmental tasks may have been overshadowed by the illness. For example, the adolescent tasks of establishing a separate identity and learning about relationships may have been disrupted. Once the patient is stabilized, these issues will need to be addressed.

If the patient has an alcohol or drug abuse dependency, this needs to be acknowledged as a problem especially since the patient usually denies the problem. Mood disorders can mask substance abuse just as substance abuse often masks mood disorders. Effective substance abuse treatment should be used concurrently with approaches for bipolar disorder (Goodwin and Jamison, 1990).

Nursing Management

ANXIETY EVIDENCED BY HYPERACTIVITY, DISTRACTIBILITY, DISORGANIZED AND UNREALISTIC THOUGHTS RELATED TO MANIC PHASE OF BIPOLAR DISORDER.

Patient Outcomes

- Slower and more controlled speech
- Organized and realistic thoughts, without delusions or hallucinations
- Demonstrates an increased ability to concentrate
- Demonstrates more controlled behavior
- Demonstrates more realistic decision making
- Complies with medication regime

Interventions

- Determine whether patient has previously been under psychiatric care for treatment of mania. If patient is not currently under psychiatric supervision, strongly encourage immediate referral and assessment. Make sure the physician and other staff are aware of the patient's history.
- Provide firm, clear limits. Describe exactly what is expected and what is not allowed. Be realistic. For instance, patient may need to have a designated area in which to pace without being disruptive to the unit.
- Administer ordered antimanic medications and monitor blood levels, adverse effects, and signs of possible toxicity.
- Assess for psychotic symptoms, and evaluate for need to administer PRN antipsychotic medications.
- Do not reinforce patient's delusional beliefs. Rather, present what is reality without arguing with the patient.

- Be consistent even if the patient produces seemingly plausible reasons and excuses. Do not participate in verbal battles—just repeat the rules. Avoid power struggles. Keep directions simple and specific.
- Use a calm, relaxed approach.
- Attempt to provide a focus to the conversation if patient jumps from one topic to another. Interrupt to slow him or her down. Bring the patient back to the chosen topic. Phrase questions so they require a brief answer. If the patient's thoughts are speeding to the point of confusion, do not encourage continued speaking, and, if possible, arrange for someone to sit quietly with patient. Supervise other caregivers who are unfamiliar with manic patients.
- Explain to staff, patients, and visitors who complain about patient's constant need for attention that the patient will feel better in a quiet atmosphere. Encourage them to limit interactions with the patient without abandoning him or her.
- Remove patient from external stimulation. If possible, place him or her in a room in a quiet area; use dim lighting. A private room is preferable. Calming music may help.
- Assess whether patient should be allowed to verbalize anger or fear. If patient becomes overly agitated, change or redirect the topic of conversation. As the mania decreases, the patient may be better able to tolerate more processing of emotion.
- Limit the patient's choices. Attempt to limit the number of objects patient has in the room. Encourage family and/or friends to take home unnecessary possessions.
- Remove hazardous objects from patient's room.
- Provide activities that require only a short attention span. If the patient becomes involved in unacceptable behavior, distract him or her into more productive ones. More complex tasks can be introduced as mania decreases.
- Do not reinforce inappropriate behaviors by giving them a lot of attention.
- Assess for activities patient can do in his or her room, such as writing or drawing.
- Provide an outlet for excessive energy. Obtain referral to physical therapy to assess whether a stationary bike or

other equipment can safely be placed in the patient's room. Supervise any physical activity.

- Support and encourage the patient's ideas that are realistic and consistent with healthcare regimen.
- Assess for any injuries, bruises, and signs of infection.
- Assess for substance abuse. Explain to the patient and family that alcohol or drug abuse can undermine bipolar treatment.
- Assist the family in dealing with any negative feelings they may have toward the patient so they can interact more constructively with him or her.
- Obtain support from peers and other resources if patient's manipulations begin to erode the nurses' ability to maintain an effective approach.

SLEEP PATTERN DISTURBANCE EVIDENCED BY INABILITY TO LAY DOWN AT NIGHT, SLEEPING ONLY BRIEF PERIODS, AND ERRATIC SLEEP PATTERNS RELATED TO MANIC/UNCONTROLLED ACTIVITY.

Patient Outcomes

- Remains alert and awake during the day
- No evidence of daytime fatigue
- Sleeps at least 5 hours per night
- Does not require naps during the day

Interventions

- Monitor sleep patterns and assess for signs of fatigue.
- Use calming techniques just before bedtime, such as warm milk, soothing music, or warm bath. Avoid stimulants such as caffeine.
- Decrease stimulation at bedtime: lights out, curtains drawn, phone unplugged. Avoid loud noises nearby and loud talking. Some patients may respond well to having someone sit quietly just outside the room until patient is asleep. This nurse can encourage the patient to remain in bed long enough to fall asleep.
- Provide ordered sleep medication if patient is unable to sleep.
- Encourage the patient to go to bed at the same time each night.

- If naps are needed during the day, encourage taking them at the same time each day.

ALTERNATE NURSING DIAGNOSES

Altered nutrition, less than or more than body requirements

Altered thought processes

Fluid volume deficit

Impaired social interaction

Ineffective individual coping

Ineffective management of therapeutic regimen, individual

Noncompliance

Risk for injury

Risk for violence; directed at others

WHEN TO CALL FOR HELP

- ✔ Out-of-control verbalizations and behavior
- ✔ Psychotic symptoms
- ✔ Patient refusing health care or refusing to take medications
- ✔ Gross interference in other patient's care that does not respond to interventions
- ✔ Symptoms of lithium toxicity
- ✔ Lab values indicating agranulocytosis in patients taking carbamazepine

---

Patient and Family Education

- Avoid health teaching until patient displays significant reduction in psychiatric symptoms and demonstrates good awareness of reality.
- Teach the family the symptoms of a manic episode so they can recognize what is occurring and not personalize the patient's interactions with them.
- Teach the patient and family the importance of continuing psychiatric medications and treatment, monitoring signs of medication adverse effects and toxicity, and noting early signs and symptoms of recurrent episodes.

- Teach patients, especially those on lithium, to maintain normal diet, fluid, and salt intake.
- Teach patients on lithium to check with their physician about withholding drug if excessive diarrhea, vomiting, or diaphoresis occurs.
- Teach the patient to make a contract with family or a trusted significant other to encourage and assist the patient to make contact with psychiatrist or counselor if there is a resurgence of symptoms. Often family members are the first to notice behavioral changes.
- Assist the family to make plans for hospitalization so they will be able to act quickly if an emergency situation arises.
- Teach patient about the process of realistic decision making and the effect on others of his or her decisions.
- Teach patient that life includes accepting periods of sadness, disappointment, and uncomfortable feelings.
- Teach patient about his or her effect on others.

Charting Tips

- Note the presence or absence of adverse effects of lithium.
- Document the amount of PRN antipsychotics given, if used.
- Document any factors that could lead to dehydration.
- Document percentage of food eaten and weight changes.
- Note changes in patient's behavior and thoughts expressed.
- Document patient's lack of compliance with healthcare regimen.

Discharge Planning

- Reinforce that it is essential that the patient continue in medical and psychiatric treatment and take prescribed medications after discharge.
- Make sure patient has appointments for required blood levels to be taken.
- Refer to social service those patients who may have alienated friends, family, and/or associates before hospitalization. Financial and legal issues may be pending

because of unwise actions, such as excessive spending sprees.

- Recommend assessing the need for transfer to psychiatric facility if patient's behavior and thought processes are not sufficiently stabilized.
- Recommend that the patient attend community support groups for bipolar disorder such as the Manic Depressive and Depressive Association.
- Recommend that the family attend support groups such as those sponsored by the National Alliance for the Mentally Ill (NAMI).

Nursing Outcomes

- Staff assigned to patient demonstrates interventions that contain patient's behavior to a safe level.
- Needed antimanic medications are administered as ordered.
- Documentation reflects appropriate assessment of behaviors and identification of adverse effects of medications.

Suggested Learning Activities

- Arrange for inservice on manic patients with a mental health professional to speak on patient management and pharmacist to speak on antimanic medications.
- Attend community support groups for bipolar disorder.
- Role play:
  - Telling an individual who persists in constantly circling the room in which area to remain.
  - Telling an individual who persists in reading aloud nonstop that it is time for breakfast.
  - Explaining the need to continue antimanic medication to an individual who does not want to be deprived of feeling elated.

10 PROBLEMS WITH CONFUSION

The Confused Patient

LEARNING OBJECTIVES

▼ *Differentiate between dementia and delirium.*
▼ *List the most common types of dementia.*
▼ *Describe common nurses' reactions to the confused patient.*
▼ *Describe effective nursing interventions for the confused patient with the following: memory deficits, unable to verbalize his or her needs, and at risk for falling.*

Confusion is not just a state of the mind seen in the elderly. It has many causes and can occur at any age. It significantly influences a patient's dignity, independence, personality, and support system and can complicate the diagnosis and treatment of a patient's illness. Confused patients are experiencing an alteration in higher-level brain functioning such as comprehension or abstract thinking. It can be caused by either delirium or dementia. Patients with delirium and dementia have difficulty remembering, learning, following directions, and/or commu-

---

Glossary

Delirium—Rapid fluctuations in mental status, memory deficits, disorientation, and perceptual disturbances over a short period of time.

Dementia—Multiple cognitive deficits *aphasia, apraxia, agnosia,* or *disturbance in executive function* such as organizing, or abstracting.

Dementia of the Alzheimer's type (Alzheimer's disease)—Progressive deterioration of memory, and/or intellectual functioning often leading to complete loss of functioning and personality. Autopsy reveals brain atrophy, senile plaques, and neurofibrillary tangles.

Nocturnal delirium (Sundowning syndrome)—Increased confusion and agitation at dusk.

Catastrophic reactions—Extreme overreaction in Alzheimer's patients to a seemingly neutral situation that requires the patient to process more information or decision making than is possible.

Prompts—Staff actions used to help dementia patient initiate self-care or other desired behaviors after loss of verbal comprehension.

Vascular dementia—Dementia caused by multiple strokes that have usually occurred at different times involving the cortex and underlying white matter.

Pseudodementia—Depression in the elderly that appears similar to dementia.

Substance-induced persisting dementia—Dementia caused by intoxication or withdrawal from a substance such as alcohol or drugs.

nicating their needs and pains. Nursing care needs to be modified to assist these patients to retain and regain those mental abilities that can be recovered and to compensate for those that can't.

Delirium is a reaction to underlying physiologic (illness, drug reaction, or exposure to a toxin) or psychologic stress. Nurses in intensive care units often see delirium induced by the disorienting and confusing environment, sensory deprivation, or sensory overload. It may also occur postoperatively. Delirium is caused by a temporary, rather than permanent, malfunction of the brain. When the underlying causative condition is resolved, the delirium generally resolves. It is a medical emergency. If left unrecognized and untreated, it could progress to dementia, coma, or death depending on the underlying cause.

Dementia is generally a permanent condition caused by a variety of factors that leads to cellular brain changes or malformations. It is characterized by slow, insidious onset affecting memory (impaired ability to learn new information or to recall previously learned information), intellectual functioning, and the ability to problem solve. Types of dementia include Alzheimer's disease, vascular dementia, substance-induced dementia, and dementia caused by other medical conditions.

Delirium and dementia are often misdiagnosed in the clinical setting. See Table 10–1, Factors That Contribute to Misdiagnosis in Dementia and Delirium, and Table 10–2, Characteristics of Delirium and Dementia.

Alzheimer's disease is the most frequently seen type of dementia, affecting over 4 million Americans. Initial changes occur so slowly that they may not be recognized. The person may be regarded as absentminded. Changes in communication, personality, and social skills occur gradually. In later stages, the individual may develop gait and motor disturbances and eventually become mute and bedridden. Death often occurs from severe debilitation, malnutrition, and dehydration. The average duration of the illness from onset of symptoms to death is 8 to 10 years.

Vascular dementia is the secondmost common form and is caused by multiple strokes. Symptoms are more variable depending on the extent, location, and timing of the strokes. Impairment is more limited and distinct de-

TABLE 10–1. **Factors That Contribute to Misdiagnosis in Dementia and Delirium**

* The symptoms of dementia and delirium are similar.
* Several causes may occur simultaneously to bring about dementia.
* Delirium occurring in a patient with a dementia can exacerbate already existing symptoms.
* Healthcare personnel may harbor unfounded beliefs that serious memory deficits, confusion, and other progressive intellectual deficits are a normal part of the aging process.
* Healthcare personnel may harbor unfounded beliefs that confusion always indicates Alzheimer's disease in an older patient.
* Confusion and behavioral changes may be the first sign of medical illness in the elderly.
* Head injuries and other conditions causing brain tissue trauma may present with symptoms similar to dementia.
* Confusion is an adverse reaction to several medications.

Source: Gorman, L, Sultan, D, and Luna-Raines, M, 1989.

TABLE 10–2. **Characteristics of Delirium and Dementia**

Delirium	Dementia
• Fluctuating levels of awareness and symptoms • Sudden onset • Clouding of consciousness • Perceptual disturbances (hallucinations, illusions) • Memory disturbance is more often to recent events • Highly distractible • Reversibility possible with treatment	• Slow, insidious onset with less fluctuation of symptoms • Deterioration of cognitive abilities • Impaired long- and short-term memory (memory impairment always present) • Personality changes • May focus on one thing for a long time • Often irreversible

pending on the area of the brain affected compared to the more global intellectual impairment of Alzheimer's disease. Evidence of strokes, such as one-sided weakness, sudden onset of loss of speech, and focal neurologic signs, such as hyperactive deep tendon reflexes, occurs with vascular dementia. Treatment of underlying hypertension and vascular disease may prevent further progression.

Etiology

Delirium can have biologic and psychologic causes. *Biologic* causes include a variety of medical conditions, exposure to toxins, and drugs. A time relationship between any of these conditions and the onset of symptoms contributes to the diagnosis. For instance, symptoms are associated with onset or exacerbation of a medical condition or introduction of a new medication. *Psychologic* causes include sensory deprivation or overload, relocation or other sudden changes, sleep deprivation, and immobilization.

Dementia can be caused by a variety of *biologic* factors including the direct physiologic effects of a medical condition, the persisting effects of a substance (drug of abuse, medication, or toxin), or multiple etiologies such as the combined effects of a stroke and Alzheimer's disease.

The etiology of Alzheimer's disease remains the focus of much research. Current theories under investigation include decrease in the activity of the neurotransmitter acetylcholine; presence in the brain of the protein beta-amyloid; and thus far unsupported theories of environmental toxins or poisons or a slow-acting virus. *Genetic* factors may also be present. There is a greater incidence of Alzheimer's in the family members of patients who acquire the disease before age 50.

Related Clinical Concerns

DELIRIUM

Medical conditions that can generate delirium include systemic infections, hypoxia, hypercapnia, hypoglycemia, and fluid and/or electrolyte imbalances (see Table 3–2,

Mental Status Changes Caused by Electrolyte Imbalance), hepatic or renal disease, thiamin deficiency, sequelae of head trauma, post-ictal states, postoperative states, and complications of cancer. There is a high rate of delirium in the final stages of terminal illness. The presence of delirium increases the risk of complications associated with a medical illness and increases the risk of mortality.

Substance intoxication delirium can occur from ingestion of alcohol, amphetamines, cannabis, cocaine, hallucinogens, phencyclidine (PCP), opioids, hypnotics, and sedatives. Substance withdrawal delirium can occur from abruptly stopping significant abuse of alcohol (formerly called "delirium tremens"), hypnotics, and antianxiety medications.

Many prescribed medications can contribute to delirium including analgesics, anesthetics, anticonvulsants, antihistamines, antiparkinson drugs, corticosteroids, gastrointestinal medications, and psychotropic medications with anticholinergic side effects. See Table 11–3, Psychotic Reactions Seen With Commonly Used Drugs.

DEMENTIA

Medical conditions that contribute to development of dementia include stroke, Parkinson's disease, Huntington's disease, AIDS, Creutzfeldt-Jakob disease, hypothyroidism, multiple sclerosis, traumatic brain injury, brain tumors, anoxia, lupus, and hepatic failure.

Lifespan Issues

CHILDHOOD TO ADOLESCENCE

Children may be more susceptible to **delirium** than adults particularly in the presence of febrile episodes and in response to some medications such as anticholinergics. Assessment may be complicated by difficulty in eliciting the signs of problems in thinking, memory, and orientation. In fact, delirium can be mistaken for uncooperative behavior. One indication of delirium may be the inability of familiar figures to soothe the child.

Dementia is rare in children and adolescents but can occur as a result of medical conditions including AIDS, brain tumors, and head injury. As with delirium, dementia can be difficult to identify in young children. Dementia in children may present as a deterioration in functioning as in adults or as a significant delay or deviation in normal development. Deterioration in school performance may be an early sign.

ELDERLY

Delirium is extremely common in the medically ill elderly. In fact, at least 10 percent of hospitalized elderly exhibit delirium on admission, and another 15 percent may develop it sometime while they are in the hospital (DSM-IV, 1994). Multiple medications, multiple chronic illnesses, use of over-the-counter medications, and impaired kidney and liver function contribute to the development of delirium. A masked depression can appear as confusion (pseudodementia). Acutely confused elderly are often inappropriately labeled as "demented" as potentially reversible conditions go undiagnosed and untreated.

Dementia in general is most common after age 85 and is often seen in residents of nursing homes. Alzheimer's disease is much more common after age 65. However, dementia is not a normal or expected part of the aging process.

Possible Nurses' Reactions

- May have a more positive attitude and take more active measures in care of patients if they believe the confusion is reversible.
- May feel very frustrated and helpless because of lack of improvement in patients with irreversible dementia, constant need to repeat instructions or break tasks down step by step, patients repeatedly asking the same question, and patients' requiring more time to provide care.
- May avoid patients to avoid feeling hopeless and helpless; may emotionally detach and give only impersonal care.
- May find themselves bored, drifting off to other thoughts, or confused if patients have considerable problems in communicating verbally.
- May be angry with patients who are ignorant of their own

pathology; may believe patients can control own behavior.
- May become impatient with negative, hostile, impulsive patients who are very slow to respond.
- May feel repulsed by poor hygiene, messy eating behaviors, incontinence, or inappropriate behaviors.

Assessment

Behavior and/or Appearance

- Disheveled, inappropriate clothing; poor grooming
- Restless, agitated, impulsive
- Wandering
- Sleep disturbance
- Impaired movement
  - Perseveration (repetitive movements)
  - Apraxia (inability to carry out motor activities despite intact comprehension and motor abilities)
  - Loss of coordination; stiff awkward movements; impairment of learned skilled movements
  - Unsteady, shuffling gait; stooped, leaning posture
  - Difficulty writing
  - Loss of ability to perform activities of daily living (ADLs)
- Types of aphasia including:
  - Echolalia (repetition of word, phrase, or syllable just said by someone else)
  - Repetitive questions
  - Palilalia (repeating sounds or words over and over)
  - Anomia (difficulty finding wanted words) that leads to paraphasia (uses similar sounding words) and circumlocution (using many words in place of the one word that is wanted)
  - Slurred speech
  - May later remember only a few key words that are used inappropriately in all situations (such as no)
  - May become mute
- Hypersexual, such as obsessive masturbation
- Hyperoral, including increased appetite
- Inappropriate eating, toileting behavior

- Difficulty sleeping
- Inability to tolerate stress, change

Mood and/or Emotions

- Emotional lability
- Depression
- Suspicion, paranoia, hostility
- Anxiety

Thoughts, Beliefs, and Perceptions

- Loss of recent and/or remote memory
- Disorientation, first to time, then place, then to person
- Impaired concentration
- Loss of abstract thinking ability
- Loss of ability to calculate
- Inability to learn and use new information
- Loss of ability to plan, initiate, sequence, monitor, and stop complex behavior
- Agnosia (failure to recognize or identify objects despite intact sensory function)
- Able to read words without knowing what they mean
- Loss of ability to read
- Confabulation
- Loss of awareness of spatial relationships; loss of awareness of own body parts and how they are organized in relation to each other
- Illusions
- Delusions, hallucinations
- Impaired insight and judgment

Relationships and Interactions

- Personality changes: accentuation or alteration of premorbid traits that affects prior relationships (e.g., caretaker role reversals); family unsure how to interact with patient
- Loss of social skills; social withdrawal
- Clinging, demanding
- Inability to sustain real relationships as memory gaps eliminate continuity; in later phases, may not recognize family or friends

- Negative, belligerent, briefly combative at times; hostility caused by brain damage or by misinterpreting events; not necessarily by the behavior of others

Physical Responses

- The patient may not verbalize or demonstrate common physical signs of pain or other symptoms such as bladder distention, constipation, dehydration, injuries, or urinary tract infections.
- Laboratory data, medication history, and possibly a drug screening should be performed to evaluate patient at the onset of confusion.

Pertinent History

- Complex medical history
- Chronic illness
- Substance abuse
- Head trauma

Collaborative Management

Pharmacologic

A great many medications cause confusion. Confused patients who are taking multiple medications may need to have each of the medications withdrawn one at a time to determine their impact on the symptoms and the underlying illness. Any medications used to treat confusion should be started at lower dosages.

Confused patients often become disruptive and may need to be controlled to protect the patient and environment. Haloperidol (Haldol) is frequently used to treat agitation and aggression. Side effects such as orthostatic hypotension must be closely monitored because the patient may not be able to verbalize how he or she is feeling.

Buspirone (Buspar) has been used successfully in patient's with Alzheimer's disease although it may take several weeks to fully take effect. Hypnotics, antidepressants (particularly the selective serotonin reuptake inhibitors used for irritability), and anticonvulsants (used for rage) are also useful. Using medications to control agitation should not replace other interventions, however. There can be a tendency to use medications to sedate the patient rather than pursue behavioral techniques. Tacrine hydrochloride (Cognex) if used very early may temporarily delay the progression of Alzheimer's disease.

Rehabilitation

A multidisciplinary approach for the patient with dementia is essential. Physical and occupational therapy, diet, speech therapy, psychiatry, social work, nursing, and medicine all need to be part of the long-term management of the patient with dementia. It is important that families use all available resources to reduce their isolation and stress.

Nursing Management

IMPAIRED VERBAL COMMUNICATION EVIDENCED BY INABILITY TO NAME OBJECTS OR SENSATIONS SUCH AS PAIN; INABILITY TO COMPREHEND VERBAL INSTRUCTIONS; INABILITY TO COMMUNICATE NEEDS; INAPPROPRIATE, DRAMATIC REACTIONS OR ACCUSATIONS, CATASTROPHIC REACTIONS RELATED TO CONFUSION, DISORIENTATION, MEMORY LOSS.

Patient Outcomes

- Demonstrates understanding of nurses and communication
- Able to communicate thoughts and needs
- Responds appropriately

Interventions

- Look directly at patient when speaking. Call patient by name frequently. Identify your name before each conversation, and refer to others by their names rather than "he" or "she."
- Keep interactions simple. Use short words and simple sentences that express one thought or question at a time.
- Ask specific questions such as "Does your stomach hurt?" rather than general ones like "How are you?"

- Reinforce speech with nonverbal techniques. For example, point, touch, or demonstrate an action while talking about it. For instance, if the patient is trying to tell you about his or her body, point as well as ask "Is this where it hurts?"
- Note in the chart or on the care plan, the phrases, key words, and techniques to which patient responds so that others can use them as well.
- If patient keeps repeating a question, try distraction and give reassurance that he or she will be cared for. Repetitive questions may indicate anxiety, and you want to be reassuring.
- If patient is searching for a particular word or trying to communicate something, guess at what it is, and ask if your guess is correct. If you are unable to determine what he or she is trying to say, focus on the feelings possibly being communicated. Always ask patient to confirm whether your determination is correct.
- If patient is reacting inappropriately, remain calm and reassure the patient you are there to help. Avoid arguing or trying to convince patient that he or she is overreacting. Clarify any information or instructions. Assist patient with the next step of a task that is the source of frustration. Try to distract patient by removing him or her from disturbing situation.
- If patient makes inappropriate accusations, such as accusing the staff of stealing his or her glasses, help look for the missing item. Remember that the patient may accuse you of stealing due to memory loss. Also, routinely check wastebaskets for missing items.

IMPAIRED MEMORY EVIDENCED BY CONFUSION, DECREASED ABILITY TO PERFORM ACTIVITIES OF DAILY LIVING (ADLs), OR INABILITY TO FOLLOW THERAPEUTIC REGIMEN; INAPPROPRIATE EMOTIONAL OR BEHAVIORAL RESPONSES RELATED TO DELIRIUM, DEMENTIA, OR OTHER COGNITIVE DEFICITS.

Patient Outcomes

- Demonstrates improved orientation to person, place, and/or time

- Demonstrates improved ability to perform ADLs
- Displays less emotional and/or behavioral agitation

Interventions

- Establish a baseline assessment of patient's mental status and functioning:
  - Observe ability to perform ADLs.
  - Use a standardized method of mental status assessment such as the Mini-Mental State Examination (see Appendix B).
  - Ask the patient orientation questions. For example, ask patient personal questions such as names of his or her children or home address. Make sure that you can verify the answers from the chart or family,
- Assess if patient is willing to discuss memory lapses. Determine emotional responses to these lapses. Do not push the discussion if the patient becomes agitated or defensive.
- Be aware that patient may try to disguise memory loss by confabulation, avoiding responding, or by speaking in a rambling style to hide the fact that no thought or information is being expressed.
- Be aware that when social skills and personality are still intact, patient may mistakenly appear stubborn and resistant rather than unable to remember.
- Do not argue with patient about what he or she remembers. Rather, focus on immediate and specific tasks to be completed. Give patient step-by-step instructions on what needs to be done. Be directive without being domineering.
- Do not make demands that the patient cannot handle nor focus on topics that clearly cause distress. Such demands will only add to the confusion and/or agitation.
- Break down complex tasks into individual steps. The seemingly simple act of brushing one's teeth can take over 10 steps. Be aware of the steps the patient can handle himself or herself and those requiring assistance.
- Establish a regular and predictable routine. Try to do things at the same time and in the same order each day, such as shave, bathe, and then eat breakfast. Communi-

cate routines to the staff to coordinate patient's care and ensure that the same techniques are used. Obtain input from the family on patient's usual routine.

- Attempt to arrange for consistent staff to care for patient.
- Keep surroundings simple. Reduce clutter. Do not leave equipment in the patient's room if possible.
- Personalize patient's room. Have the family bring in photos and favorite objects.
- Place a large visible clock and calendar in the patient's room. Cross each day off calendar daily. Place large signs on the wall noting where patient is and special events such as when the family is coming and the next upcoming holiday.
- Write lists of daily activities or tasks patient needs to do if still able to read and comprehend. Put labels on possessions and patient's name on his or her door in large letters.
- Avoid an overstimulating environment. In the hospital, patient's room should be close enough to nurses' station to monitor safety yet far enough away to avoid noise. Restrict the number of people visiting at one time.
- If patient tends to wander, make sure all staff are aware of this problem and can bring him or her back to the unit. Consider using alarms, if available, if patient is at high risk to leave the area. Monitor all exits. Draw a large red octagon shaped stop sign, and hang it by the exit. At home, make sure exits are monitored. Have the family notify neighbors of the problem, and elicit their assistance to monitor for wandering. Make sure the patient always has some form of identification stating that he or she is confused. Maintain photos of the patient to be shown if he or she is missing.
- Provide some form of night light. If the bathroom is connected to his or her room, leave the bathroom light on. Otherwise, use reflective tape in the shape of arrows to direct the patient to the bathroom door. Encourage the use of a bedside commode.

RISK FOR INJURY EVIDENCED BY FALLS AND BUMPING INTO OBJECTS. RELATED TO PROBLEMS IN GAIT, VISION, HEARING, LACK OF COORDINATION, CONFUSION, OR LACK OF UNDERSTANDING OF ENVIRONMENTAL HAZARDS.

Patient Outcomes

- Remains injury free
- Demonstrates appropriate actions to avoid injury

Interventions

- Be aware of factors that increase risk for falls. See Table 10–3, Causes of Increased Risk of Falls and Injuries.
- Keep side rails up and bed in lowest position at all times.

TABLE 10–3. **Causes of Increased Risk of Falls and Injury**

• Stiff, awkward movements caused by damage to areas of brain that control muscle movement: ○ Difficulty getting out of bed   ○ Stooped or leaning posture and shuffling gait as disease progresses   ○ Apraxia, with inability to make or coordinate movements   • Overmedication: Changes in drowsiness, walking, posture, stiffness, agitation, falling, increased postural hypertension   • Visual problems: ○ Cataracts   ○ Increased near or farsightedness   ○ Inability to distinguish between similar color intensities (may have difficulty identifying railings that are same color as walls; may stumble into walls of color intensity similar to that of floor)   ○ Poor depth perception   ○ Blurred vision (may be side effect of medication, anticholinergic action)   • Hearing problems: May not hear approaching machinery, or people   • Agnosia: May bump into furniture, not recognizing what it is   • Diminished or absent pain perception: ○ Inability to recognize or communicate injury (for example, patient may walk on broken leg)   ○ Only manifestation may be change in behavior   ○ May burn self while smoking   • Sundowning syndrome (increased confusion at night) with night restlessness, wandering   • Any factor, including concurrent delirium, that increases confusion and disorientation

Source: Gorman, L, Sultan, D, and Luna-Raines, M, 1989.

- Even with side rails up, be aware that patient may get out of bed. Keep area around bed free from clutter. Make sure that there is always a clear path to the bathroom since that is the place the patient will most often attempt to go. Make sure that patient uses the bathroom before going to bed at night. Plan administration of medications such as laxatives and diuretics so that they are not given in the evening. Recognize that the patient with dementia may have sleep pattern disturbances and become more confused at night.
- Make rounds frequently for those at high risk for falling. Keep the patient's door open, and make sure all staff know this patient is at risk.
- Use restraints only after all other methods are ineffective. In some instances, restraints can increase confusion in the elderly.
- If the patient has an unsteady gait, have him or her take your arm instead of the reverse while walking. Make sure the patient has access to any needed equipment such as walkers or wheelchairs. Provide instruction as appropriate within the patient's ability to understand. Ensure that any furniture or objects the patient leans on for support are sturdy and well balanced. Railings in hallways and bathrooms are very helpful. The patient may need prompts to perform simple actions, such as walking.
- Make sure the patient receives adequate exercise within limitations of his or her abilities and condition.
- If the patient wears glasses or a hearing aid, make sure that these are in place before any activity. Be sure to check that the hearing aid battery is good.
- Ensure that the room is adequately lighted for any activity and that the call light is within reach when patient is in bed, in bathroom, or up in chair.
- Check the patient routinely for bruises, cuts, or burns.
- Use colored, waterproof tape along the area of the bathtub where patient is to stop filling with water. Decorative markers that stick to the bottom of the shower or tub can compensate for spatial disorientation.
- Use brightly colored materials in the room, if possible.
- Be aware that the patient may try to pull out catheters or intravenous tubing. Try to reduce risk of the patient's

pulling out the tubes by reducing discomfort associated with tubes. For instance, use the smallest-size nasogastric tube or cover the IV site with a large bandage to avoid the patient's pulling on the tubes. Wrist restraints or monitoring by a family member may be required to avoid injury.
- Be aware of medication interactions that could add to confusion and the risk for falls.

SELF-CARE DEFICITS, ALTERED NUTRITION; LESS THAN BODY REQUIREMENTS, and FLUID VOLUME DEFICIT EVIDENCED BY WEIGHT LOSS, ELECTROLYTE IMBALANCE, INCREASED CONFUSION, OR OTHER SIGNS OF DEHYDRATION. RELATED TO IMPAIRED RECOGNITION OF HUNGER AND THIRST, MEMORY LOSS, IMPAIRED MOVEMENTS.

Patient Outcomes

- Receives adequate nutritional and fluid intake
- Displays ability to recognize signs of hunger and thirst
- Demonstrates ability to feed self

Interventions

- Assess the patient's ability to feed and care for self (see Fig. 10–1).
- Provide assistance, as needed, for dressing and personal hygiene.
- Assess patient's ability to feed self. Provide assistance as needed. Determine how much patient can safely do independently. Perhaps just opening containers or cutting meat prompts all that is needed to promote independence. Provide verbal cues to keep patient on track.
- Determine patient's food preferences, and provide these foods, if possible. Encourage the family to bring familiar foods from home, if appropriate.
- Make sure that dentures are in place and that they fit correctly before serving a meal.
- Allow hot foods to cool to prevent burn injury.
- Simplify the meal routine. The patient may be able to cope with only one food or one utensil at a time. Provide finger foods if utensils are difficult to use.

Self-Care Checklist

Ambulation:

Independent with steady gait _____

Uses cane _____ walker _____ wheelchair _____

Needs staff to accompany when walking _____ assist sitting/getting up _____

assist in/out of bed _____ assist up/down stairs _____

Effective techniques for assistance

Resists using necessary equipment/assistance: Yes _____ No _____

If yes, nursing approach: _____

Feeding:

Independent _____   Adequate nutritional intake _____

Difficulty swallowing _____   Needs staff to locate dining area _____

Provide assistance prompts _____   Feed patient _____

Effective techniques for assistance

Requires special feeding routine: Yes _____ No _____

Requires special food/supplements: Yes _____ No _____

If yes, describe: _____

Fluid intake:

Independent _____

Adequate amount _____

Needs staff to monitor daily amount of fluid intake _____

Provide prompts to drink _____ hold cup while drinking _____ drink with straw _____

Effective techniques for assistance _____

Toileting:

Independent: Yes _____ No _____

If no, words/behaviors patient uses to express need to toilet: _____

Diarrhea _____ Constipation _____ Frequency _____ adult diapers _____

Uses bedpan _____ urinal _____ commode _____ defecation _____

Needs assessment of frequency/circumstances of urination _____ before going to bed _____

Needs staff to take to toilet at scheduled times (every hour _____

Effective technique to encourage patient to use toilet _____

Bathing/Hygiene

Independent: _____

Areas of skin breakdown _____

Areas of paralysis _____

Needs staff to provide assistance and prompts _____

Wash certain body areas (list) _____

Full bath _____

Mouth care _____

Effective means for assistance _____

Dressing/Grooming

Independent _____

Hearing aid _____ Glasses _____

Needs staff to provide assistance and prompts _____

Change clothes _____

Provide grooming (for example, comb hair) _____

If yes, specify steps that require assistance or if total care is needed: _____

Effective techniques for assistance _____

201

- Reduce distraction during mealtimes. For instance, turn off the television or radio.
- Assess regularly for signs of dehydration. Offer fluids regularly.
- Make sure that patient can see his or her food and hear your instructions.
- Consider liquid supplements if eating solid food is too difficult.
- Assess for constipation.
- For patient with end-stage dementia, family may face decision on whether to pursue aggressive nutrition intervention if patient refuses to eat or is unable to swallow. Provide support for the family in attempting to weigh these difficult options. Consider offering ethics consultation or hospice assistance, if appropriate.

ALTERNATE NURSING DIAGNOSES

Altered family processes
Altered thought processes
Ineffective management of therapeutic regimen, individual
Sensory or perceptual alteration
Sleep pattern disturbance

Patient and Family Education

- Provide the patient with simple instructions based on his or her current ability to comprehend.
- Teach the family techniques to control uncooperative and aggressive behavior.
- Give the family information about the disease so that they can better understand that the patient has no control over his or her behavior.
- Teach the family or caregivers about the need to avoid stress and fatigue for the patient as this can increase behavior problems.
- Encourage family to obtain material and newsletters from the Alzheimer's Disease and Related Disorders Association (ADRDA). Also encourage them to obtain a copy of *The 36-Hour Day* by Mace and Rabins.
- Alert families to signs of caregiver abuse.

- Teach the family or caregivers to build in support systems to maintain a balance in their lives.
- Teach the family about the emotional strain created by caring for the confused patient. Educate them that, with Alzheimer's disease in particular, the family may go through a mourning process for the person that their loved one used to be. This process is complicated because the patient looks the same but no longer has the same personality. Adult children must be prepared to reverse roles and become caretakers.

Charting Tips

- Document any changes in levels of confusion, memory, behavioral routines, or consciousness.
- Document which activities the patient cannot do.
- Document if patient is able to start an activity but requires a prompt to continue. Document words or physical directions that work as a prompt.
- Document stimulus that causes the patient to have catastrophic reactions, such as too much noise or too many demands at the same time.
- Document the patient's response to medications.
- Document any techniques that have been effective in calming patient.

WHEN TO CALL FOR HELP

✔ Sudden onset of confusion
✔ Episodes of patient's becoming physically combative
✔ Severe agitation unresponsive to medication or other interventions
✔ Delirium that does not remit or gets worse

Discharge Planning

- Be sure that the family has the needed information on financial resources and legal information for power of attorney if patient is unable to care for himself or herself.
- Report all indications of abuse.

- Assist the family or caregivers to set a plan to provide them with needed rest and recreation. Encourage family and caregivers to seek out support of friends or clergy. Encourage attendance at local support groups.
- If the care demands become too much, families need to consider placing the patient in a nursing home or day-care. Provide information on any specialized programs in the community and suggestions for what to look for in a facility. Provide families with support to make this difficult decision.
- Give specific information on this patient's management to home health agencies and nursing homes.
- Give information from local Alzheimer's Disease and Related Disorders Association on treatment programs, research, and facilities.

Nursing Outcomes

- Selection of appropriate interventions allows the patient to function at the highest possible level.
- Documentation reflects nursing interventions for cognitive symptoms.
- Consistency of approach is demonstrated among staff.
- Staff provides respectful care to patient.

Suggested Learning Activities

- Attend classes and inservices on Alzheimer's disease and other dementias.
- Attend Alzheimer's Disease and Related Disorders Association support groups.
- Choose a common activity of daily living such as brushing teeth. Write down all the steps required to accomplish the task in the order in which they are to be done. Compare lists with others present.
- Role play to gain information about how a confused patient feels:
  - Player number 1 is told that she cannot have the key to leave the room unless she can recite back the words said to her. Player number 2 states 12 unrelated words. If the player is unable to recite them (which he or she probably can't), repeat this exchange up to three

times. Then have the players discuss the feelings they had during the exercise.

○ Choose a common word such as *door*. Tell the others present about the door to your home without using the word (as if you cannot remember it).

○ Read *The 36-Hour Day* by NL Mace and PV Rabins.

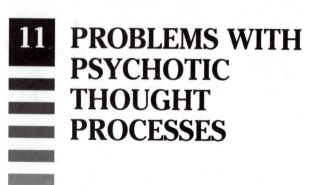

11 PROBLEMS WITH PSYCHOTIC THOUGHT PROCESSES

The Psychotic Patient

LEARNING OBJECTIVES

▼ *Differentiate between schizophrenia and other psychoses.*
▼ *Describe effective interventions for the hallucinating and delusional patient.*
▼ *Describe possible nurses' reactions to the psychotic patient.*
▼ *Discuss specific interventions for the patient experiencing intensive care unit psychosis.*

Caring for a patient who is hearing voices, believes that the staff is trying to kill him or her, or exhibits other bizarre behavior can be confusing, disorienting, frightening, and disarming for the nurse. While nurses in the psychiatric setting may frequently see psychotic patients (over 50 percent of hospital beds for the mentally ill are filled with schizophrenics, Berkow, 1992), nurses in other settings

Glossary

Hallucinations—Sensory experiences that are very real to the patient but that do not exist in external reality occuring while the patient is awake and when no one else has a similar experience.

Delusions—False, fixed beliefs that cannot be corrected by feedback and are not accepted as true by others in the same culture.

Psychosis—Severe distortion of and withdrawal from reality accompanied by severe disorganization of the personality.

Schizophrenia—A severe thought disturbance characterized by impaired reality testing, hallucinations, delusions, limited socialization, and the diagnosis requires the symptoms to last at least 6 months.

Delusional disorder—Persistent suspicions, persecutory ideation, and delusions or delusional jealousies with resentment, anger, and sometimes grandiosity without other signs of psychotic thoughts or mood disorders. Patients are usually able to maintain daily functioning.

Good reality testing—The ability to accurately identify and evaluate events. Absence of delusions, hallucinations, and other distorted perceptions.

Poor reality testing—Defects in a person's ability to assess accurately external events and interactions with others.

Schizoaffective disorder—Symptoms of major depressive disorder or the manic phase of bipolar disorder as well as some of the symptoms of schizophrenia.

may be unprepared for managing the psychotic patient. These patients are often feared and shunned by health-care workers.

Hallucinations and delusions can be frightening for both the patient to experience and the nurse to observe. Even those hallucinations that begin as fairly innocuous experiences can become frightening or accusatory to the patient (see Table 11–1). The subject of delusions are varied. Some common delusions are described in Table 11–2.

Hallucinations, delusions, or other psychotic thought disorders occur in a primary psychiatric disorder such as schizophrenia, delusional disorder, brief psychotic disorder due to an episode of extreme stress, or severe depressive disorder. They can also be caused by physiologic changes or drug and alcohol use or withdrawal. Whether or not the etiology of the symptoms is known, the basic interventions are similar.

Psychotic thought disorders lead to severe distortion of and withdrawal from reality accompanied by major personality disorganization. This disorganization leads to hallucinations, delusions, and bizarre behavior such as catatonia (assuming inappropriate postures or becoming completely immobile), or echolalia (repetition of words heard).

TABLE 11–1. **Recognizing Hallucinations**

Affected Sense	Example
Visual	"I watch gypsies bring different babies to my apartment each night."
Auditory (most common)	"The voices are calling me a prostitute."
Tactile	"When I touched my arm, I could tell my arm is made of stone."
Olfactory	"I don't want to stay in that room. I can smell the odors of the people who died there."
Gustatory	"I taste milk in my mouth all the time."
Kinesthetic (bodily or movement sense)	"It feels as if the rats in my head are eating up my brain."

TABLE 11–2. **Recognizing Delusions**

Delusion	Example
Grandeur (belief of exaggerated importance)	"I am Napoleon Bonaparte."
Paranoia (belief of deliberate harassment and persecution)	"The FBI is following me and wants to kill me."
Reference (belief that the thoughts and behavior of others is directed toward self)	"Those people on the TV show are talking to me."
Physical sensations (belief that parts of body are diseased, distorted, or missing)	"I have no blood in me."

Schizophrenia, a psychiatric diagnosis characterized by changes in cognitive, perceptual, affective, motor, and social domains, is one of the commonest forms of psychosis. Schizophrenics have psychotic episodes, but not all psychotic episodes are due to schizophrenia. Many people erroneously define schizophrenia as multiple personality disorder. The word *schizophrenia* actually refers to splits between different components of the personality, for example, what the patient says does not match the emotion shown. Patients with multiple personalities usually do not display psychosis and be long to a different diagnostic category called *personality disorders*.

Onset of schizophrenia usually occurs in late teens to mid-thirties though onset at older ages can occur. Schizophrenia is a chronic, disabling condition though symptoms can be controlled with appropriate medication management. Though all socioeconomic and cultural groups are affected, schizophrenics tend to cluster in the lower socioeconomic levels because of their difficulty maintaining employment and functioning in society.

Patients without a psychiatric illness who experience sensory deprivation or overstimulation can become psychotic. A common example is referred to as *intensive care unit (ICU) psychosis*; however, the patient does not need to be physically located in the intensive care unit to experience this problem. Psychologic stress, sleep deprivation, sensory overload, and immobilization all contribute to the critically ill person's developing personality changes, hallucinations, and delusions. Physiologic changes, such as hypoxia, renal failure, and response to medications also contribute. The elderly are particularly vulnerable because they may already have diminished senses. Though it may be impossible to completely prevent ICU psychosis, nursing actions such as maintaining a patient's sleep-wake cycle, providing frequent reality orientation, personalizing care, and explaining what is happening can all play a role in reducing the effects.

Etiology

No one single cause of schizophrenia has been identified. *Genetic* theories recognize possible hereditary tendencies as there is a higher incidence in families with one schizophrenic parent or sibling. *Biologic* theories have received increasing attention. Some causes may be brain dysfunction in the limbic system and prefrontal cortex, as well as biochemical disruption in neurotransmitters such as dopamine.

Psychologic theory focuses on deficits caused by severely inadequate parenting throughout development, with special recognition of the devastating impact of deprivation during the first years of life. These individuals are thought to have never achieved the ability to trust others, the ability to tolerate anxiety and feelings, internal cohesion, and consistent identity. Thus, under stress the individual's anxiety escalates to panic leading to a breakdown of personality and loss of the ability to discriminate between what is happening inside and outside of the person. *Cognitive* theories indicate that the schizophrenic has problems with attention or information processing. The person is unable to filter stimuli leading to disorganization of mental functioning.

Family theory has examined communication patterns that present unrealistic and unworkable expectations for the susceptible individual.

Other types of psychotic disorders may develop in individuals with fragile egos who become flooded with anxiety under severe stress. Unacceptable thoughts and feelings may overwhelm the person's weakened defense mechanisms leading to hallucinations, delusions, and other psychotic behaviors in which the forbidden thoughts/feelings may be symbolically expressed.

Related Clinical Concerns

Certain physical conditions and medications, drug and alcohol withdrawal, and sleep and sensory deprivation cause some type of brain dysfunction that may result in psychosis. Examples of physical conditions include brain tumors, head injuries, high fever, septicemia, AIDS, encephalitis, epilepsy, and hepatic encephalopathy. See Table 11–3 for the types of psychotic reactions caused by medications.

Disorders, medications, and environmental factors can alter cerebral perfusion and chemistry to create biologic states that mimic some psychiatric disorders, including exhibiting psychosis and thought disorders. The combination of medications, sensory and sleep deprivation, fear and anxiety, and illness make the patient in an intensive care unit at risk of experiencing psychotic episodes. If this occurs, a thorough assessment is essential to accurately determine the underlying cause.

A patient with a psychotic disorder may also misuse drugs and/or alcohol as a way to self-medicate for uncomfortable symptoms. These medications could contribute to intensifying psychotic symptoms and confuse the diagnosis and treatment.

Lifespan Issues

CHILDHOOD

Though rare, schizophrenia has been identified in children. Symptoms of inappropriate affect, hallucinations, and mutism have been identified. Although not true, it is often confused with autism, which is the most severe developmental disability of childhood. Children with psychotic dis-

TABLE 11–3. **Psychotic Reactions Seen With Commonly Used Drugs**

Generic Name or Drug Category	Reaction
Amphetamines	Hallucinations, paranoia
Albuterol	Hallucinations, paranoia
Anticholinergics (Atropine, Scopolamine)	Confusion, delirium, hallucinations
Anticonvulsants	Confusion, delirium
Antidepressants	Hallucinations
Antihistamines	Hallucinations
Benzodiazepines	Rage, paranoia, hallucinations
Beta-blockers (Inderal/Timoptic)	Confusion, hallucinations
Ciprofloxacin (Cipro)	Delirium, psychosis
Corticosteroids (Prednisone, Decadron)	Confusion, paranoia
Cyclosporine	Hallucinations
Digitalis	Nightmares, confusion
Disulfiram (Antabuse)	Delirium, psychosis
Histamine H2 receptor antagonists (Tagamet, Pepcid, Zantac)	Hallucinations, paranoia
Interferon	Delirium, paranoia
Meperidine (Demerol)	Agitation, nightmares, hallucinations
Methylphenidate	Hallucinations, paranoia
Opioids	Hallucinations, nightmares
Procaine derivatives (Pronestyl)	Confusions, psychosis
Promethazine (Phenergan)	Hallucinations
Pseudoephedrine (in cold remedies)	Hallucinations
Sedatives or hypnotics	Confusion, hallucinations
Sulfonamides	Confusion, hallucinations
Tamoxifen	Delusions
Thyroid hormones	Hallucinations
Trimethoprim-sulfamethoxazole (Bactrim)	Hallucinations, delusions
Zidovudine (AZT)	Paranoia, hallucinations

Source: Reference Med Letter: Drugs that cause psychiatric symptoms. Med Let 35:65, July 23, 1993, adapted with permission.

orders can be treated with antipsychotic medications though side effects of sedation and weight gain are a concern.

Children of the mentally ill are at high risk for being victims of abuse. They are also more likely to take on more responsibility to care for the household. Because so many schizophrenics are homeless, their children may be living on the streets.

ADOLESCENCE

Diagnosis of schizophrenia is more common in adolescence. Teens may be more likely to experiment with drugs in an effort to self-medicate to deal with distressing symptoms of anxiety and hallucinations.

ELDERLY

Elderly schizophrenics often have fewer and less severe symptoms, especially hallucinations and delusions, though symptoms of emotional flattening and loss of motivation often continue. These patients often do not verbalize pain or discomfort leading to undertreatment of medical conditions. The first signs of physical illness in these patients may be changes in ability to perform activities of daily living. They are also more prone to the nonreversible drug side effect of tardive dyskinesia (constant involuntary movements). See Chapter 20 for further discussion. With the elderly living longer and the mentally ill less likely to be institutionalized, it is believed that there will be an increase in the number of these patients in nursing homes and retirement settings.

New onset of psychotic behavior in the elderly must be closely assessed to rule out physical illness or medication toxicity. Because the elderly may already have some sensory deprivation, illness, and use a variety of medications, the simple fact of being hospitalized can increase anxiety and can make them at risk for confusion and psychosis. It is essential that the elderly be kept oriented to the unit to help prevent confusion. Symptoms can easily be confused with dementia, which could lead to inappropriate treatment.

Possible Nurses' Reactions

- May avoid these patients because the nurse feels he or she lacks knowledge or experience with psychotic patients.
- May feel strangely uncomfortable or detached because of patient's lack of emotional connectedness.
- May feel frustrated and angry that patient cannot do more self care. May have unrealistic expectation of patient.
- May feel afraid because of patient's bizarre behavior. May fear violence and personal harm.
- May feel confused when usual predictable responses do not occur and patient treats nurse as if he or she were someone else.
- May ignore patient's complaints because "he's crazy."
- May feel rejected if patient's extreme mistrust or fear of others is not understood.
- May feel he or she has to control patient's bizarre behavior to be effective.
- May feel unable to intervene, leading to the nurse's giving up on the patient.

Assessment

Behavior and/or Appearance

- Strange, bizarre appearance; poor grooming
- Disheveled; eccentric clothing
- Unusual gestures, mannerisms, facial grimaces, posturing
- Neglect or difficulty performing activities of daily living
- Incoherent, repetitive speech; mumbling; found talking to self
- May not answer questions; frequently asks that questions be repeated; responds only to part of question
- May be watchful of others or withdrawn
- Unpredictable behavior; childlike behavior
- Socially unacceptable behavior and speech
- Uses words only patient seems to understand
- Marginal functioning, such as being unable to maintain employment

- Eyes moving as if watching something not visible to others
- Head positioned as if listening

Mood and/or Emotions

- Inappropriate emotions to situation such as crying when others are laughing
- Displays contradictory emotions at same time
- Flat affect
- Highly anxious, panic
- Outburst of rage
- Unpredictable changes in mood
- Difficulty controlling emotions

Thoughts, Beliefs, and Perceptions

- Impaired ability for abstract and/or logical thinking
- Loose associations (ideas shift rapidly from one subject to another that are unrelated)
- Hallucinations
- Sensory distortions such as seeing objects or people change in size and shape
- Delusions
- Extreme sense of worthlessness
- Overwhelming, inappropriate guilt
- Decreased recognition of own body sensations, such as hunger, pain, and urge to urinate
- Depersonalization (sense of feeling separated from body)
- Suspicious
- Extreme ambivalence
- Impaired decision-making ability
- Inability to problem solve
- Altered sense of self; uncertain where own body stops and external objects and people begin

Relationships and Interactions

- Dependent on others for basic needs
- Fear and distrust of others
- Unable to maintain close relationships
- Poor eye contact
- Lack of social skills

- Interactions seem cold and detached
- Withdrawn

Physical Responses

- Complaints of unusual or bizarre symptoms
- Blunting of pain

Pertinent History

- Psychiatric hospitalizations
- Ongoing or periodic outpatient psychotherapy
- Substance abuse
- Childhood behavior problems such as being isolated or described as "odd"
- Minor infractions of law
- History of suicide attempts

Collaborative Management

Pharmacologic

Though they are not cures, antipsychotic (or neuroleptic) medications can reduce and control many of the symptoms of psychosis. See Chapter 20 for detailed discussion of these medications. Antipsychotics are especially effective in managing agitation, combativeness, and belligerence. New antipsychotics, such as risperidone and clozapine, are particularly effective in treating social withdrawal and flat affect. These are now being used in schizophrenics refractory to other antipsychotics. They have fewer extrapyramidal side effects than the older antipsychotics, but clozapine can cause agranulocytosis. Hallucinations may take longer to treat and delusions may not respond. Schizophrenics may need to remain on these medications for the rest of their lives, and symptoms can recur if they stop taking them. Antipsychotics can be given on an occasional basis to manage acute agitation, such as might be seen in ICU psychosis or a drug reaction. They control the symptoms until the problem resolves or the cause can be treated. See Table 20–3 for appropriate drug selection based on the patient's symptoms, as some drugs are more sedating than others.

Nursing Management

ALTERED THOUGHT PROCESSES EVIDENCED BY INABILITY TO EVALUATE REALITY; HALLUCINATIONS, DELUSIONS RELATED TO SCHIZOPHRENIA OR OTHER PSYCHOSES.

Patient Outcomes

- Demonstrates clear communication to others
- Maintains reality orientation
- Demonstrates improved ability to participate in treatment plan

Interventions

- Determine if patient's behavior is a chronic problem or if this is a new onset. If a chronic problem, determine patient's baseline behavior, medications taken, and what psychiatric care he or she is receiving. If a new problem, determine possible causes.
- Be aware that short frequent contacts will help build trust and help the patient feel more secure.
- Focus on the present reality rather than the future or past. Speak simply and focus on concrete subjects. Keep directions simple, and give only one step of the direction at a time. Avoid theoretic or philosophical topics.
- Provide a quiet, nonstimulating environment.
- Use one form of communication at a time. For example, avoid using a lot of hand motions while speaking.
- Be aware that even though much of psychotic speech seems to be unclear, communication may be symbolic. The patient is usually not aware consciously of this symbolism.
- Avoid giving choices to severely disorganized patients since having to make choices may be too anxiety provoking.
- If possible, problem solve with the patient about ways to cope with anxiety.
- Provide frequent reality orientation; for example, review where he or she is, the date, and so on.
- Arrange for the same staff to care for patient, if possible.
- Find ways to provide structure in patient's day. Give pa-

tient a schedule of daily activities, and try not to deviate from it.

- Make sure patient is taking and swallowing prescribed antipsychotic medications. Recognize that hallucinations and especially delusions may take weeks to months to diminish fully once the medication is started.
- Patient can easily misinterpret what you are saying, so obtain frequent feedback from patient to ensure that he or she understands what you are saying.
- Monitor patient's decisions. Poor judgment may indicate an exacerbation.
- Ask the physician to arrange for a psychiatric consultation.
- For the patient who may be reacting psychotically to the stressful hospital environment:
  - Ensure that the patient is able to get adequate rest and sleep.
  - Make sure patient is oriented to the time of day.
  - Explain equipment and noises and their significance to patient.
  - Call patient by name, and personalize his or her care.
  - Encourage family to bring in personal belongings such as photographs.
  - Vary stimuli around the patient; for example, turn on music or TV at times.
- If the patient is hallucinating:
  - Ask patient directly about his or her hallucinations. For instance, you may say "Are you hearing voices? What are they saying to you?"
  - Watch patient for cues that he or she is hallucinating, such as eyes darting to one side, muttering, or watching a vacant area of the room.
  - Avoid reacting to hallucinations as if they are real. Do not argue back to the voices.
  - Do not negate patient's experience but offer your own perceptions. For instance, you may say "I don't see the devil standing over you, but I do understand how upsetting that must be for you."
  - Focus on reality-based diversions and topics such as conversations or simple projects. Tell patient, "Try to not listen to the voices right now. I have to talk with you."

- ○ Be alert to signs of anxiety in the patient, which may indicate hallucinations are increasing.
- If the patient is having delusions:
  - ○ Be open, honest, and reliable in interactions to reduce suspiciousness.
  - ○ Respond to suspicions in a matter-of-fact and calm manner.
  - ○ Ask patient to describe the delusions, for instance, "Who is trying to hurt you?"
  - ○ Avoid arguing about the content, but interject doubt where appropriate, for instance, "I don't think it would be possible for that petite girl to hurt you."
  - ○ Focus on the feelings the delusions generate, such as "It must feel frightening to think there is a conspiracy against you."
  - ○ Once patient describes delusion, do not dwell on it. Rather, focus conversation on more reality-based topics. If patient obsesses on delusions, set firm limits on amount of time you will devote to talking about them.
  - ○ Observe for events that trigger delusions. If possible, discuss these with patient.
  - ○ Validate if part of the delusion is real, for instance, "Yes, there was a man at the nurse's station, but I did not hear him talk about you."

RISK FOR VIOLENCE EVIDENCED BY AGITATION, AGGRESSIVE BEHAVIOR RELATED TO DELUSIONS AND HALLUCINATIONS.

Patient Outcomes

- Able to maintain control of own behavior
- Demonstrates less anxiety
- Does not cause harm to self or others

Interventions

- Reassure patient that he or she is safe and the staff will provide protection. Be aware that the psychotic patient is more timid and frightened than dangerous.
- Be aware of signs that indicate tension level is increasing.
- Reinforce the patient's ability to remain in control and control his or her own behavior. If patient is able to understand that the hallucinations are not reality, reinforce

that these are his or her own thoughts and not coming from others.

- If patient is hearing voices, encourage him or her to tell you what they are saying to be prepared for what patient will do.
- Monitor patient's behavior closely. If having hallucinations or delusions that are very frightening, be aware that patient could inadvertently harm self or others. For instance, the patient has to protect himself or herself from the "monster" in the room or voices saying to kill oneself. Be aware that patient could feel pressured to bizarre behaviors possibly inflicting harm on himself or herself or others. Observe closely if this occurs, and seek out additional assistance.
- Avoid putting patient on the defensive so that he or she feels a need to protect himself or herself. Avoid ultimatums.
- Be aware that patient may interpret even the most innocent behavior as threatening. For example, turning up the thermostat could be distorted as turning on poison gas, which could generate an extreme reaction.
- Ask the patient if he or she is hearing "command" hallucinations, such as voices commanding to act a certain way. If these commands are for dangerous behavior, monitor the patient closely.
- Administer ordered antipsychotic medications. Consider injectable ones for faster onset of action. Patient may need these medications administered frequently (rapid tranquilization) until behavior is controlled. Monitor closely for side effects including postural hypotension and extrapyramidal symptoms.
- Determine if use of touch calms patient or adds to his or her distress. Ask the patient's permission to be touched.
- Set limits on destructive behavior. Let the patient know what behavior is and is not allowed. Reinforce to staff that everyone must support the same approach.
- If patient is out of control, use restraints only as last resort. See Chapter 8 on managing violent behavior and restraint application. For the psychotic patient, restraints can represent a relief from the tremendous anxiety and loss of control being experienced, or it can significantly increase anxiety and persecution delusions.

Have adequate, trained staff available to manage potential violence.
- Maintain a nonstimulating environment. Use a calm voice with relaxed, nonthreatening body language.

ALTERNATE NURSING DIAGNOSES

Ineffective individual coping
Risk for injury
Risk for self-mutilation
Self-care deficit
Sleep pattern disturbance
Social isolation

WHEN TO CALL FOR HELP

✔ Self-mutilation
✔ Suicide threats or attempts
✔ Aggressive behavior escalating to violence
✔ Hallucinations or delusions with increasingly violent, bizarre content
✔ Patient's inability to care for self
✔ Increasing staff anxiety and fear over patient's behavior

Patient and Family Education

- Teach patient signs of escalating symptoms.
- Teach the patient effective interventions to control anxiety and fears, such as distracting himself or herself to other topics.
- Review with patient ways to validate whether what is being experienced is real, such as asking others if they see or hear the same things.
- Make sure family or caregivers are aware of signs of escalating symptoms, and provide suggestions for managing them. For chronic psychotic disorders, give the family written information on the diagnosis or suggest appropriate reading, such as *Surviving Schizophrenia Family Manual* by EF Torrey.
- Teach the importance of taking prescribed medications and ways to manage side effects.

- Teach the importance of informing the physician of new symptoms, delusions, physical symptoms, and pains.

Charting Tips

- Document patient's behavior and content of delusions and hallucinations.
- Document the administration of medications, side effects, and patient's response to the medication.
- Document efforts to control patient's behavior.
- If restraints are needed, document the type used and appropriate monitoring provided.
- Document the family response to patient.

Discharge Planning

- Determine if the patient has been followed for psychiatric care. If so, reinforce the need to continue in treatment. Reinforce to the family or caregivers their responsibility for getting the patient to follow-up appointments. Give patient and family referrals for psychiatric care if needed.
- Reinforce to the family their need for emotional support. Refer to appropriate programs or support groups, such as local chapters of the National Alliance for the Mentally Ill.
- If this patient has a chronic psychiatric disorder, determine patient's functional ability. He or she may need referrals to programs to assist with employment skills and living arrangements.
- If patient has difficulty functioning in society, he or she may need to be transferred to a psychiatric hospital or need more protected living arrangements, such as a halfway house, group living home, or day treatment program.
- Reinforce need to continue follow-up medical care.

Nursing Outcomes

- Staff provides appropriate, nonjudgmental care.
- Staff is able to set limits to control patient's behavior.
- Medications are administered appropriately.
- Staff and patients remain safe and free from injury.

Selected Learning Activities

- Arrange for an inservice by mental health professionals on schizophrenia or paranoia.
- Arrange to view the education film *World of Schizophrenia.*
- Arrange to visit a group living situation or long-term psychiatric facility.
- Contact the National Alliance for the Mentally Ill, 1901 Fort Myer Drive, Arlington, Virginia, for information on support programs for families of the mentally ill. If a local chapter is available, arrange to attend a meeting.
- Discuss with colleagues the occurrence of ICU psychosis in your intensive care unit. Examine its environment, and problem solve with staff about ways to improve the environment.

The Manipulative Patient

LEARNING OBJECTIVES

▼ *Identify types of manipulative behaviors.*
▼ *Identify some possible nurses' reactions toward manipulative patients.*
▼ *Describe "staff splitting" and characteristic manifestations.*
▼ *Define confrontation and limit setting as therapeutic responses.*
▼ *List effective nursing interventions to deal with manipulative patients.*

The word *manipulation* usually conjures up negative images of pushy, untrustworthy individuals who are only concerned with getting what they want with no regard for other people's feelings, priorities, or needs. However, manipulation can be viewed more accurately as a tool that is not inherently bad and that can be used in either constructive or maladaptive ways. For instance, constructive manipulation is an effective technique for a charge nurse making assignments to ensure the best use of nursing

Glossary

Adaptive manipulation—Skillful management or use of oneself to impact or change a situation to one's best advantage. It is goal oriented, used only when appropriate, considers others' needs and welfare, and is only one of several coping mechanisms used.

Maladaptive manipulation—Similar to an addiction and not goal directed, it is the predominant, continuous controlling of others whether or not it is appropriate, effective, or attains specific goals.

Splitting—An unconscious defense mechanism found in certain manipulative people that causes them to experience others only in the extremes of love or hate, good or bad.

Staff splitting—An unfortunate staff response to a patient which leaves the staff arguing and not coordinating with each other. The staff members whom the patient treats well think highly of the patient others do not.

Personality disorder—A group of psychiatric disorders in which specific, pervasive patterns of inflexible, enduring maladaptive thinking about one's self and the environment cause difficulties in interpersonal relationships and the ability to do work.

Borderline personality disorder—A psychiatric disorder in which there is a chronic state of instability with changes in relationships, self-image, and mood.

Antisocial personality disorder—A psychiatric disorder in which there is a pervasive pattern of disregard for and violation of the rights of others. They rarely feel motivated to change.

personnel to meet patients' needs while considering the nurses' preferences and learning needs.

Some people use maladaptive manipulation strategies during periods of stress to avoid uncomfortable, anxiety-arousing feelings and to gain a sense of security. The patient may use manipulation to compensate for feeling overwhelmed, out of control, and frightened by illness, hospitalization, or personal or occupational concerns. People who consistently use maladaptive manipulation regardless of the circumstances may have a personality disorder, most notably a *borderline* and *antisocial personality* disorder. The person with borderline personality disorder manipulates to gain nurturance, whereas the person with an antisocial personality disorder manipulates to gain power, possession, or some other material gratification. Individuals with personality disorders characteristically exhibit dysfunctional behavior-thinking-relating patterns rather than specific symptoms. They operate using ingrained behavior patterns that have been effective for them, and they may not be aware of their manipulative behavior, the cause-and-effect relationship between their actions and resulting consequences, or the possibility of alternative, effective approaches. This type of manipulative behavior can be either blatant or insidiously covert. The manipulative person may appear superficially pleasant. However, the person being manipulated often recognizes the impact or results even if unable to describe clearly how they occurred.

The first sign of a patient's use of maladaptive manipulative behavior may be the staff's growing frustration and anger. Manipulative patients may, unconsciously, project their own thoughts and feelings onto staff and come to experience the staff or some (even one) of the nurses as a mirror image of themselves. As a result, the patient perceives these staff members as being manipulative, unreliable, and even verbally abusive. When the patient feels threatened, he or she tries to control the situation by manipulating, attacking, or avoiding the staff.

Two effective techniques for working with manipulative patients are *confrontation* and *limit setting*. Both of these techniques need to be used consistently with concern for the patient. Although the word *confrontation* is usually associated with hostile, antagonistic battles, it is used effectively as an intervention to dispassionately point out to the patient a discrepancy in words, actions, or feelings. For instance, "You said you have not seen a doctor before coming to the ER, but you have a bottle of prescription drugs dated last week. Where did you get that?" *Setting limits* is teaching and maintaining boundaries of the nurses' and the patient's roles and acceptable behaviors. This may mean telling a patient what he or she may or may not do under certain conditions or in certain situations.

Despite protests, manipulative patients will feel more secure and less out of control when their behavior is contained. Using these techniques, nurses can alleviate much of the patient's insecurity and help to create the appropriate boundaries of acceptable behavior. Before being successful at using these techniques, however, you need to feel comfortable being assertive and being in the role of an authority figure. The nurse's past experiences with authority figures and individual personality influence one's ability to master these techniques. It is important to realize, however, that no one can completely control another's behavior.

Manipulative patients who unconsciously block painful feeling by *splitting* their perceptions of people into the extremes of all good or all bad can have a very disruptive, divisive effect on the staff. *Staff splitting* is a possible response to splitting when the patient idealizes certain staff members, treating them as all worthy and good while viewing others as all bad and criticizing and devaluing them. The staff may respond similarly, each one either intensely liking or disliking the patient and eventually becoming alienated from each other (see Table 12–1).

Etiology

According to *psychologic* theory, manipulative patients do not trust other people to like or accept them, to be responsive to them, or be responsible toward them. Consciously or unconsciously, they rely on manipulative behavior to demand that others supply what they need and want.

TABLE 12–1. **Warning Signs of Staff Splitting**

A manipulative patient can have a devastating effect on the staff and functioning of the unit. Staff group behavior that can indicate that staff splitting has occurred includes:

* Diagnostic uncertainty with contradictory evaluation of patient.
* Groups of staff members feel emotionally isolated from one another. For instance, two or more staff members become suspicious of the motives and behaviors of other staff members toward the patient.
* Lunch hour and coffee break dominated by discussion of the specific patient.
* The nucleus of an in-group believe that only they can help the patient.
* Loss of morale and confusion in the out-group.
* Blurring of staff-client role boundaries (for instance, patient and staff discuss another staff member, staff share personal information with patient).
* Split in- and out-groups make accusations: "ins" accuse "outs" of being cold and insensitive; "outs" accuse "ins" of being too permissive and gullible and of spoiling patient.
* Splits between departments in a hospital structure.

Source: Adapted from Lego, S, Borderline personality disorders. In Varca-rolis, E, Foundations of Psychiatric Mental Health Nursing. WB Saunders, Philadelphia, 1994. Reprinted with permission.

Manipulative behavior in healthcare settings may reflect the patient's ongoing, habitual mode of interaction, or it may be an escalation of milder, more common control mechanisms. In the hospital setting, the patient may regress and have unrealistic expectations that his or her every need will be instantly gratified. Disappointment turns to fury and an increase in manipulative behavior.

Chronic manipulative behavior may result from childhood dilemmas if parents undermined attempts toward independence and autonomy. These individuals have come to suspect that any person or institution may try to control them, rendering them powerless and vulnerable to attack. Even being cooperative can be viewed as giving in or being weak, negatively affecting self-esteem. Authority figures are seen as being stronger and having too much control over the patient's life. The patient may seek ways to equalize the power by controlling staff, not complying with medical regimen, and making excess demands. Suicidal gestures may be a frantic attempt to regain control or block painful feelings of helplessness or dependence. Fear of rejection and abandonment or expectation of increased responsibility are also triggers for self-destructive acts.

Learning theory focuses on manipulative behavior that may have been learned in childhood based on adult role models, peers, and even the media.

Family theory suggests that manipulative behavior may have been developed, especially in younger years, as the only way to cope with a severely dysfunctional family.

Related Clinical Concerns

This patient may rely on sedatives, analgesics, or other substances to reduce feelings of anxiety. These may also trigger reduced inhibitions and increased aggressive responses.

Lifespan Issues

CHILDHOOD TO ADOLESCENCE

Manipulative behavior begins in the earliest years, partly as a way to test out responses from caretakers. Toddlers have temper tantrums and quickly learn whether or not they can get their way. Children of all ages mimic the manipulative behavior of parents and siblings, such as making promises that are not kept. Or they may try getting permission from one parent after receiving a no from the other. They also learn from their peers. They may try to get privileges or possessions by saying that all their friends have these already.

Disturbed, maladaptive manipulative behaviors manifested in conduct disorders are seen in childhood and adolescence. Those who rely on deceitfulness can also display cruelty to animals or other children, destructiveness of property, and serious violations of rules. This can evolve into antisocial personality disorder in adulthood. They may have experienced more severe deprivations such as multiple rejections, neglect, and/or abuse.

ADULTHOOD

People who have successfully used manipulative behavior as children tend to become more proficient as they grow older. They tend to flourish in systems where they are able to manipulate. People who are extremely manipulative and exploitative may violate laws and end up in the criminal justice system. Those who exhibit strong manipulative tendencies but are able to stay within legal confines may become successful in using people, personally and professionally, for their own goals.

ELDERLY

As people age and become more dependent on other people for assistance in activities or socialization, they may resort more frequently or aggressively to manipulative behaviors to get their needs met. If guilt has been a favorite ploy, declarations such as "I don't want to be a burden" may be intended to stir guilt and get attention.

Possible Nurses' Reactions

- May feel angry, frustrated, or resentful for being tricked; lowered self-esteem if unable to stop the manipulation; or embarrassed or humiliated.
- May feel helpless in relieving patient's apparent distress or when attempting to get patient to conform to nurse's expectations of reasonable conduct.
- May feel vulnerable and afraid of patient's attacks.
- May take manipulations personally and react defensively, especially when challenged in authority or position.
- May reject patient as the experience of coping with personal reactions is too draining and demoralizing.
- May avoid patient, spend minimal time needed to provide physical nursing care, or assign a different nurse to the patient each day.
- May compensate by becoming overcontrolling or engage in power struggles with patient.
- May experience desire for revenge, retaliation; may become punitive, want to counterattack by insulting, hurt-

ing, or embarrassing patient. May secretly hope things go wrong for patient.
- May experience guilt about negative feelings toward patient.
- May become overinvolved, or overattached and desire to rescue patient.
- May feel total responsibility for patient's improvement or lack of improvement.
- May be punitive in setting limits or confronting the patient or may be inconsistent or hesitant in enforcing rules for fear of patient's reaction.

Assessment

Behavior and/or Appearance

- Frequent disregard of rules
- Argumentative
- Can be superficially charming and entertaining
- Demanding; the more staff try to cater to demands, the more they escalate
- Impulsive and unpredictable; lacks ability to tolerate frustration; can easily become out of control
- Uses threats to get demand met
- May use intimidation to control or feel superior
- Frustration causes more intense manipulative behavior
- Destructive toward self, others, property without taking responsibility
- Lies, cheats, steals
- Intense manipulation around medication; overuse of medication
- Noncompliant with healthcare treatment
- Undermines treatment of other patients such as encouraging them to ignore doctor's recommendations or suggesting alternate treatments

Mood and/or Emotions

- Anger predominates. Behavior can be cutting, sarcastic, and vicious.
- Anxiety rises rapidly to panic, which precipitates impul-

sive actions. May not experience anxiety unless facing a threat to self-image or self-esteem.
- Views self as very vulnerable and frightened, even when being intimidating, or as totally invulnerable to harm or negative consequences resulting in reckless behavior.
- Labile moods and emotions. The more patient is in crisis, the more frequently moods and emotions may fluctuate over the course of a day. May appear resistant to depression or may have periodic depressive reactions.
- May have inflated or diminished self-esteem. If inflated, denies or distorts information that would lower self-esteem.

Thoughts, Beliefs, and Perceptions

- Thinking can contain gross distortions of some specific events or people while maintaining accurate perception and good reality of others.
- Projects own thoughts and feelings onto others, resulting in feelings of fear and manipulation by others.

Relationships and Interactions

- May seek or avoid attention
- Exploitative with little real concern for others; limited capacity for empathy; demonstrates caring only to get own needs met
- Quick to recognize vulnerable areas in others
- Limited ability to see others for who they really are; distorted perceptions of how others experience self
- Needs to feel either in control or helpless and vulnerable. (Life is seen as a seesaw competition. If someone else is up, then patient feels down.)
- Does not feel a sense of obligation to reciprocate favors or helpful acts
- Devalues others to feel good about self
- Sees others as attacking or dangerous
- Feels and acts as if he or she were entitled to having needs met without comparable effort or cost
- Becomes a "special patient" to the staff
- Blames others for mistakes and problems without taking personal responsibility; confuses taking responsibility with being blamed, worthless, and vulnerable to attack

- Belief of being superior; cannot admit to lack of knowledge and has great difficulty asking for assistance and information; obtains information by using indirect manipulation; unable to accept suggestions or criticism

Physical Responses

- Physical complaints that cannot be substantiated with testing
- Magnifies any subjective symptoms that cannot be measured
- With documentable disability, usually requires more frequent medication and higher dosages; recovery takes longer than usual

Pertinent History

- Erratic, impulsive behavior with marked instability; frequent changes in jobs, relationships, and physicians
- Drug or alcohol abuse
- Long history of many physical complaints

Collaborative Interventions

Multidisciplinary Team Communication

When staff members have extremely different experiences with the same patient, infighting amongst each other can occur when discussing care for the patient. These variations in experiences can occur between individuals in the nursing staff, between shifts, between nurses and physicians, or between all staff and administrators. To overcome this staff splitting, the group needs to recognize the patient's dynamics and cooperatively share their different perceptions to gain a more complete picture of the patient. They need to identify whom the patient sees as "all good" or "all bad" and how this affects interactions.

Once they have identified the problem behaviors, it is essential to formulate a united, consistent care plan. Each staff member should monitor the intensity of his or her individual reactions to the manipulative behavior. This will help to avoid becoming entrapped into feeling the need to be special or the only one who can help or avoid getting caught in power struggles. A supportive and coordinated multidisciplinary team approach helps neutralize the manipulative patient's ability to identify vulnerability in team members and discord in the healthcare organization.

Pharmacologic

If the patient is given tranquilizers to reduce anxiety, there is a risk for drug dependence and power struggles.

Nursing Management

INEFFECTIVE INDIVIDUAL COPING EVIDENCED BY NONCOMPLIANCE WITH RULES AND TREATMENTS RELATED TO IMPULSIVE, MANIPULATIVE BEHAVIOR.

Patient Outcomes

- Decreased use of maladaptive, manipulative behaviors
- Complies with treatment regimen and hospital rules
- Uses effective coping patterns
- Demonstrates more adaptive methods of dealing with stress, such as using problem-solving skills

Interventions

- Carefully assess patient's mode of interaction and frequency over time before labeling behavior as "manipulative."
- Determine if the patient is using manipulation to indirectly express a need, anxiety, or distressful emotion. Active listening and empathetic responses to underlying issues can help diminish the patient's anxiety and need to control others.
- Approach patient in a calm and matter-of-fact manner, using a neutral tone of voice.
- Provide feedback to patient who may not be aware that manipulative behaviors are being used. State specific observations about his or her style of interactions without arguing. If patient argues or denies, calmly repeat your

observation without becoming defensive. Describe options and consequences. Follow through consistently with consequences.
- Don't state consequences that you do not have the authority to exercise.
- State which behaviors are not acceptable without personally rejecting the patient.
- Help patient identify when using manipulative behavior becomes an attempt to control anxiety. Encourage patient to identify triggers for anger and frustration.
- Encourage patient to verbalize feelings instead of acting them out. Ask the patient to identify what he or she is experiencing and what feelings and thoughts preceded the behavior.
- Evaluate if patient's manipulative behavior increases or decreases when not reinforced by nurse's attention. Be aware that even in those instances when ignoring provocation is effective over time, there may be an initial escalation to test responses.
- Avoid power struggles and attempts to out-manipulate the patient. Point out that the patient is undermining own care. State explicitly that the patient will not be forced to accept treatment and that each individual is responsible for the outcome of the treatment.
- Explain as early as possible rules and regulations and the reasons for them. If allowable limits are not stated, patient may push and test until they are clarified. If he or she attempts to break the rules, review firmly the stated expectations.
- Include the patient in decisions about limits, and provide opportunities for personal decision making to enhance sense of control. When all rules are rigid, the patient may feel a greater need to rebel. Be careful not to allow patient to dictate nursing decisions.
- Written contracts defining both staff and patient expectations can be most effective. Specifically define any consequences of patient's continued manipulation and lack of cooperation. Contracts can be signed by nurse and patient.
- Describe in detail on care plan the limits set and the consequences of breaking them. In periodic staff meetings

and multidisciplinary case conferences, give current information and promote agreement about the patient, which will enable staff to work more consistently and cohesively.

- Make sure all staff are aware of limits and consequences. Confront colleagues who are observed not following the treatment plan.
- Consult with physician when patient seems to exaggerate complaints of pain or becomes preoccupied with timing of medications. The physician may decide to convert a PRN order to low doses of regularly administered medications to avoid power struggles.
- Assess for signs of substance abuse and/or withdrawal if patient has such a history and/or shows symptoms.

IMPAIRED SOCIAL INTERACTION EVIDENCED BY ATTEMPTS TO UNDERMINE, CONTROL AND INFLUENCE, AND CAUSE CONFLICT RELATED TO SPLITTING, DISTORTED PERCEPTIONS OF OTHERS, IMPULSIVITY, AND ANXIETY.

Patient Outcomes

- Uses acceptable methods to interact with others to communicate and obtain needs
- Positively responds to confrontation and limit setting
- Tolerates frustration and waiting
- Does not reject or denigrate the staff as "bad" when they are unable to respond in desired manner
- Develops a more trusting relationship with at least one staff member by sharing personal thoughts and feelings

Interventions

- Maintain assertive, centered, firm but fair, and eventoned stance when patient tries to manipulate or undermine you.
- Tell the patient that he or she may understand events and interactions differently than the staff does.
- Direct patient who complains about staff member to discuss the problem with implicated staff person. Do not allow yourself to be used as an intermediary; do not take sides.
- Use "I" statements indicating how patient made you feel.

Avoid becoming defensive, which can escalate manipulative behavior.

- Confront the patient with your perception that he or she is trying to put you down. This can have an impact even if patient denies it.
- Take time to think about effective responses and to diminish the intensity of your reactions if patient is trying to manipulate. Use stress reduction techniques.
- Role play or discuss situation with other staff, if necessary.
- Return to original topic if patient tries to divert topic to a personal attack.
- Be aware of patient interactions that can increase staff divisiveness by blaming, accusations, or comparisons. Monitor your own responses.
- Provide praise and reinforcement when patient communicates directly and openly about needs and concerns.
- Use kind but firm approach. Clarify that setting limits is constructive and caring rather than punitive.
- Establish from the beginning that you take all of the limits very seriously. More flexibility can be introduced later as the patient takes more responsibility.
- Find neutral actions and topics for conversation. This will help to present you as a person interested in the patient and not just a rule keeper.
- Be aware that patient may need to test limits repeatedly to see whether there are repercussions and to be reassured that the staff will follow through on the consequences.
- Let patient know immediately that threats or verbal abuse are unacceptable, that you expect these will never be repeated, and state the consequences of repeated abuses.
- Confront patient when he or she attempts to undermine other patients' treatment.
- Do not allow patient to manipulate, flatter, seduce, bargain, or intimidate staff into granting him or her special status. Do not accept gifts or favors or share personal information, especially about any current difficulties.
- Never agree to keep a secret with a patient. Remind patient that the entire health team needs to be aware of patient's concerns in order to offer the best care.

- Assess interactions with family. If patient uses same approaches with them, family members may need information on changing their response.

ALTERNATE NURSING DIAGNOSES

Anxiety
Defensive coping
Noncompliance
Powerlessness
Self-esteem disturbance

WHEN TO CALL FOR HELP

✔ Threats or actions of physical harm to others or self, including suicidal threats or gestures
✔ Undermining own or other's health care and unresponsive to nursing interventions
✔ Repeated violation of agency rules
✔ Evidence of staff splitting
✔ Noncompliance, which jeopardizes patient's health status, such as refusing to take medications

---

Patient and Family Education

- Teach patient to ask directly for what he or she wants and needs in words, not actions. Teach problem-solving skills.
- Help patient recognize that his or her desires may not require immediate action and that he or she may not always get desired responses.
- Explain the consequences of manipulative behavior.
- If a patient will not take responsibility for own actions, explain how his or her behavior contributed to the unwanted response or consequences and that taking responsibility is not the same as being blamed.
- Teach patient that understanding of one's own behavior and developing improved interactions are the avenues for developing stable support networks.
- Involve family in patient education. The same skills used in working with the patient may be helpful for the family.

Charting Tips

- Describe specific manipulative behaviors objectively, rather than just labeling the patient as manipulative.
- Develop a detailed treatment plan so that the team can respond consistently. Chart patient's responses to interventions.
- Document usage of PRN medication, reason for use, and patient's response.

Discharge Planning

- Begin discharge planning as early as possible, to decrease last-minute impulsive and inappropriate decisions the patient might make without consideration for consequences.
- Inform the family and patient together of patient's health-care needs to reduce manipulative behavior with family.
- Inform referring agencies of patient's behavior and short-term treatment planning goals.

Nursing Outcomes

- Staff demonstrates appropriate consistent interventions and responses to manipulative behavior.
- Documentation reflects consistent implementation of treatment plan by all involved nursing staff.
- Any staff conflict is resolved in a timely manner.
- Staff does not become split when caring for the patient.
- Staff demonstrates appropriate limit setting with realistic consequences.

Suggested Learning Activities

- Take classes in assertiveness training, stress reduction, and nonviolent crisis intervention.
- Attend inservice on caring for patients with borderline or antisocial personality disorders.
- List manipulative behaviors that would be difficult for you to handle. Write down possible reasons. Role play constructive interventions and responses.

- In a group role-playing situation, have one person act as the patient and interact with half the group separately as if they were the most wonderful, helpful nurses and the other half of the group as if they were the most hateful, harmful, inadequate, and inept nurses. Then have both groups come together and discuss their observations of the patient's behavior and their feelings about the patient. Finally have each half group discuss their observations and feelings about the people who are in the other group.

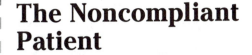

The Noncompliant Patient

LEARNING OBJECTIVES

▼ *Identify factors that contribute to a patient's noncompliance with treatment plans.*
▼ *List the principles of adult education that contribute to effective patient education.*
▼ *Identify nursing interventions to reduce noncompliance in the patient whose cultural beliefs impede compliance.*
▼ *List some nursing staff reactions to the noncompliant patient.*

*C*ompliance and *noncompliance* are terms that are used to describe patient behavior in response to information given about his or her health care. What makes a patient follow, change, or ignore health teaching is complex and may not always be related to the amount and quality of information provided. Nurses need to be aware that noncompliance is a symptom of an underlying problem and not the actual problem and that labeling behavior as "noncompliant" can have negative connotations, such as blaming or criticizing a patient who is not following instruction. Once you have identified that the patient is noncompliant, you need to investigate what the illness and treatment mean to the patient as well as the other variables that influence the patient's willingness to comply.

The cost of noncompliance is greater than can actually be documented. Besides factors such as the cost of medications purchased but not taken or taken incorrectly, poor results of diagnostic tests caused by poor preparation, and more severe illness from not following recommended treatments, both patients and healthcare providers can experience a great deal of frustration.

Although not the only reason for noncompliance, inadequate or inappropriate patient education is among the most common. When teaching adults, the nurse needs to incorporate principles of adult learning. Adults have different learning needs than children do. Adults are goal oriented. The goals need to be clearly identified and at-

---

Glossary

Noncompliance—Patient's failure to follow therapeutic recommendations.
Compliance—Patient's accurately following a prescribed regimen of treatment.
Ineffective management of therapeutic regimen—A pattern of regulating and integrating into daily living a program for treatment of illness and the sequelae of illness that is unsatisfactory for meeting specific health goals.

tainable, and they need to consistently be made aware of their progress toward their goal. Adults need to understand how the education will benefit them. Adults tend to learn better when they understand the rationale for what they are learning, apply what they learn immediately, and can compare what they are learning to knowledge from past experiences. Learning is inhibited when authoritarian teaching methods are used. Interpersonal relationships with teachers are important.

Etiology

There are many dynamics that contribute to noncompliance. For example, although the patient may fully understand the information and consequences of not following recommendations, he or she has the right to choose not to follow that advice. The patient's decision is in keeping with the principle of autonomy. In this situation, it is the healthcare provider's responsibility to ensure that the patient has all the information he or she needs to make that decision and then the responsibilty of making the decision remains with the patient.

Other major factors contributing to noncompliance include:

- *Denial:* This may be a conscious or unconscious method of believing that he or she is not sick. By not checking blood sugars, the patient's diagnosis of diabetes can be blocked out of his or her mind.
- *Power struggles:* At times the patient who feels a lack of control over his or her body uses noncompliance as a way to maintain some control over a sense of destiny or over healthcare providers.
- *Counterdependence:* The patient could be concerned that following recommendations would increase dependency on others. Since dependency can enhance feelings of loss of identity, noncompliance becomes a statement of independence and individualism.
- *Loss of coping mechanisms:* Often health teaching involves asking the patient to give up habits that are part of the person's usual coping strategies. For example, smoking, diet changes, or exercise may need to be altered or avoided. If the patient has not yet developed

alternative coping mechanisms, the anxiety created by the loss of these habits may be overwhelming.

- *Conflict with self-image:* Noncompliance may be a method of self-protection against the threat of an altered body image, particularly in those individuals whose health and activity are a source of pride. Taking medication or imposing limitations on activity may represent a threat to the individual's self-image.
- *Fatalistic viewpoint:* A patient may believe there is no point to following instructions because of the belief that nothing will change the outcome.
- *Hidden benefits of illness:* Some people may consciously or unconsciously perceive benefits from the sick role, such as attention, avoidance of responsibility, controlling the destiny of another, or maintaining stability in a rocky relationship.
- *Self-destructive behavior:* A patient could be consciously or unconsciously participating in a wish to die or hurt himself or herself, possibly reflecting depression or suicidal tendencies. It could represent behaviors associated with a serious personality disorder.
- *Psychiatric disorder:* Psychiatric illness or altered thought processes may make consistent compliance with a health routine impossible.
- *Family influence:* Family members may discourage or undermine compliance because they are using denial, lack the understanding of the treatment, or unconscious need to maintain the patient in sick role.
- *Lack of economic resources:* If the patient has insufficient funds or no insurance, he or she may need to decide between eating or feeding the family and buying needed medications.
- *Lack of social resources:* Lack of funds, fear of being dependent on others, or lack of social contacts may cause the patient to miss appointments because there is no transportation to get there.
- *Unsatisfactory relationship with healthcare team:* If the patient perceives the doctors or nurses as cold, uncaring, not knowledgeable, or authoritarian, he or she may resent or ignore instructions. This may stir up in the patient such issues as resentment of authority and

feeling unrecognized as an individual. This patient may minimize or distort information given due to his or her emotional response. Long waits and uncomfortable waiting areas may also contribute to the poor relationship.

- *Lack of trust in information given:* Patient may not believe health information given because it has not proved useful in the past. Also, with the increase in media reporting of conflicting reports of studies, patients may think the information isn't trustworthy enough to warrant a change in lifestyle.
- *Cultural beliefs:* Cultural or religious beliefs may influence the way the patient views his or her illness and the treatments that are acceptable. For instance, women in some cultures may not allow a male healthcare provider to examine their breasts or a Jehovah's Witness may not accept a blood transfusion.
- *Inability to read or understand instructions:* Some patients may be too embarrassed to acknowledge that they cannot read English. This may apply to those who speak another language or even to those who do speak English. Literacy rates in the United States are dropping so some patients who function well in society may not be able to read. Also, be aware that some patients will not admit that they do not understand language that is too technical or that contains too much jargon. To be understood by the majority, patient education materials should be written at the average reading level, which for most adults is the fifth to eighth grade level.
- *Uncomfortable side effects:* Patients may be noncompliant due to real or perceived side effects, especially with medications. The patient may be less likely to report them if they are more embarrassing such as impotence or incontinence. In addition, incorrect beliefs like fear of becoming dependent on medications may cause some to not take medications.

Noncompliance can become part of a negative cycle as the patient feels embarrassed or guilty for not following through and then begins canceling appointments to avoid healthcare providers.

Related Clinical Concerns

When patients are dealing with an acute crisis, the majority of their energy will be focused on just coping with the situation at hand. They will not be able to concentrate on learning until the crisis has subsided or they have made adaptations to deal with the situation. During this time, instruction should involve only what is absolutely necessary. You'll need to be prepared to repeat much of the information provided as the patient may not remember what he or she was told.

Any physical or mental problem that impairs cognition will also interfere with learning.

Lifespan Issues

CHILDHOOD

Following a particular treatment plan can be difficult for ill children and their family. Medications may affect behavior, alertness, or school performance. Incorporating a child's medical care into family life can create many stressors, contributing to noncompliance since the child may not be able to be responsible. It can be time-consuming and difficult to administer. Working parents and single-parent families may not have the time to be able to supervise the child or take him or her for follow-up care. Because the child may not be able to communicate his or her needs, medical care can be difficult to monitor.

Parental noncompliance could have legal and ethical ramifications. Parents who refuse to give a child needed medical attention could be accused of negligence or even abuse. Parental autonomy to make decisions for their child may be overridden if it is determined the child is placed at some risk. In these extreme situations, legal intervention would be required.

ADOLESCENCE

Adolescents are particularly vulnerable to problems with compliance. Their attitude is often related to struggles with maintaining independence and rebelling against adult authority. In addition, any medical regimen that impacts body image will put additional demands on the teenager. Also because the adolescent does not want to appear different from his or her peer group, complying with instructions may be particularly difficult. For example, a diabetic adolescent who is eating lunch with friends may be fearful to expose his or her dietary restrictions.

ELDERLY

Noncompliance is an extremely important issue for the elderly who experience more chronic illness than the general population. Chronic illnesses often require multiple medications and are often combined with over-the-counter drugs. Some elderly see more than one specialist and have a variety of prescriptions from the physicians they see or may be given contradictory treatment advice. They may become easily confused. Decreased muscle mass and increased fat stores may make individuals more prone to drug side effects. The elderly patient may need more assistance and time to explain instructions. If living alone, the elderly patient may have limited support for encouragement or reminding. Hearing and vision deficits as well as limited manual dexterity due to arthritis can present other problems. In addition, cognitive impairments including poor short-term memory may inhibit the patient's compliance by causing him or her to forget instructions or how many pills have already been taken.

Possible Nurses' Reactions

- May become angry or frustrated because the time spent with patient seemed fruitless.
- May criticize or judge patient who does not follow instructions.
- May judge one's self as inadequate or incompetent when patient does not follow instructions.
- May feel responsible for patient's noncompliance. Nurse may have difficulty recognizing that ultimately the responsibility for one's health care belongs to the patient.

Assessment

Behavior and/or Appearance

- Does not follow rules or instructions demonstrated by:
  - Refusing to take or change medications
  - Continuing unhealthy habits
  - Missing medical appointments
  - Altering medical regimen
  - Challenging the necessity or helpfulness of treatments
  - Leaving hospital against medical advice
  - Arguing without constructive resolution
  - Indicating understanding or agreement with treatment plan and then not following through
  - Hiding inability to read or comprehend educational material

Mood and/or Emotions

- Anger
- Depression
- Resentment
- Irritability
- Anxiety

Thoughts, Beliefs, and Perceptions

- Religious or cultural beliefs in contradiction with compliance actions
- Believes healthcare should be obtained only when symptoms are blatant or impairing needed activity.
- Suspicions concerning motivations of healthcare professionals
- Lack of confidence in own abilities
- Denial of healthcare needs
- Psychotic thought process or suicidal thoughts

Relationships and Interactions

- May avoid sharing information with others about medical regimen
- Tendency to manipulate or control others
- Family not providing needed support
- Inconsistent relationship with healthcare team; at times

may be very critical of them and other times more positive toward them
- Following instructions from only one particular nurse

Physical Responses

- Deterioration of health due to lack of compliance
- Blood or urine tests showing drug levels inconsistent
  with reported medication intake; discrepancies in other
  tests

Pertinent History

- Poor outcomes from previous medical treatment
- Poor relationships with past healthcare providers
- Noncompliance in earlier healthcare treatments

Collaborative Management

Multidisciplinary Team Communication

To ensure the best chance for patient compliance, a team
approach is essential. All healthcare providers should be
consulted to ensure a cohesive treatment plan and approach that the patient understands. This is a pivotal nursing responsibility since they coordinate most of the care
provided both in the hospital and in the home. Discrepancies in instructions from physicians, physical or occupational therapists, pharmacists, or other healthcare providers need to be discussed so that the patient is not left to
choose whose advice to follow.

Nursing Management

NONCOMPLIANCE EVIDENCED BY FAILURE TO ADHERE TO MEDI-
CAL REGIMEN, FAILURE TO KEEP APPOINTMENTS RELATED TO HEALTH
BELIEFS, CULTURAL INFLUENCES.

Patient Outcomes

- Verbalizes beliefs that influence noncompliance
- Demonstrates adherence to treatment plan
- Expected therapeutic goals realized

Interventions

- Develop a trusting relationship with patient. Communicate interest and openness to patient's needs and beliefs.
- Assess the degree of noncompliance and the underlying reason for it. One common area of noncompliance is in using medications. Many prescriptions are never filled or filled and never used. When seeing a patient in the hospital or in the home, always review the medications the patient has, how they are being taken and his or her understanding of why the drug is necessary. Check expiration dates, name of the physician who ordered the drugs, and instructions on the labels. Analyze whether the patient is taking more than one drug for the same reason, especially if they were ordered by different physicians.
- Encourage the patient to share beliefs or traditions that impact health care. Demonstrate to patient your interest in learning about these. Do not criticize or belittle these beliefs; rather, communicate your respect for them.
- Ask the patient to share rationale for avoiding the prescribed treatment. Resolve any misunderstanding the patient may have about the treatment, its side effects, or its potential outcome. Avoid insisting that the patient give up his or her beliefs. Never argue with patient about the value of the beliefs. Instead, explain any negative outcomes that these beliefs may cause with his or her condition.
- In critical situations the patient may need to be confronted more directly with life-threatening consequences of noncompliance (e.g., taking insulin).
- Enlist assistance of family, friends, caregivers, or, if beliefs are based in a particular culture, others with whom the patient may relate to, to explain the consequences of these actions on his or her health status.
- Talk with family members about their beliefs about patient's illness to determine their role in noncompliance.
- Obtain feedback from patient to ensure that the patient understands the instructions given. Use an interpreter if needed.
- If appropriate, negotiate the best compromise with the patient. Have him or her commit to one or two areas in which he or she will comply rather than expecting the patient to give up all his or her beliefs completely.

- Identify one staff member who has the best relationship with patient to provide information.
- Recognize that it may be impossible to alter the patient's strong cultural or religious beliefs. Understand that in some cases illness, or even death, may be more acceptable and a higher priority than giving up one's beliefs.

INEFFECTIVE MANAGEMENT OF THERAPEUTIC REGIMEN (INDIVIDUALS) EVIDENCED BY ACCELERATION OF ILLNESS SYMPTOMS OR VERBALIZED DIFFICULTY WITH REGULATING OR INTEGRATING PRESCRIBED REGIMENS RELATED TO COMPLEXITY OF THERAPEUTIC REGIMEN OR HEALTHCARE SYSTEM.

Patient Outcomes

- Identifies factors that contribute to noncompliance
- Demonstrates adherence to treatment plan
- Expected therapeutic goals realized

Interventions

- Encourage patient to share factors that contribute to noncompliance. Ask the patient to explain the rationale for actions taken or not taken.
- Avoid using medical jargon or abbreviations that may confuse or intimidate. Encourage open communication so that the patient will tell you when he or she does not understand something.
- Have patient perform a return demonstration or verbalize his or her routine to determine patient's understanding and determine areas of noncompliance.
- Assess whether other methods of teaching would be more appropriate, such as videos, role playing, pamphlets with more pictures, or pamphlets written at a lower reading level. Minimize any distractions during teaching sessions.
- Incorporate principles of adult learning in educating adult patients. For example, explain rationale, avoid lecturing or belittling the patient, involve patient in discussion, and allow patient to identify ways teaching can be incorporated into his or her lifestyle.
- Ensure that the patient is in the best physical and emotional state for learning to occur. Remember to repeat information that was previously given when the patient

was dealing with the acute crisis. Avoid teaching if patient in pain or has other discomforts.

- Assess role of family in patient's healthcare regimen. Determine who provides care for patient at home, and determine the caregiver's role in the noncompliance. Observe caregiver's technique if appropriate, and provide information as needed.
- Determine patient's understanding of using the healthcare system. Review ways to get appointments, arrange additional care such as home care, and how to contact healthcare providers. As needed, check with social service agencies to provide needed transportation, equipment, or other services.
- Help identify ways patient can individualize information. For example, if a patient works rotating shifts or travels extensively, you will need to focus your teaching on how to adapt the treatment plan to best fit into his or her lifestyle.
- Identify ways to reinforce patient's self-esteem and sense of competency. Provide positive reinforcement and recognition of patient improvement.
- Incorporate rewards as part of the teaching. For an adult, rewards may include those activities that increase self-esteem and a sense of control.

INEFFECTIVE INDIVIDUAL COPING EVIDENCED BY NOT DO-ING, PARTIALLY DOING, OR REVAMPING TREATMENT PLAN RELATED TO ANXIETY ABOUT ILLNESS, INADEQUATE COPING MECHANISMS.

Patient Outcomes

- Verbalizes anxieties and concerns
- Verbalizes acceptance and commitment to the treatment plan
- Demonstrates adherence to healthcare regimen
- Expected therapeutic goals realized

Interventions

- Encourage the patient to discuss worries and concerns regarding the illness. Determine patient's understanding of the illness, prognosis, and treatment plan. If patient's understanding is not accurate, review the appropriate information about the condition with him or her.

- Encourage the patient to express feelings verbally rather than act them out through noncompliance.
- Repeat and reinforce teaching. The patient's learning ability may be impaired due to anxiety or physical status.
- Give patient some control in treatment regimen. Seek his or her ideas for adaptations that can be made. Identify other areas in patient's life where he or she can exert control. Consider negotiating a contract with the patient to reinforce compliance.
- For the patient who is impatient and perfectionistic, point out the need to develop realistic expectations of behavior changes. For example, he or she may not be able to lose weight and give up smoking at the same time.
- Approach the suspicious patient with the expectation of compliance. Keep directions clear and simple, and always be honest.
- Reinforce that the patient is ultimately responsible for his or her own health.
- If major life changes must be made, break down expected changes into achievable steps that may be easier to accept and master. Develop a way patient can chart own progress.

ALTERNATE NURSING DIAGNOSES

Altered thought processes
Anxiety
Decisional conflict
Ineffective management of therapeutic regimen, families
Knowledge deficit
Powerlessness
Self-care deficit

WHEN TO CALL FOR HELP

- ✔ Patient refuses to comply with medical regimen with life-threatening implications.
- ✔ Family or caregiver abuses patient or interferes with patient's compliance.
- ✔ Patient uses folk remedies or alternative health practices that complicate current medical condition.

> ✔ There is evidence of suicidal or psychotic thinking as reason for noncompliance.
> ✔ There is increased staff conflict over dealing with patient's noncompliance.

Patient and Family Education

- Determine appropriate materials available to assist in patient education including pamphlets, videos, closed-circuit health education channels in the hospital, or flip-charts.
- Determine if appropriate educational materials are available from pharmaceutical and medical equipment companies. Many times they have excellent materials available at no charge.
- Identify appropriate times to provide education to patient and family. Realize that at times the patient may not be ready for teaching when the nurse is available. Other alternatives need to be identified.
- Identify other resources, such as diabetes educators, ostomy nurses, pharmacists, or dietitians, to assist in teaching. Be sure to coordinate teaching so that no conflicting information is given.

Charting Tips

- Document all identified factors that contribute to noncompliance.
- Use objective, nonjudgmental terms to describe behavior.
- Document the teaching plan and patient goals to ensure that all healthcare team members are providing the same information.
- Document all teaching given and patient and family response to the education.
- Document patient's verbalized reason for and effects of noncompliance.

Discharge Planning

- Refer the patient for home health follow-up to evaluate home situation and its influence on compliance. Inform home health nurses of concerns regarding patient's compliance and any effective or ineffective strategies you have used.

- Identify practical issues that inhibit compliance such as lack of transportation or lack of funds or insurance. Then seek out potential resources for assistance. Involve social worker, case manager, or community resources advisor for assistance.
- Refer to support groups, community education programs, or volunteer support programs, such as Reach for Recovery, or ostomy visitors. These people may provide needed reinforcement or role models for motivation and support.
- Ensure that the patient and caregivers have adequate information for follow-up appointments and future treatment and that they have needed phone numbers and resources to call for more assistance.
- Refer patient for follow-up counseling if persistent noncompliance is related to inadequate coping skills or psychiatric disorder.

Nursing Outcomes

- Staff provides needed education to patient and family.
- Staff identifies factors contributing to patient noncompliance.
- Teaching plan is effective.
- Staff remains objective and nonjudgmental while caring for patient.

Suggested Learning Activities

- Obtain education materials from nursing organizations or pharmaceutical or medical equipment companies.
- Attend support groups and community education programs that emphasize patient education.
- Arrange an inservice by members of frequently seen cultural groups to discuss alternative attitudes toward illness and treatment.

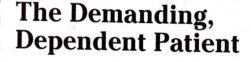

The Demanding, Dependent Patient

LEARNING OBJECTIVES

▼ List the possible causes of underlying anxieties that could escalate a patient's demanding, dependent behavior.
▼ Select effective interventions for a patient who consistently needs to be the center of attention.
▼ Identify possible nurses' reactions toward demanding, dependent patients.

Both demanding and dependent patients can consume an enormous amount of nursing resources. When patients exhibit these behaviors, it is essential to identify the problems early so that efforts are not counterproductive and resources are not drained. Setting baseline behavior goals help the patient contain or deal with his or her needs to a tolerable degree for both the staff and the pa-

Glossary

Interdependence—Having the capability for a normal balance between dependent and independent behaviors.

(Healthy) narcissism—An adequate amount of self-love, acquired during early childhood, providing a healthy self-esteem without negating the needs of others.

Hidden dependency—Dependent behavior that is not obvious. May try to coerce others into behaving in ways that meet his or her needs.

Entitlement—An unreasonable expectation that others will provide especially favorable treatment and automatic compliance.

Regression—An individual's response to overwhelming anxiety by moving back to a much earlier, more comforting phase of childhood.

Dependent personality disorder—Behavior characterized by a pervasive and excessive need to be taken care of leading to submissive and clinging behaviors; fears of separations; a severe lack of self-confidence; difficulty making everyday decisions and difficulty expressing disagreement.

Narcissistic personality disorder—Behavior characterized by a pervasive pattern of an inflated sense of self-importance, need for admiration, and lack of empathy for others.

Histrionic personality disorder—Behavior characterized by pervasive and excessive expression of emotion and attention-seeking behavior.

tient and prevent dysfunctional behavior from interfering with the planned healthcare regime.

The *demanding* patient consistently wants more than the nurse can or should give and asks for more than is reasonable. A request is usually expressed as an emergency, with absolute insistence that it is a legitimate, rightful claim. The *dependent* patient wants to be taken care of in more ways than is normal for an adult. Unable to function independently or with self-reliance, this individual has a sense of helplessness and powerlessness and either actively or passively expects others to take responsibility to meet his or her needs, make personal decisions, and provide support.

When a person is hospitalized, a dependent relationship occurs because basic rules of living, such as when to eat, are set by others. An adult with healthy coping mechanisms can usually adjust to this dependency role appropriately. However, the response is not so predictable in individuals who have consistently learned to use maladaptive coping mechanisms throughout their lives or in those whose situational stress have exhausted their normal coping abilities. When the patient deviates too much from commonly expected behaviors, misunderstandings and battles can be generated between the patient and staff. Maladaptive responses can include growing resentment at feeling so helpless, regression to a clinging neediness more characteristic of earlier years in life, fighting and refusing to follow rules, covert expressions of the need to be cared for with an overemphasis on physical symptoms, or relentless demands for affection.

Patients with certain types of personality disorders, particularly dependent, narcissistic, or histrionic types, normally exhibit a relentless demand for attention and need to be dependent on others. These individuals believe that their views are correct and that others must adapt to them. Because these behaviors are long-standing, they are very resistant to change. Additionally, the stress of illness and hospitalization can cause other individuals who normally function without the need to be demanding and dependent to exhibit these behaviors. This may occur when there is a growing resentment at being helpless or when normal coping mechanisms have been exhausted. This behavior can also be a normal temporary response in an individual faced with adjusting to a chronic illness, such as quadriplegia. An individual may express his or her intolerance for the dependent role by fighting, refusing to follow rules and meet expectations, or by overemphasizing physical symptoms.

Etiology

Psychologic theories examine early developmental experiences that inhibit successful independence contributing to demanding or dependent adult behavior and may even result in a personality disorder. For instance, a child may learn that to be heard and acknowledged, he or she must persist in making demands on parental attention. Both inadequately met needs and overindulgence during the first 18 months of life can discourage independence. If the child was not allowed to ask directly for what is needed, he or she may learn to get needs met by having physical symptoms, particularly if extra attention is received only during early bouts of illness, when physical care provided the only expressions of support and nurturing. If the child assumed the caretaker role for an ill parent, he or she may view illness as the main vehicle for obtaining care and assistance.

Patients who feel unloved and worthless or who are afraid to be alone may make frequent requests for the nurse to do things in an attempt to get attention. With attention given, the patient's anxiety decreases, and he or she becomes less demanding.

In hidden dependency, the patient can be very controlling, intimidating, dominating, or, possibly even, an overly caring caretaker. The patient does not seem obviously dependent but attempts to coerce others to behave in ways designed to meet his or her needs.

Patients with chronic personality disorders have a limited repertoire of coping skills and can respond to anxiety by becoming more dependent and demanding, regardless of whether such behavior is appropriate to the situation.

Related Clinical Concerns

Independent decision making and initiative taking can be adversely affected by dementia, depression, hearing and other sensory problems, and limited intellectual abilities.

Dependent individuals may use drugs as a method of coping with intolerable feelings of helplessness, which can lead to a pattern of substance dependency.

Lifespan Issues

CHILDHOOD

Growing independence is gained by changing from environmental to self-support. Infants are expected to be totally dependent. Younger children are still expected to be dependent in the areas where they have not yet matured to the point of being able to do for themselves. As children age and physical, psychologic, cognitive, and social spheres develop, they are expected to do age-appropriate tasks, make decisions, and interact and exhibit independent behaviors.

ADOLESCENCE

Adolescents can have an inflated sense of self and self-importance with little empathy for others as a natural part of trying to form their own identities; however, this does not mean they will develop a personality disorder. This age group may be influenced more by their peers who are supports against the pressures of the adult world and its expectations. Parents can become confused by the frequent vacillation between responsible behavior and childlike dependency, especially in earlier adolescent years.

ADULTHOOD

Dependency can be manifested in fears of leaving home of origin, difficulties maintaining jobs, and remaining financially dependent on parents. Brief periods of dependency during times of stress can be normal.

ELDERLY

As individuals age, there can be an accompanying increased dependence based on losses in agility, speed, or strength of prior abilities. Some elderly face illnesses along with the loss of prior support systems. Old friends and relatives can become preoccupied with their own growing limitations or even have died. Elderly who are treated as children incapable of making independent decisions and behavior can eventually respond with dependent and demanding behaviors.

For an elderly individual with a narcissistic personality disorder, adjusting to physical and occupational limitations can be particularly difficult, often straining family relationships.

Possible Nurses' Reactions

- Nurses have different tolerance levels for demanding, dependent behaviors. Patient may be considered difficult by one nurse but not by another. The extremes of these behaviors are usually considered difficult by all.
- May experience frustration and anger with the constant demands.
- May expect thanks or reward for meeting patient's needs.
- May feel guilty about not meeting all the patient's stated needs and question own competence. May try to avoid the patient.
- May not recognize that giving too much for patients who can do for themselves is detrimental to patients' emotional and physical health.
- May confuse appropriate limit setting with being overly harsh and withholding.
- May be punitive or may hesitate to be firm with patients because of anger and fear about being punitive. It may also seem easier to just give in to the patient's demands.
- The nurse with strong dependency needs or who is inexperienced may initially overidentify with patients and try to meet all of their demands. May resent giving so much and not being appreciated.

Assessment

Behavior and/or Appearance

- Intrudes into personal space and time of others
- Unkempt appearance, either actual inability to provide self-care or an unconscious attempt to get others to provide care
- Demanding assistance although able to do things for self

- Manipulative behavior, such as:
  - Arguing or begging
  - Crying, clinging
  - Calling nurse "mean," "hardhearted," "a bad person," "incompetent"
  - Dwelling on health problems and medical history
  - Complaining of feeling used and victimized by others
  - Constantly seeking attention, suggestions from others
- Disregard of hospital rules
- Regression; wanting to be totally taken care of, fed, repeatedly reassured, or comforted
- Frequent use of call lights
- Repeated visits to nurses' station
- Demands to have physician called several times each day
- Use of family visits to demonstrate helplessness; gets relatives to make demands on staff

Mood and/or Emotions

- Frequently angry; may be expressed in passive-aggressive behavior
- Fears being alone or abandoned
- Anxiety

Thoughts, Beliefs, and Perceptions

- Believes that each request is an actual problem requiring instant attention
- Low self-esteem with chronic feeling of helplessness and inadequacy
- Resistant to interpretations that point out reason for behavior (may experience this as an attack)

Relationships and Interactions

- Self-absorbed and little interest in others concerns or problems
- Frequently clings to others
- Sometimes nagging
- Fights or reverses roles and becomes a helper to others if unable to tolerate or acknowledge own dependency needs
- Dependent relationships with significant others, where other person makes all decisions, answers for patient

- Others dislike caring for or being with patient for long periods

Physical Responses

- Overconcern about health and preoccupied with symptoms
- Frequent requests for and preoccupied with medications, especially for pain or anxiety
- Adverse drug interactions if prescriptions taken from several different doctors who are not aware of each other's involvement

Pertinent History

- Long history of medical problems, some of which linger atypically for an unusually long time or do not quite match patterns of usually diagnosed diseases; does not respond to usual treatments
- Goes from one doctor to another in search for diagnosis and treatment for complaints that show no physical basis
- Multiple hospitalizations
- Unnecessary surgery

Collaborative Interventions

Pharmacologic

Multiple medications, perhaps from different prescribing doctors, can generate a host of problematic adverse effects. Psychiatric medicines may also be used. Confusion and lethargy in the elderly, which can lead to more dependent behavior, can be due to overmedicating or too many types of medications. A pharmacologic review can be helpful in these instances.

Nursing Management

POWERLESSNESS EVIDENCED BY DEMANDING, DEPENDENT BEHAVIORS RELATED TO ANXIETIES GENERATED BY ILLNESS, DISABILITY, AND/OR HOSPITALIZATION.

Patient Outcomes

- Displays less demanding, dependent behavior and conveys needs more directly and appropriately
- Provides increased amount of self-care as physical condition permits
- No longer exaggerates physical complaints to gain attention, support, and concern

Interventions

- Assess baseline:
  - Consult with family or significant other to determine if behaviors are normal for the person.
  - Evaluate if the patient is demanding in all situations or only in specific ones and if he or she exhibits this behavior only with certain people.
  - Identify the specific behaviors the patient uses to express dependency.
  - Determine whether the patient's helplessness is consistent with his or her medical problem or if more independent when not in view of others.
- State limits and rules in advance. Discourage unnecessary or excessive time spent at the nurses' station. Discourage asking for nurses' assistance when the patient is aware the nurse is on break, at lunch, or leaving at the end of the shift.
- Assess the required amount of assistance the patient needs and provide help when it is needed. Point out, diplomatically, unreasonable demands: "We're concerned about your overall well-being. In our experience, patients feel more effective and better about themselves when they do as much as they can. Let's discuss what you're realistically able to do right now and what the nurses need to provide."
- Make an extra effort to communicate concern.
  - Demonstrate active listening. Sit down rather than stand up during the talk. Repeat statements or reflect feeling being expressed, as necessary.
  - Be consistent. If you have told patient that you will speak with him or her at a specific time and are unable to do so, explain reasons and reschedule.
  - Give feedback to demonstrate that you understand

what patient is asking for, feels, or needs. Encourage patient to describe his or her fears and anger over the loss of control.

- Explain that identifying each situation as an emergency makes it difficult to determine what is an actual emergency.
- Determine if the patient has had previous bad experiences with healthcare providers or institutions. He or she may need reassurance that proper treatment is being given.
- Give support and reassurance to allay fears when first attempting behaviors that will lead to more independence. Assure the patient that you will be available if needed.
- Assist patient to distinguish between how feeling helpless versus being helpless. Provide a progress list of at least one new activity per day, however small, that he or she can do independently.
- Encourage the patient to identify and verbalize real sources of anger. Ask how he or she usually handles anger. Suggest ways to redirect anger into positive activities.
- Encourage patient to make independent choices. Accept different preferences and opinions.
- Do not take an overly directive approach as it can reinforce dependency.
- Identify and point out patient's strengths; provide praise whenever used.
- Determine whether some of the patient's expressed needs are better met by other professionals.

INEFFECTIVE INDIVIDUAL COPING EVIDENCED BY DEMANDING, DEPENDENT BEHAVIOR RELATED TO CONTINUOUS AND ONGOING PERSONALITY DISTURBANCE THAT HINDERS ABILITY TO DO HEALTHCARE TASKS EFFECTIVELY AND COMMUNICATE CONCERNS APPROPRIATELY.

Patient Outcomes

- Uses less dependent behavior with fewer unnecessary demands for nurses' attention
- Uses appropriate methods to gain attention and support

- Verbalizes appropriate degree of health concerns
- Makes informed choices
- Initiates and carries through tasks

Interventions

- Obtain history from patient and significant others to determine patient's baseline style of interaction prior to illness or hospitalization. Those who have displayed demanding and dependent behaviors as a lifelong pattern may need a different approach.
- Be aware that patients who have long-standing, ingrained, demanding, dependent patterns will be resistant to change. Be patient, and explain limit setting as often as needed.
- Determine realistic expectations for behavioral changes, and expect that any changes will occur in small gradual steps.
- If the patient becomes upset because you aren't presently able to spend time with him or her, determine a convenient time and assure patient that he or she will have your undivided attention.
- Assess whether the patient is inappropriately using the volunteers or other healthcare workers or is interacting inappropriately with visitors or other patients.
- Do not personalize remarks made by patients who need to feel superior. If the patient only wants to speak with the charge nurse or doctor, let those individuals explain the limits of their availability.
- Be aware when patients are using seductive behaviors to gain attention, control, or unnecessary assistance. Mild behaviors can be ignored to discourage future use. Persistent behaviors need firm confrontation.
- Assess for the use of manipulative behaviors to gain attention or dependence. Encourage methods to increase self-esteem that can decrease the patient's need for approval from others.
- Analyze behaviors to determine what needs the patient may be expressing when he or she asks the staff to perform tasks that could easily be done independently.
- Point out to the patient ways in which he or she has control of some situations.

- Assess the cause of a problem with independent decision making. If it is due to a lack of information, provide all the information you can. If the patient always has difficulty making decisions, teach effective problem-solving skills.
- Recognize your own tolerance for demanding, dependent behavior. Ask for assistance or temporary reprieve if necessary. For extremely dependent patients, strive for a balance between rotating staff to help decrease dependency on one nurse and providing consistent nursing care.
- Be especially diplomatic in correcting patient's behavior. Narcissistic patients may react to criticism or defeat with rage, disdain, or counterattack. If this occurs, help the patient regain a perspective on feedback and response.
- Maintain your own perspective when receiving praise from dependent or histrionic patients as well as the devaluing or ignoring of your efforts and contributions by more narcissistic patients, who tend to take all the credit.
- Praise independent functioning. Reassure the patient that he or she will not be forgotten nor abandoned by the staff when more independent. Reward less demanding behavior by spending more time with the patient.

ALTERNATE NURSING DIAGNOSES

Anxiety
Decisional conflict
Impaired social interaction
Self-care deficit
Self-esteem disturbance

WHEN TO CALL FOR HELP

✔ When the patient is "burning out" staff with insatiable, unreasonable requests
✔ When the patient's demands or needs for assistance become so unrealistically prolonged that it impairs staff's ability to adequately care for other patients
✔ When the patient is not getting good medical care because of staff anger
✔ If the patient seems resistant to all interventions attempted

Patient and Family Education

- Teach decision-making skills, such as problem identification, listing possible solutions, considering possible outcomes of each, and evaluating each outcome. Teach the patient to draw upon past experience and intuition when making decisions. Point out potential stumbling blocks such as choices that lower self-esteem or violate values or goals. Caution the patient that there may not be a perfect solution. Teach the concept of collaborative decision making.
- Teach the patient to recognize personal strengths.
- Explain to the patient that in delegating personal decision making to another, one still can retain personal responsibility for one's own life. He or she will have to live with the consequences of the decision.
- Teach the patient to distinguish situations that require immediate attention from those that don't. Explain that identifying each situation as an emergency makes it difficult to determine what is an actual emergency.
- Teach the patient to identify which problems require assistance. Teach the patient to use frustration as a time for problem solving.
- Teach relaxation techniques.
- Teach the family members to identify when they are promoting dependent behaviors and to examine alternatives. Teach approaches that staff have found effective.
- Teach the patient the differences between providing good nursing care and catering to excessive demands.

Charting Tips

- Document specifics of demands and their frequency. Note if they occur at similar times or events.
- Document actual patient responses to specific interventions listed in the treatment plan. Avoid subjective opinions about the behaviors.
- Document frequency of requests for PRN medications.
- Document details of unusual physical complaints.

Discharge Planning

- Anticipate increased dependency and demanding behavior as discharge becomes imminent; reduce anxiety by discussing concerns as early as possible.
- Anticipate that discharge will probably be a difficult time if the patient will be going to a facility with different caretakers and less staff.
- Assess what services patient will need at home, and discuss arrangements with patient and family.
- Ensure that patient has specific plans for follow-up appointment with physician.
- Remind patient who is about to be transferred to an extended care facility to continue to use the methods learned for expressing needs.
- Discuss with the next caregivers the interventions that have been effective.
- If the patient's behavioral patterns continue to significantly impair health care and the patient is distressed about this, discuss the possibility of seeking psychotherapy.

Nursing Outcomes

- The nurse responds effectively to communications expressed by demanding dependent behavior. The nursing staff demonstrates reasonable expectations and goals for modifying the patient's behavior.
- The nurse is able to set realistic limits on patient demands.
- Staff provides consistent treatment plan.

Suggested Learning Activities

- Role play some of the following situations, and then discuss how you felt:
  - Demands from a patient who wants a room change in order to have a better view
  - A patient who will talk only with the doctor or charge nurse

  ○ A capable individual asking you to change his or her shoes three times within 10 minutes
- For a thoughtful description of the development of problems with narcissism read *The Drama of the Gifted Child,* by A. Miller.

13 PROBLEMS WITH SUBSTANCE ABUSE

The Patient Abusing Alcohol

LEARNING OBJECTIVES

▼ *Identify factors that contribute to the etiology of alcoholism.*
▼ *Formulate appropriate nursing interventions for patients with alcoholism.*
▼ *Describe common nurse's reactions to the patient abusing alcohol.*
▼ *Identify indications of successful recovery from alcoholism.*
▼ *Describe the characteristics of codependency.*

Alcohol remains the most used and misused drug in America. Alcohol use is socially accepted throughout our culture and is included as part of celebrations, religious rituals, and social occasions, and often used as a relaxant. According to the *Diagnostic and Statistical Manual of Mental Disorders*, Fourth Edition (DSM-IV), nearly 90 percent of all American adults have used alcohol at some time in their life.

Glossary

Alcoholism—A complex progressive disease characterized by significant physical, social, or mental impairment directly related to alcohol dependence and addiction.

Alcohol intoxication—Excessive use of alcohol that leads to maladaptive behavior and at least one of the following: slurred speech, uncoordination, unsteady gait, nystagmus, impairment in attention or memory, and stupor.

Blackouts—Lapses of memory resulting from persistent heavy drinking. During blackouts the person may appear to function normally while drinking but cannot recall events afterwards.

Dual diagnosis—Diagnosis of both a substance dependency and a major psychiatric disorder.

Tolerance—The need for increasing amounts of a substance in order to achieve desired effect.

Detoxification—The process of withdrawal of alcohol from the body through supervised medical intervention to prevent complications.

Codependency—Maladaptive coping behaviors that prevent individuals from taking care of their own needs because they are preoccupied with the thoughts and feelings of another. Also known as "enabling behavior."

Korsakoff's syndrome—Severe memory impairment related to thiamin deficiency from long-term alcohol use. Characterized by confabulation and inappropriate cheerfulness.

Moving from social use of alcohol to alcoholism can occur very quickly in some people and over many years in others. For many years alcoholism was viewed as a defective character trait, a weakness, or moral flaw. Since the 1950s, it has been suggested that alcoholism is a complex disease that responds to proper treatment.

Studies indicate that about 7 percent of Americans are dependent on alcohol at any one time while 14 percent report alcohol dependence at some time in their life (DSM-IV, 1994). This includes daily or binge drinking that negatively affects the way one lives. Five times as many men as women are reported to have a drinking problem; however, it is suggested that women are more secretive in their drinking behavior, and, therefore, it may be underreported. Alcohol is often used along other substances, especially in younger individuals, often to alleviate or enhance the effects of other drugs.

Alcohol is a central nervous system depressant that produces mind-altering and mood-altering effects. Twenty percent of alcohol consumed is absorbed directly into the bloodstream through the stomach. The remainder moves through the digestive system and is absorbed more slowly. Drinking rapidly on an empty stomach or consuming drinks with higher alcohol content will lead to a more rapid rise in blood alcohol level. One ounce of distilled liquor, 5 ounces of wine, and 12 ounces of beer have equivalent amounts of alcohol. It is known that given the same amount of alcohol, women have higher blood alcohol concentrations than men, even when size is taken into consideration. This is due to differences in fat and body water content, making women more prone to long-term effects of alcohol.

Alcoholism has a tremendous impact on the person, the family, and society. Many alcoholics experience physical disorders such as gastritis, esophagitis, cirrhosis of the liver, and pancreatitis and emotional disorders such as depression and anxiety. In addition, some chronic conditions can be exacerbated including hypertension, diabetes, and heart disease. Patients with major psychiatric disorders may also have a problem with alcohol. Their drinking may be used as a way to self-medicate for the psychiatric symptoms or could be unrelated. Spouses and, especially, children are particularly vulnerable to be victims of alcohol-related abuse. They may experience violence or emotional and physical neglect, and they may blame themselves for the alcoholic's abusive state. Alcoholism is truly a family crisis.

Innocent members of society can also be victims of alcohol-related traffic accidents, violence and other crimes perpetrated during alcohol use.

Etiology

Because alcoholism runs in families, there is currently support for the *genetic* and *biologic* theories as the cause of alcoholism. Studies show that children of alcoholic parents are four times more likely to develop alcoholism with sons being at greater risk (DSM-N, 1994). The risk remains even if the children are not raised in the same home as the alcoholic parent. One current theory suggests that there is an inherited deficiency in some neurotransmitters that leads to a greater tendency to develop dysphoria or feelings of discomfort. Alcohol then becomes learned as a way to relieve these uncomfortable feelings. Also, because it is known that cross tolerance develops when an individual moves from alcohol to barbiturates and/or benzodiazepines, it is believed that a specific neurotransmitter is involved.

There are a number of *psychologic* factors that are recognized as contributing to alcohol abuse. One of the most important looks at the link between depression and alcoholism. Alcoholics may have a higher incidence of depression and low self-esteem. Alcohol becomes a way to relieve those feelings. Each time a drink makes the person feel better, it reinforces this behavior. Difficulty managing anxiety and low self-esteem has led to identification of common coping styles (see Table 13–1).

Alcohol use can severely affect the dynamics of the family relationship. Family members use protective behaviors, sometimes called "codependent" or "enabling behaviors," to control or hide the alcoholic's behavior so that a sense of normalcy can be maintained. Affected family members care for and attempt to control the behavior of the alcoholic at the expense of their own needs. The family does

TABLE 13–1. **Common Coping Styles of Alcoholics**

Coping Style	Definition	Behaviors
Denial	Person minimizes or does not acknowledge the problem or the results of the problem even when strong evidence is presented.	• "I only have 2 drinks a day, I could stop any time." • Refuses to admit drinking problems that are obvious to others. • Family may participate in denial by covering up the problems created by the drinker.
Projection	Blames others for their drinking and behavior.	• Avoids taking responsibility for own unacceptable behavior. • "My brother is the one with the problem. He drinks more than I do." • "I'd stop if everyone would leave me alone."
Rationalization	Justifies intolerable behavior by giving plausible excuses.	• Excuses reinforce denial. • "My kids are always in trouble. They make me drink." • "I only drink beer."
Minimizing	Avoids conflict by reducing the impact of the behavior.	• Places less value on the behavior and the impact of the problem. • "You worry too much." • "I'm not hurting anyone."
Manipulation	Plays one person against another in order to get one's way or cover up or avoid a problem.	• Convinces one or two people that he/she will improve if they will help. • If he/she fails it is the fault of the helper.

TABLE 13–1. **Common Coping Styles of Alcoholics**
(Continued)

Coping Style	Definition	Behaviors
Grandiosity	Maintains a sense of superiority and irresponsibility particularly evident when intoxicated.	• Lacks concern for others feelings.

not realize this type of behavior reinforces the drinking patterns and dysfunctional behavior. Examples of survival behavior include minimizing the drinking, finding excuses for the drinker's alcohol use, attempting to control their drinking by diluting bottles or pouring out liquor, covering up for the drinker's unacceptable behavior, and blaming themselves for the drinking. Family members and friends of the person abusing alcohol are at an increased risk of emotional or physical abuse.

Social and *cultural* factors may also contribute to the development of alcoholism. Certain cultural groups have higher incidences of drinking problems, which may represent an increased acceptance of heavy alcohol use. One's social circle may play a role in how alcohol is used as one observes its use by friends or family to avoid problems, become a risk taker, and so on.

Related Clinical Concerns

Some individuals have less tolerance to alcohol and become intoxicated much more easily. This is sometimes referred to as an *allergy to alcohol*. Whether this contributes to the development of alcoholism is unclear.

Alcohol is toxic to many major organs, especially the heart and liver. The patient with heart disease who abuses alcohol is at increased risk of complications. Liver metabolism may be compromised and, therefore, drugs metabolized by the liver may need dosage adjustments.

Lifespan Issues

CHILDHOOD TO ADOLESCENCE

Alcohol use by children and adolescents has shown an alarming increase in recent years. Access to alcohol from the home or from friends can make it readily available. The Carnegie Council (1989) found that 92 percent of U.S. high school students have used alcohol and 15 percent are considered heavy drinkers. As with adults, children learn from parents, peers, or television and movie images that alcohol can be a defense against feelings of depression, low self-esteem, or anxiety. It may also represent an acting out against parental authority or enhance a sense of closeness with peers. Children who grow up in a home where one or both parents have an alcohol abuse problem may have an increased risk of abusing alcohol. However, even those children who intensely dislike their parents' drinking behavior may use alcohol as a coping mechanism because they have not learned more appropriate ones. Children and adolescents who become intoxicated are at an increased risk of injury related to motor vehicle and bicycle accidents because they usually do not drink in the home. They are also at increased risk of alterations in growth and development because of nutritional deficiencies and because they often do not learn to deal effectively with normal anxiety and other uncomfortable emotions.

ELDERLY

It is estimated that 10 percent of emotional problems in the aged are caused by alcohol and drug abuse (DSM-IV, 1994). However, it is often unrecognized and undertreated, especially in women. Because alcohol abuse is often a life-long pattern, the elderly may continue their earlier struggles with alcohol. As they face increasing problems, such as isolation, loss of spouse, and changes in health status, with less reserve, they may resort to alcohol use. Because society does not generally view the elderly as an at-risk group, alcoholism often goes undiagnosed. King (1994) notes that one-third of elderly alcoholics begin drinking heavily after age 60. Alcohol may produce significant health problems in the elderly, particularly if they have impaired liver function. Mental changes from alcohol use may be confused with dementia. The brain in the elderly is more susceptible to the depressant effect of alcohol, and therefore, depression may mask the signs of alcoholism. Other signs might be unexplained falls, poor nutrition, and self-neglect. Use of multiple medications with alcohol can exacerbate alcohol's effects.

Possible Nurses' Reactions

- May view alcohol abuse as a personality defect or weakness rather than a health problem.
- May avoid, criticize, or reject the patient. This may trigger guilt feelings, and the nurse may try to make up for these feelings by being overly sympathetic.
- May have feelings of disgust for the patient.
- May have unresolved feelings related to a past family or personal history of substance abuse.
- May feel helpless to facilitate change especially in a patient with a long history of alcohol problems.

Assessment

Behavior and/or Appearance

- Signs of intoxication include smell of alcohol, slurred speech, loud talking, loss of inhibition, loss of coordination, and poor judgment
- Sudden onset of signs of withdrawal
- Frequently talks or brags about alcohol use
- Exhibits extremes of behavior from euphoria to irritability
- Justifies drinking or the need to drink (see Table 13–2)
- Refuses to discuss drinking or lies about drinking
- Drinks large quantities of alcohol
- Needs to drink more to get same effect
- Unable to stop drinking once he or she starts
- Overreacts when questioned about drinking pattern
- Reports drinking a much smaller amount than is accurate

TABLE 13–2. **CAGE Questionnaire**

To determine the patient's perception of his or her drinking problem, you may ask the following questions. Two or more affirmative answers strongly suggest dependence on alcohol.

1. Have you ever felt you should cut down your drinking?
2. Have people annoyed you by criticizing your drinking?
3. Have you ever felt bad or guilty about your drinking?
4. Have you ever had a drink first thing in the morning to steady your nerves or get rid of a hangover?

Source: Mayfield, D, McLeod, G, and Hall, P: The CAGE Questionnaire: Validation of a new alcoholism screening instrument. Am J Pyschiatr 131:1121, 1974, with permission.

Mood and/or Emotions

- Depressed
- Remorse after a binge
- Low frustration tolerance
- Anxiety
- Low self-esteem

Thoughts, Beliefs, and Perceptions

- Evidence of defense mechanisms of denial, rationalization, projection, and/or minimizing
- Thinking about alcohol supply and plans to obtain it
- Blackouts
- Hallucinations

Relationships and Interactions

- Dependent
- Resentful of authority
- Manipulates others to avoid confrontation, conflict
- Blames others for drinking
- Argues with family about drinking

Physical Responses

- Blood alcohol level (0.08 to 0.10 is legal limit to define intoxication in most states) or positive polydrug panel (may be negative depending on time since last consumption). Blood level is less useful in the elderly because of altered metabolism

- Amylase may be elevated if liver damage is present. Blood sugar may indicate hyper- or hypoglycemia. Serum magnesium may be low from alcohol damage to the nervous system. Hemoglobin may be low if bleeding is present
- May have signs of gastrointestinal bleeding, ascites, or jaundice
- May be underweight and show signs of malnutrition
- Korsakoff's syndrome from prolonged thiamin deficiency creates a secondary dementia marked by ataxia, confabulation, and peripheral neuropathy
- Withdrawal symptoms may occur 8 to 24 hours after last alcohol use. Analgesics and/or recovery from anesthesia can precipitate an acute withdrawal reaction. This emphasizes the importance of quick diagnosis to institute detoxification
- Alcohol-related delirium is a medical emergency with a 20 percent mortality rate if left untreated. Complications include pneumonia, dehydration, electrolyte imbalance, respiratory failure, and status epilepticus (see Table 13–3)

Pertinent History

- Previous history of a alcohol or polydrug use
- Psychotic, depressed, or manic behavior
- Blackouts, seizures, or delirium
- Alcohol-related police record, possibly including motor vehicle violations or accidents, physical violence, or child or spouse abuse
- May have history of being abused as a child
- Erratic work record due to alcohol
- One or both parents has history of alcohol problems

Collaborative Management

Pharmacologic

Protocols for detoxification from alcohol include pharmacologic treatment to prevent or reduce the development

TABLE 13–3. **DSM-IV Criteria for Diagnosis of Alcohol-Related Syndrome**

Alcohol abuse—Maladaptive pattern of alcohol use that is manifested by one or more of the following within the same 12 months:

1. Inability to fulfill major role obligations at work, school, and home
2. Recurrent legal or interpersonal problems
3. Reduction or absence of important social, occupational, and recreational activities
4. Participation in physically hazardous situations while impaired, for example, driving a car, exacerbation of a symptom

Alcohol dependence—Maladaptive pattern of alcohol use leading to impairment by 3 or more of the following occurring at any time the same 12 months:

1. All criteria for alcohol abuse
2. Presence of tolerance to drug
3. Presence of alcohol withdrawal syndrome
4. Ingestion of alcohol to relieve or prevent withdrawal
5. Taking more alcohol over longer period of time than intended
6. Unsuccessful or persistent desire to cut down or control use
7. Great deal of time spent in getting, taking, and recovering from alcohol

Alcohol withdrawal—Cessation of alcohol use which has been heavy and prolonged and has at least 2 of the following within several hours to a few days:

1. Autonomic hyperactivity (high blood pressure, tachycardia, fever)
2. Hand tremor
3. Insomnia
4. Nausea and or vomiting
5. Anxiety
6. Transient visual, tactile, or auditory hallucinations or illusions
7. Grand mal seizures

TABLE 13–3. **DSM-IV Criteria for Diagnosis of Alcohol-Related Syndrome** (*Continued*)

Alcohol-induced delirium—An organic mental disorder with symptoms in excess of the usual withdrawal (formerly called "delirium tremens") or intoxication symptoms that occurs after cessation or reduction of long-term heavy drinking or during intoxication. In someone with a history of substance use symptoms, includes

1. Impaired consciousness
2. Changes in cognition including memory, language, disorientation, hallucinations (especially tactile such as feeling bugs crawling on one's body)
3. Develops over short period of time (hours to days) and fluctuates over a day.

Source: Adapted from DSM-IV, 1994.

of alcohol-related delirium. Sedation with longer-acting central nervous system depressants is substituted for the shorter-acting alcohol. Benzodiazepines such as diazepam (Valium) and chlordiazepoxide (Librium) are the drugs of choice because they have anticonvulsant actions and are relatively safe. The drugs are usually administered on a routine basis and then tapered down by 20 to 25 percent per day until withdrawal is complete. Detoxification may be done in an alcohol treatment unit, hospital, or at home, if adequate supervision is available. Other medications including oxazepam (Serax) may be used if patient has liver disease. Anticonvulsants may also be needed.

Multivitamins, thiamin, and magnesium therapy is indicated in chronic alcoholics to prevent neurologic complications.

Disulfiram (Antabuse) has been used for chronic alcohol abuse. This drug inhibits impulsive drinking because it produces an extremely uncomfortable physical reaction when alcohol is ingested. The drug is taken daily and stays in the system for 5 days after the last dose. If the patient is exposed to alcohol while the drug remains active, he or she may experience headache, tachycardia, nausea, vomiting, flushing, sweating, and changes in blood pressure as well as potentially serious reactions including shock and cardiac arrythmias. Because of the risks involved with using this drug, the patient must have the ability to understand the reaction if alcohol is ingested and give informed consent. The patient must be instructed to avoid inhaling substances that could contain alcohol such as paint or wood stains and refrain from using any substances with alcohol including those with hidden sources such as some mouthwashes, elixirs, skin preparations, or colognes. The drug metronidazole (Flagyl) may cause a disulfiram-like reaction when alcohol is also ingested.

Naltrexone may also be used to prevent the euphoria associated with alcohol intake.

12 Step Program

The 12 Step program of Alcoholics Anonymous (AA) is generally accepted as part of every alcoholic's treatment program. AA's philosophy mandates that the individual become sober and never drink or use mood-altering substances again. The person acknowledges that he or she is powerless over alcohol, is always considered recovering, and is never cured. One drink could cause a downward spiral to heavy drinking.

AA uses sponsors who have been sober for longer periods to support new members. The alcoholic needs to attend regular, even daily, group support meetings and work on the 12 Step program. AA chapters are in virtually every community in the United States. The only requirement for membership is the desire to stop drinking. Alcoholics Anonymous has been the model for other self-help groups including Gamblers Anonymous and Cocaine Anonymous. Family members of alcoholics can participate in self-help groups following the same model including Al-Anon for spouses and friends, Al-a-Teen for adolescents and Adult Children of Alcoholics (ACoA).

Nursing Management

INEFFECTIVE DENIAL EVIDENCED BY LACK OF ACKNOWLEDGMENT OF ALCOHOL ABUSE RELATED TO IMPAIRED ABILITY TO ACCEPT CONSEQUENCES OF OWN BEHAVIOR.

Patient Outcomes

- Acknowledges own drinking problem
- Express feelings while under nurse's care
- Demonstrates problem-solving skills
- Abstains from alcohol and drug use or significantly reduces intake
- Asks for assistance with drinking problem

Interventions

- Help patient identify disturbing feelings by listening to concerns and helping him or her put labels on possible emotions. Patient may have used alcohol to deny feelings and needs assistance to identify them.
- Foster problem solving. Explore with the patient, the coping mechanisms that are more appropriate than alcohol to deal with the specific causes of stress and/or anxiety.
- Talk with patient about the normal range of personal emotions.
- Discuss behavioral inconsistencies.
- Maintain a positive attitude. Communicate that patient *can* overcome his or her problems.
- Work with patient to set realistic small goals for abstaining from alcohol and managing his or her problems. This may require structured planning for how to get through the next day without a drink. Encourage use of readings and meditations.
- Reenforce the Alcoholics Anonymous philosophy of "one day at a time." This means setting a goal of not drinking today rather than thinking about not drinking for the next year.
- Develop a trusting relationship. When the patient feels safe with a staff member, encourage examination of the negative consequences of his or her behavior. Recognize that this relationship could become too threatening to the patient and he or she may try to sabotage it or reject the nurse. This is all part of the struggle to face one's problems.
- If patient states "I could stop drinking any time," have him or her identify what could be done right now to stop. Look for windows in denial that might indicate the slightest insight and focus.
- Set limits on manipulative behavior. Some patients may

have learned to be very charming. The goal of these behaviors is to avoid dealing with the real problems.

RISK FOR INJURY EVIDENCED BY DISORIENTATION, LACK OF CO-ORDINATION, OR AGGRESSIVE OR DISRUPTIVE BEHAVIOR RELATED TO ACUTE ALCOHOL INTOXICATION, WITHDRAWAL, AND/OR DELIRIUM.

Patient Outcomes

- Remains free from injury while under care of the nurse.
- Sleeps at least 6 hours at night.
- Has reduced incidence of medical complications.
- Exhibits appropriate behavior.

Interventions

- Monitor vital signs, seizures, and changes in mental status closely for 5 days after withdrawal from alcohol.
- Monitor closely for signs of withdrawal, and report to physician to begin early treatment. With appropriate management, severe complications can be prevented. Recognize that the patient may be using several drugs so that signs of alcohol withdrawal may be masked or delayed.
- Follow agency policy and/or protocol for detoxification for high-risk patients.
- Maintain a quiet, calm environment. Use a soft voice and calm, supportive approach to reassure patient.
- Keep a night light on. Institute fall precautions. Encourage staff or family to stay with patient to ensure safety.
- Avoid restraints if at all possible by adequate use of medication.
- If the patient has pain from another medical condition, such as trauma or surgery, be sure to treat the pain. Do not withhold analgesia for fear that it will reinforce addictive tendencies.
- Promote use of relaxation techniques and herbal teas to reduce tension and help with possible insomnia.
- Monitor for complications including cardiac arrythmias or diabetes.
- Monitor food intake. Encourage fluids and a high-carbohydrate diet. Discourage use of dehydrating foods and/or fluids such as coffee, tea, and chocolate. Administer vitamins, as ordered.

INEFFECTIVE FAMILY COPING: COMPROMISED EVIDENCED BY OVERRESPONSIBLE BEHAVIOR TO CONTROL THE ALCOHOLISM RELATED TO ANXIETY IN THE FAMILY SYSTEM.

Patient and Family Outcomes

- Demonstrates assertive response when faced with abusive behavior
- Expresses feelings about the impact of alcohol on the family
- Demonstrates reduced number of behaviors that take responsibility for patient's drinking
- Attends support group meetings

Interventions

- Recognize that alcoholism is a health problem that affects all family members. Monitor response of all family members to patient's behavior.
- Give feedback to individuals about overresponsible behavior. Encourage them to recognize the signs and feelings associated with it. Explain how efforts to contain the patient's drinking merely delays the needed confrontation.
- Assist family members to set limits on the urge to "rescue" the patient. Give suggestions on coping mechanisms to reduce the stress. They need support to accept that they are not responsible for patient's drinking or behavior.
- Educate family members about availability and purpose of group support programs. Talk to them about meeting with a chemical dependency specialist for assistance. Participate in a planned intervention technique under the supervision of the specialist when the patient is confronted by family and friends with his or her drinking problem.
- Give person permission to take care of own needs first.
- Teach the family assertive responses to abuse or criticism from others, especially the patient.
- Encourage them to express emotions, both positive and negative.

- Reenforce that ultimately the individual with the drinking problem can only control his or her own behavior.
- Recognize that family members may unconsciously sabotage patient's recovery in order to maintain the security of the status quo. Remain as objective as possible, and avoid becoming involved in family conflicts.
- Prepare patient for changes in relationships with family and friends that may occur once he or she has stopped drinking. There may be some individuals who no longer like the patient when sober. Patient needs to reexamine these relationships.

ALTERNATE NURSING DIAGNOSES

Altered nutrition, less than body requirements
Alterated thought processes
Noncompliance
Risk for violence
Sleep pattern disturbance

WHEN TO CALL FOR HELP

✔ Escalation of aggressive, belligerent behavior to violence
✔ Need to apply restraints
✔ Intoxication
✔ Complications including seizures, cardiac arrythmias, bleeding, high temperature
✔ Inadequate staff available to manage behavior
✔ Sudden change in mental status

Patient and Family Education

- Reinforce strategies to avoid exposure to alcohol. For example, caution patient to avoid contact with drinking friends. Teach patient to avoid his or her old habits that included drinking, and remove all alcohol from the home. Teach patient and family to read labels of products purchased. Avoid products with alcohol in them such as mouthwashes and cough syrup. Avoid any mood-altering substance that could be used as a substitute for alcohol.

- Provide information about the addictive process and how it affects all aspects of one's life. Review "one-day-at-a-time" philosophy.
- Provide dieting information on good diet, vitamins, and so on.
- Provide information to patient and family on managing potential seizures.
- Provide health teaching on the potential of gastrointestinal bleeding and liver disease. Encourage them to avoid using products containing aspirin.
- Educate the patient and family on hazards of drinking in pregnancy and the effects of alcohol on driving and on the job.
- Teach strategies to replace alcohol with more healthy activities such as sports, hobbies, and journal keeping.
- Reinforce relaxation measures.
- Prepare patient for need to develop social contacts who do not drink.
- Reinforce education to family on avoiding overresponsible responses.
- Prepare the patient for the fact that intense emotions may be more painful without alcohol. He or she may need extra help at these times.
- Remind patient to tell every physician seen about his or her history to ensure that doctor will prescribe medications appropriately.

Charting Tips

- Document vital signs and any evidence of symptoms of withdrawal and delirium.
- Describe in detail the description of the patient's level of consciousness and mental status.
- Document the patient's response to the medications being used for withdrawal.
- Document the family's response to patient behavior.
- Document any observations of continued alcohol use.
- Document any actions taken to prevent violent behavior.
- If restraints are necessary, document the type, the time in restraints, reason they were applied, the patient's response to treatment, when limbs were released, and the care given while in restraints.

Discharge Planning

- Provide information to patient and family on location and phone numbers for local chapters of AA, Al-Anon, Al-a-Teen, or ACoA, as needed.
- Encourage the patient to continue counseling or provide referral to alcohol counseling programs.
- Encourage the patient to follow up with medical appointments
- Arrange for follow-up home health visits for patients being discharged from alcohol treatment to home.
- If appropriate, involve patient's employer in treatment plan.
- Provide information to referring agencies, such as home health agencies or nursing homes, on patient's drinking patterns and the treatment program.

Nursing Outcomes

- Staff creates a safe environment for all patients.
- Staff is free from injury.
- Staff demonstrates nonjudgmental approach in working with patient.
- Staff sets appropriate limits on manipulative behavior.

Suggested Learning Activities

- Attend AA, Al-Anon, Al-a-Teen, or ACoA meeting.
- Arrange an inservice from staff of a chemical dependency program.
- Obtain information from the National Council of Alcoholism, Mothers Against Drunk Drivers, or similar organizations.
- View and discuss popular movies on alcoholism, such as *Days of Wine and Roses, The Lost Weekend*, and *When A Man Loves A Woman*.
- Read and discuss the book *It Will Never Happen to Me* on the origins of the group for Adult Children of Alcoholics and books on codependency such as *Beyond Codependency* by Melody Beattie.

The Patient Abusing Other Substances

LEARNING OBJECTIVES

▼ *Differentiate between substance abuse and dependence.*
▼ *Identify common reactions of the nurse to the substance abuser.*
▼ *Describe important nursing considerations of abusing amphetamines, cocaine, hallucinogens, nicotine, opioids, and sedatives.*
▼ *Identify nursing diagnoses and interventions in caring for the substance abuser.*

Using mind- and mood-altering substances is probably as old as the human race. Today, many people use medications or other substances to relax, sleep, and increase energy. Prescription and over-the-counter psychoactive substances, such as caffeine, cigarettes, alcohol, painkillers, tranquilizers, and common cold treatments are both socially acceptable and commonly used. So, it is interesting that we accept these substances to help us feel better

---

Glossary

Binge—Pattern of periodic intervals of heavy use of substances with intervals of no or little usage.

Cross tolerance—State in which the effect of a substance is reduced because the individual has become tolerant to a similar drug.

Detoxification—Process of withdrawal from a drug from the body through supervised medical intervention to prevent complications.

Drug tolerance—Need for higher and higher doses to achieve same desired effect.

Flashback—Transient recurrence of a disturbance in perceptions associated with hallucinogens that are reminiscent of those experienced when taking the drug. Sometimes referred to as a "hallucinogen persisting perceptual disorder."

Polypharmacy—Taking more than one substance at any given time.

Substance abuse—The maladaptive and consistent use of a drug accompanied by recurrent and significant adverse consequences often related to physical hazards, multiple legal problems, and recurrent social and interpersonal problems.

Substance dependence—Cluster of cognitive, behavioral, and physiologic symptoms indicating that the individual continues use of the substance despite significant substance-related problems.

Withdrawal—Negative physiologic and psychologic reactions that occur when the drug is reduced or no longer taken.

but loathe people who are dependent on or abuse drugs. People who eventually become substance abusers also take drugs to feel better, possibly as a way to avoid some problems and stressors. Eventually though, the need to obtain and use the drug negatively affects all aspects of the person's life including family, job, friends, and other responsibilities. Many people who use drugs retreat to the company of others who share their lifestyle, beliefs, and drugs.

There is a significant difference between substance dependence and substance abuse. According to the DSM-IV, *substance dependence* is characterized by a pattern of repeated self-administration of a drug that usually results in tolerance, withdrawal, and compulsive drug-taking behavior. *Substance abuse* is characterized by compulsive use in which the individual continues to use the drug even in the face of problems including inability to fulfill major role obligations at work, school, or home; recurrent use in situations in which it is physically hazardous; recurrent legal problems related to the substance use; and/or recurrent social or interpersonal problems related to drug use.

Substance abuse is a major health problem and for individuals in all ages and socioeconomic groups; however, abuse rates are highest in the 18- to 24-year-old group (DSM-IV, 1994). Patterns of use vary related to cost and availability. It is difficult to say which substance is the most abused because often more than one drug at a time is used to control side effects.

The economic impact of drug abuse is tremendous, including crime, medical costs, accidents, and loss of workdays in addition to the resulting family and work dysfunction. Drug abuse during pregnancy may have lifelong consequences for the offspring. Babies born to mothers using cocaine or heroin may be born physically dependent on these substances and require detoxification at birth. They are often of low birth weight and have multiple problems including possible brain damage.

Nurses are believed to have a 50 percent higher rate of substance dependency than the general population (McAndrew, 1994). Sisney (1993) estimates 420,000 registered nurses in this country abuse drugs and/or alcohol. Stressful jobs, tendency to perfectionism yet feeling inadequate, and knowledge about and access to drugs increases the risk of substance abuse in this population. Because they don't fit the image of a "junkie," nurses often minimize or deny their problem. Many states have now developed Diversion Programs to provide treatment and rehabilitation confidentially.

Etiology

The causes of drug abuse are similar to those of alcohol abuse; however, because of the wide range of drugs abused, there are some differences. *Biologic* theories look at the role of specific neurotransmitters. Various drugs activate slightly different areas of the brain or brain circuits. Cocaine use has been studied in more depth than some of the other drugs, and it is believed that there may be a deficiency of dopamine and norepinephrine which creates more of a craving for that drug. With opioids, it is theorized that there may be some abnormality in opioid receptors and endorphins.

Psychologic theories view drug dependence as an attempt to adapt to severe emotional distress. Low self-esteem and anxiety become masked under the influence of the drug. Drugs relieve feelings of depression and dependency and may be used to suppress anxiety, particularly after a traumatic event such as rape or violent crime. As with alcoholism, the person may also be fixated in the oral stage of development and seek ingestion of substances as a way to meet those needs (psychoanalytic theory). Individuals with tendencies toward antisocial behavior and difficulties with impulse control and frustration tolerance may use substances as a way to control anxiety that contributes to antisocial behavior. In addition, the role of the family and tendency to codependent relationships (see the preceding subsection on alcoholism for complete discussion) also exist with substance abuse. Drug abusers use many of the same coping mechanism that alcoholics do including denial, projection, and manipulation (see Table 13–3).

Sociocultural views recognize that certain drugs may be

more likely to be used depending on peer group, income, or culture. Acceptable behavior within a group, access to specific drugs, and status related to specific drugs may all be influencing factors. For example, crack cocaine has spread quickly within the low-income groups due to its easy availability and low cost.

Related Clinical Concerns

There is no evidence to suggest that an individual will become drug dependent by taking analgesics for pain. In fact, McCaffery and Ferrell (1994) report that less than 1 percent of individuals who take analgesics for a painful condition become addicted to that substance. Individuals who have developed a drug tolerance will require larger amounts of medications to relieve pain.

Individuals with a substance abuse problem may experience withdrawal symptoms when hospital admission prevents them from taking the addictive substance. This is an important consideration when analyzing assessment findings. For instance, when a patient that has been hospitalized and NPO for 2 days experiences headaches and irritability, it may be related to caffeine withdrawal. In certain instances, withdrawal symptoms for more potent substances can increase the risk of complications. For example, the confusion resulting from amphetamine withdrawal may cause a postoperative patient to attempt to get out of bed, tear out tubes and intravenous lines, and, possibly, fall.

Lifespan Issues

CHILDHOOD TO ADOLESCENCE

Children and adolescents today are at high risk for exposure to substance use and abuse due to easy availability of drugs in the schools and community. Peer pressure, experimentation, curiosity, and rebellion as well as trying to find ways to cope or escape from problems may be part of the etiology. Children as young as 7 years old have been identified as using a variety of drugs including crack and inhalants. Drug use often begins while experimenting with peers. When the child experiences a sense of well-being and power, drug use continues. The child may then become drawn into the drug culture, possibly into a gang, which provides a support system for continued use.

Recent studies indicate that adolescents who abuse drugs have a higher incidence of psychopathology and suicidal ideation, particularly in boys (Deykin and Buka, 1994). In addition, children with a history of attention deficit disorder and/or conduct disorder have been found to be prone to amphetamine use as adults. Amphetamines counteract some of the symptoms of these disorders.

ELDERLY

Substance use and abuse in the elderly are complicated because they routinely take a greater number of prescribed and over-the-counter drugs and have diminished tolerance to many drugs. The individual, family, and health professionals often deny this problem in the elderly. This may be because children are reluctant to accuse a parent or because symptoms are masked or mistakenly attributed to the use of another drug the person is taking. The older adult is more likely to abuse prescribed tranquilizers, sedatives (especially benzodiazepines), and opioids. Falls, unexplained accidents, increased lethargy, loss of memory and attention span, and unexplained confusion may be signs of a drug abuse problem. Use of illicit drugs is relatively uncommon in the elderly, but it may increase in the future as young and middle-age addicts grow older.

Possible Nurses' Reactions

- May have strong negative feelings, viewing the patient as weak, immoral, or responsible for his or her own problems.
- May fear the patient's manipulative, provocative behavior and potential for criminal and/or violent behavior.
- May tend to minimize patient's concerns or discomforts because of resentment or fear of being manipulated.
- May have a rescue fantasy of being the one to help this patient. The nurse may then become repeatedly disappointed when the patient returns to drug use.

- May view the patient as hopeless to be cured.
- May allow personal or family experience with substance abuse to influence response to the patient.

Assessment (see Table 13–4)

Behavior and/or Appearance

- May talk frequently about drugs or brag about using drugs
- May have an in-depth knowledge of drugs and how they work
- Dramatic behavior changes, for instance, may be suddenly euphoric, drowsy, more outgoing
- Wears sunglasses indoors
- Unpredictable behavior
- Grandiosity, overconfidence
- Disheveled appearance
- In children and adolescents, loss of interest in school, drop in grades

Mood and/or Emotions

- Mood swings
- Low frustration tolerance, angers easily
- Angry outbursts
- Anxiety, especially associated with discussion of drug use
- Emotional reactions related to change in medication regimen, particularly changes in analgesics
- Depressed; verbalizes self-deprecating thoughts

Thoughts, Beliefs, and Perceptions

- Denies impact of drug use
- Rationalizes that he or she can stop using any time
- Persistent belief that drug is for medical use only
- Obsessive thoughts about drug use and access to drug supply
- Suicidal ideations

Relationships and Interactions

- Change in circle of friends and isolation from family
- Blames others for need to use substances and other problems
- May become more isolated as fears of exposing habit to others increases
- Charming, charismatic, or manipulative with others

Physical Responses

- Needle tracks (raised marks from repeated IV injections) may be seen in antecubital space, wrist, feet, behind knees or in tattoos
- Recent injection sites may be red and swollen
- Abscesses and ulcerations may be present
- There is evidence of drug(s) in urine testing. Each drug varies as to how long it remains in the body. Check with the laboratory for specifics
- Pupil response varies from constricted to nonreactive with different drugs

Pertinent History

- History of withdrawal symptoms, overdosage, complications from past drug use
- Psychiatric disorders
- Family history of drug or alcohol abuse
- Criminal record and other legal problems
- Daily or binge drug abuse or dependence
- History of eating disorders

Collaborative Management

Pharmacologic

Medications are used in detoxification programs for many drugs including opioids, barbiturates, sedatives, and tranquilizers. They are used to control withdrawal symptoms and discourage continued use of the abused substance. Most are used for only short periods until withdrawal is complete; however, in some cases they may be used for longer periods to control cravings for the drug.

TABLE 13–4. Comparing Commonly Abused Substances

Drug	Intoxication	Overdose	Withdrawal	Nursing Considerations
Amphetamines, including dexedrine and methamphetamines	*Signs:* Euphoria, high energy, impaired judgment, anxiety, aggressive behavior, paranoia, and delusions (often seen with long-term use)	*Signs:* Ataxia, high temperature, seizures, respiratory distress, cardiovascular collapse, coma, death *Treatment:* Supportive	*Signs:* Depression, agitation, insomnia, vivid dreams followed by extreme lethargy *Treatment:* Antidepressants, counseling, suicide precautions	• Used in weight reduction programs and to treat benzodiazepine abuse. • May cause a paradoxical reaction in children. • Remains in urine for up to 3 days.
Cannabis, including marijuana and hashish	*Signs:* Euphoria; intensified perceptions; impaired judgment and motor ability; increased appetite; weight gain, sinusitis, and bronchitis with	*Signs:* Extreme paranoia, psychosis *Treatment:* Antipsychotics	*Signs:* None	• Most widely used illicit drug. • Remains in urine for up to 7 days. • May exacerbate psychiatric symptoms in mentally ill patients. • May negatively affect fertility.

298

| Cocaine, including crack | *Signs:* Euphoria, grandiosity, sexual excitement, impaired judgment, insomnia, anorexia; nasal perforation associated with inhaled route; psychosis associated with long-term abuse | *Signs:* High temperature, seizures, transient venospasms possibly causing MI or CVA, coma, death
 Treatment: Supportive | *Signs:* Fatigue, depression, anxiety, suicidal behavior
 Treatment: Support counseling, antidepressants | chronic use; anxiety; paranoia; red conjunctiva

 • Crack is smoked or injected IV; has a rapid onset and high dependency rate.
 • Cocaine is inhaled, snorted or injected IV.
 • High risk of acquiring HIV, hepatitis, bacterial endocarditis, and osteomyelitis from shared IV needles or promiscuous sexual relations.
 • May be used to control appetite. |

• May therapeutically reduce nausea and vomiting, intraocular pressure, and stimulate appetite.

TABLE 13-4. Comparing Commonly Abused Substances (Continued)

Drug	Intoxication	Overdose	Withdrawal	Nursing Considerations
Hallucinogens, including LSD and mescaline	*Signs:* Dilated pupils, diaphoresis, palpitations, tremors, enhanced perceptions of colors, sounds, depersonalization, grandiosity	*Signs:* Panic, psychosis with hallucinations, cerebral tissue damage, death *Treatment:* Diazepam or chloral hydrate; quiet environment antipsychotics	*Signs:* None	• Flashbacks can occur for up to 5 years. • Could precipitate a psychiatric disorder in susceptible persons.
Inhalants, including glue, gasoline, and paint thinner	*Signs:* Euphoria, impaired judgment, blurred vision, unsteady gait	*Signs:* Psychosis with hallucinations, cardiac arrhythmias, CNS depression, coma, cerebral tissue damage, death *Treatment:* Supportive	*Signs:* None	• Most available substance for younger children. • May be difficult to detect specific substance used. • Particularly irritating and or flammable substances can cause trauma and burns in nose, mouth, and airways.

Substance	Signs	Signs	Signs / Treatment	Comments
Nicotine, including cigarettes, chewing tobacco, and nicotine gum or patch	*Signs:* Produces a sense of anxiety reduction, relief from depression, and satisfaction	*Signs:* None	*Signs:* Insomnia, depression, irritability, anxiety, poor concentration, increased appetite *Treatment:* Transdermal nicotine patches in decreasing doses, nicotine gum and clonidine for severe anxiety, behavioral modification	• Since most medical facilities do not allow smoking, inpatients may experience withdrawal symptoms. • Less than 25% of individuals are successful with first attempt to quit. • Monitor for weight gain. • Monitor for hypotension with clonidine.
Opioids, including heroin, morphine, meperidine, and codeine	*Signs:* Euphoria, drowsiness, impaired judgment, constricted pupils	*Signs:* Dilated pupils, respiratory depression, seizures, cardiopulmonary arrest, coma, death *Treatment:* Naloxone, supportive	*Signs:* Yawning, insomnia, anorexia, irritability, rhinorrhea, muscle cramps, chills, nausea, and vomiting, feelings of doom and panic	• High risk of acquiring HIV, hepatitis, bacterial endocarditis, and osteomyelitis from shared IV needles. • Monitor for hypotension with clonidine

TABLE 13-4. **Comparing Commonly Abused Substances** (*Continued*)

Drug	Intoxication	Overdose	Withdrawal	Nursing Considerations
Opiods (Continued)			*Treatment:* Detoxification, possibly with clonidine for severe anxiety and naloxone, or burenorphine to block euphoria *Signs:* None	• Have adequate staff available since behavior is unpredictable and patient may become violent. • May consider using four-point restraints. • Drugs remain in urine for several weeks.
Phencyclidine (PCP, angel dust)	*Signs:* Impulsive behavior, impaired judgment, belligerent, assaultive behavior, ataxia, muscle rigidity, nystagmus, hypertension, numbness or diminished response to pain	*Signs:* Hallucinations, psychosis, seizures, respiratory arrest, stroke *Treatment:* Gastric lavage; cranberry juice or ammonium chloride to acidity urine (if awake); quiet environment; haloperidol or diazepam; fluids		

	Signs	Signs / Treatment	Signs / Treatment	
Sedatives, hypnotics, and anxiolytics including barbiturates and benzodiazepines	*Signs:* Slurred speech, labile mood, inappropriate sexual behavior, loss of inhibitions, drowsiness, impaired memory	*Signs:* Hypotension, nystagmus, stupor, cardiorespiratory depression, coma, death *Treatment:* Benzodiazepine antagonist (flumazenil); induce vomiting, if awake; activated charcoal; cardiorespiratory support	*Signs:* Insomnia, hand tremor, agitation, nausea and vomiting, anxiety, tinnitus (with benzodiazepines), seizures, and cardiac arrest *Treatment:* Detoxification using gradually reduced dosages of a similar drug, anticonvulsants, and support and counseling	• Avoid using phenothiazines because they can potentiate the effects of PCP. • Abrupt barbiturate withdrawal can be life-threatening. • Alcohol will potentiate drug effects. • Cross-tolerance may develop between alcohol and other CNS depressants. • Detectable in blood and urine. • Shorter-acting benzodiazepines have a greater risk of producing addiction and more severe rebound anxiety than longer-acting ones.

Methadone, a synthetic narcotic that resembles morphine and heroin but does not produce the euphoric effects, is used daily on a long-term basis to treat heroin addiction. Both physical and psychologic dependence are maintained on methadone, but the euphoric effects of heroin are blocked. Patients usually make daily trips to a methadone clinic to obtain the drug.

Naltrexone also reduces the euphoric sensation from narcotics, and clonidine decreases discomfort during narcotic withdrawal.

Despiramine, bromocriptine, amantadine, and phenylalanine and tryosine are used to decrease craving during cocaine withdrawal.

Dual diagnosis patients may require medications for treatment of their psychiatric diagnosis, but efforts are made to avoid sedatives and tranquilizers. Patients with anxiety or psychotic disorders may be using illicit drugs as a way of controlling hallucinations or anxiety.

12 Step Program

The 12 Step program has been used to treat substance abuse and includes groups such as Narcotics Anonymous, Cocaine Anonymous, and Pills Anonymous. The philosophy mandates that the individual remains free from the substance and acknowledges that he or she is powerless over the chemical. Individuals need to attend group meetings routinely. Sponsors who have been drug free for longer periods provide support for new members. Family members can also participate in self-help groups following the same model.

Counseling

Drug rehabilitation also includes counseling to restore physical and emotional stability, identify the person's usual coping mechanism and work to adopt more effective ones, and develop a sense of self-worth and self-esteem.

Nursing Management

INEFFECTIVE DENIAL EVIDENCED BY LACK OF ACKNOWLEDGMENT OF SUBSTANCE ABUSE PROBLEM RELATED TO IMPAIRED ABILITY TO ACCEPT CONSEQUENCES OF OWN BEHAVIOR

Patient Outcomes

- Acknowledges substance abuse problem
- Abstains from substance use
- Participates in treatment plan

Interventions

- Convey acceptance of patient. Avoid criticizing, preaching to, or attacking the patient to get his or her attention.
- Promote trust by listening to concerns and treating him or her as an individual.
- Give patient specific feedback on any behavior that appears drug related. Identify defense mechanisms such as blaming others or rationalizing behavior. Encourage personal responsibility for own behavior.
- Provide information on treatment approaches, such as Cocaine Anonymous (CA) or Narcotics Anonymous (NA).
- Help patient identify and share the possible emotions he or she is feeling.
- Help patient see link between substance use and personal and medical problems. Give the patient the opportunity to identify these, if possible.
- Assist patient to identify ways drug use effects daily life. Encourage being specific and honest.
- Set limits on manipulative behavior, and make realistic consequences for this behavior. Recognize that patient may exhibit charming, charismatic behavior, making limit setting more difficult. Never cover up for the patient or act entertained by drug use.
- Recognize that the drug effects may overwhelm the patient's motivation to stop. However, do not ignore signs of patient intoxication. Become familiar with your institution's policies for suspected drug use such as conducting a room search or confiscating drugs.
- If patient indicates that he or she wants to participate in a treatment program, immediately contact appropriate resources, such as a social worker, to facilitate admittance to a program.

INEFFECTIVE INDIVIDUAL COPING EVIDENCED BY ANXIETY, WITHDRAWAL SYMPTOMS, INABILITY TO FUNCTION WITHOUT DRUGS IN RECOVERY RELATED TO INADEQUATE COPING SKILLS TO MANAGE STRESSORS WITHOUT DRUGS

Patient Outcomes

- Participates in treatment plan
- Demonstrates alternate coping mechanisms to deal with stress that do not involve drugs
- Verbalizes need to continue in treatment
- Abstains from substance use

Interventions

- Help patient to focus on getting through each day without drugs rather than the overwhelming thought of never using them again.
- Give reinforcement for ability to delay gratification and tolerate frustration. Provide information on possible coping mechanisms to reduce stress and tolerate discomfort. Review alternative ways to cope with anger. Role play dealing with stressful situations.
- Explain the long-term physical effects of drug use, such as short attention span, that will impact daily life.
- Prepare patient that family and friends may have difficulty relating to him or her when not using drugs. For instance, friends may seem to abandon the patient because of no longer wanting to participate in their drug-related activities. The patient will need to prepare to accept this and work on changing these relationships or developing new ones.
- Help the patient discuss realistic future plans and life changes to make when no longer using drugs. Help to identify steps to achieve these goals.
- Encourage participation in support groups or visits or phone contacts with sponsors.
- Monitor if visitors are bringing in drugs.

RISK FOR INJURY EVIDENCED BY DISORIENTATION, LACK OF CO-ORDINATION, OR AGGRESSIVE OR DISRUPTIVE BEHAVIOR RELATED TO SUBSTANCE INTOXICATION, OVERDOSE, OR WITHDRAWAL

Patient Outcomes

- Remains free from injury
- Reduced incidence of medical complications related to substance abuse
- Sleeps at least 6 hours a night

Interventions

- Recognize that many people who abuse drugs can function in society fairly well. Early signs of withdrawal may occur during hospitalization with no access to drug supply. Suspicious symptoms should be assessed carefully so treatment can be instituted as early as possible.
- Determine which substances the patient has been using. Take a careful history from patient or family and friends (if applicable). Obtain ordered urine and blood for drug screening, and carefully monitor the patient's clinical condition and behavior. Recognize that many patients are using more than one substance including alcohol.
- Institute fall and seizure precautions, as appropriate.
- Recognize that many substance abusers have poor nutritional habits due to anorexia, emotional changes, or inadequate intake. Monitor food and fluid intake. Encourage adequate fluids and nutrition.
- Administer ordered medications to ease symptoms, and monitor for adverse and therapeutic effects. Monitor for signs of aggressive, agitated behavior. Avoid restraints if at all possible.
- Promote rest and sleep by maintaining a quiet environment and encouraging use of relaxation techniques and herbal teas.
- Patients with painful medical conditions need to have analgesics. The substance-abusing patient may need higher doses of analgesics and benefit from a regular dosing rather than per schedule.

ALTERNATE NURSING DIAGNOSES

Altered thought processes
Impaired social interaction
Knowledge deficit
Risk for infection
Self-care deficit
Self-concept disturbance

WHEN TO CALL FOR HELP

✔ Escalation or onset of aggressive, belligerent behavior or violence

✔ Change in level of consciousness unrelated to underlying medical condition
✔ Need to apply restraints
✔ Inadequate staff available to manage behavior
✔ Suspected criminal activity related to drug use, selling drugs

Patient and Family Education

• Encourage patient to inform healthcare providers about drug use since this information will influence drug and dosage selections for needed medical treatments.
• Teach family members about need to adjust some aspects of their relationship with patient. Help them to identify possible behaviors that could be reinforcing substance use. Give them specific feedback if you observe any of these behaviors.
• Encourage patient to establish new routines and activities that do not involve drug use. This may include avoiding old circle of friends and developing hobbies or new interests.
• Provide information on risks of exposure to HIV, hepatitis, and other infections. Encourage patient who is at risk to obtain blood tests to determine exposure, and teach health practices to reduce risk to self and others.
• Help patient recognize potential fears and changes that may occur when he or she changes his or her life to live without drugs.
• Provide information on the health impact of specific substances patient is abusing.
• Provide information on treatment of substance abuse to patient and family.
• Educate on effects of drugs on pregnancy, on the job, or operating mechanical equipment.

Charting Tips

• Document behavior associated with intoxication, overdose, or withdrawal.
• Document any indications of inappropriate drug use.

- Describe patient behavior after visits from family or friends.
- Describe response to treatments.
- Describe pain or anxiety behaviors and need for analgesics or tranquilizers.

Discharge Planning

- Provide referral information on clinics, hotlines, halfway houses, drug treatment programs, and counseling that assist drug abusers.
- Inform referring agencies of patient's history.
- Arrange for follow-up home health visit to reinforce drug treatment program, as needed.
- Encourage follow-up medical appointments.

Nursing Outcomes

- Staff demonstrates nonjudgmental approach in working with patient.
- Staff sets appropriate limits on patient's behavior.
- Staff demonstrates appropriate level of involvement with patient.
- Staff creates safe environment.

Suggested Learning Activities

- Attend Cocaine Anonymous or Narcotics Anonymous meeting (check first which meetings are open to the public).
- Arrange an inservice from staff of chemical dependency program.
- Visit drug treatment programs such as a methadone clinic.
- View and discuss popular movies on drug abuse such as *Man with the Golden Arm*.

14

PROBLEMS WITH SEXUAL DYSFUNCTION

The Patient With Sexual Dysfunction

LEARNING OBJECTIVES

▼ *Define sexuality and sexual health for adults.*
▼ *Differentiate the major sexual dysfunctions found among males and females.*
▼ *Identify therapeutic interventions for sexual dysfunction.*
▼ *Distinguish among levels of nursing education and appropriate assessment and intervention strategies.*

Human sexuality is a complex phenomenon encompassing biologic, psychologic, and sociocultural aspects. Biologic aspects include the anatomy and physiology of sexual development and sexual activities; psychologic aspects include gender identity, sexual self-concept, and

Glossary

Sexual dysfunction—A change in sexual health or function, which the individual views as unrewarding or inadequate. Sexual dysfunction is usually related to one or more of the following: lack of knowledge or incorrect information; biologic or physiologic causes, such as diabetes, drug or alcohol use, hormonal disorders; change in or loss of body part; ineffective coping or poor relationships; or organic problems (impotence, premature ejaculation, vaginismus, and orgasmic dysfunction).

Sexual response cycle—Includes excitement, plateau, orgasm, and resolution. Each of these stages is affected by gender, age, culture, experience, and expectation.

Sexually transmitted diseases—Any disease that can be contracted by sexual contact; also called *venereal diseases*. Symptoms range from merely annoying to life-threatening.

Female sexual dysfunction—Includes inhibited desire, orgasmic dysfunction, and vaginismus.

Male sexual dysfunction—Includes inhibited desire, erective incapacity, premature ejaculation, ejaculatory incompetence, and ejaculatory pain.

Dyspareunia—Persistent genital pain in either a male or female before, during, or after sex.

Impotence—Erectile dysfunction or inability to attain or maintain an erection sufficient to complete intercourse.

Premature ejaculation—Persistent and recurrent ejaculation with minimal sexual stimulation and before the person wishes it.

Vaginismus—Involuntary spastic constriction of the lower vaginal muscles.

valuing one's self as male or female; and sociocultural aspects include sexual orientation learned from the value systems of family, peers, and community. All these aspects are interrelated, influencing the individual to experience and value self as masculine or feminine, seeking and giving affection and striving to meet basic needs for love and belonging.

A sexually healthy person has the following characteristics:

- Behavior agreeing with gender identity (persistent feeling of oneself as male or female)
- Ability to participate in loving and committed relationships
- Physical ability to find erotic stimulation pleasurable
- Ability to make decisions about sexual behavior that are compatible with values and beliefs, cultural norms, and social mores
- Ability to make adjustments in sexual functioning appropriate to limitations and changes resulting from illness, injury, or other events such as unavailability of a partner

Human sexuality can be healthy, satisfying, and enriching, or it can be the source of physical and mental distress. Sexuality encompasses a person's feelings about himself or herself and how to interact with others. Sexuality and sexual behaviors are influenced by age, knowledge, marital status, resources, values, social, spiritual and cultural norms, and emotional and physical health.

Society today allows people to experience various types of adult relationships. Once believed to be the legal and moral right of only the married, many individuals now consider sexual activity to be acceptable for any consenting adult. More people are involved in relationships not considered acceptable just a decade or two ago, such as premarital, open marriages, remarried or blended families, the never-married adult, single-parent families, and lesbian and gay men's relationships. Sexual preferences are considered a matter of personal choice, and homosexuality is no longer considered a mental illness.

All aspects of human sexuality may be affected by acute and, especially, chronic illness. Ill health is one of the greatest detriments to sexual expression not only because it focuses energies toward recuperation but also because it often lowers an individual's sense of personal worth and attractiveness, and indirectly, sexual desire.

The most common dysfunctions in women are arousal and/or orgasmic dysfunction. Common dysfunctions in men are impotence and premature ejaculation. A diagnosis of sexual dysfunction is used when an individual identifies a problem with sexuality (not when the caregiver is uncomfortable with the patient's sexual preference) or when antisocial sexual behavior results in harm to others. Individuals have the right to make choices regarding their sexual options and should be offered education about them, such as appliances and strengthening exercises for cord-injured patients; however, they do not have the right to inflict discomfort or harm to others. Changing social norms for sexual behavior have recently made deviations from "traditional" sexuality more acceptable. Some individuals who adopt alternative modes of sexuality (homosexuality) experience little or no conflict internally or externally and thus may not be subject to problems of sexual dysfunction. However, some members of society continue to harbor extreme discomfort with less traditional sexual expression.

Competence and success in handling problems with sexual dysfunction depend on the nurse's knowledge and experience and the nurse's comfort with his or her own sexuality. It can be difficult for some nurses to assess a patient's sexual problems or intervene for inappropriate sexual behavior. It may be useful in these situations to confer with nurse colleagues, especially a nurse specialist or a mental health practitioner with training in sexual counseling.

Nurses should not feel as if they need to be sex therapists. They can, however, help resolve those sexual problems created by the patient's illness and the limitations it creates. To be prepared to deal with this aspect of care:

- Be knowledgeable about sexuality and sexual norms.
- Use this knowledge to understand others' behavior and reactions to sexuality in health and illness.
- Be aware of differences in cultural and individual attitudes and perspectives regarding sexuality.

- Assist patients' adaptation to and optimal health regarding their sexuality.
- Make appropriate referrals for those patients with more complex sexual dysfunction.

Etiology

The human sexual response cycle stages (excitement, plateau, orgasm, and resolution) describe the type of responses people have during sexual activity. Sexual dysfunction can occur at any of these stages.

There is seldom one single cause of unsatisfying or inadequate sexual experiences. *Physiologic* causes include disruption of neural pathways as in spinal cord injury or prostate surgery; impaired circulation as in diabetes or peripheral vascular disease; hormonal changes as in testicular or ovarian dysfunction.

Psychologic causes include unresolved internal conflicts, low self esteem, discordant relationships with current and/or past partners, feelings of dependency or abandonment.

Sociocultural factors include cultural or religious myths or beliefs that inhibit sexual activity.

Related Clinical Concerns

Sexual dysfunction may be a temporary concomitant of an illness or treatment, or it may be a permanent consequence of chronic illness or injury. Sexual problems associated with illness can be classified into four groups:
- Lack of interest in or desire for sexual activity
- Physical incapacity for or discomfort during sexual activity
- Fear of precipitating or aggravating a physical illness through sexual activity
- Use of illness as an excuse to avoid feared or undesired sexual activity

Surgical procedures resulting in changes in sexual functioning include urologic procedures for prostatic hypertrophy; intestinal surgery for colitis, ileitis, or Crohn's disease; and most other fecal or urinary diversion surgery for neoplasms. Loss of external or internal body parts or functions, relocation of orifices, such as hysterectomy, mastectomy, colectomy, and cystectomy, and amputations can all lead to changes in both physical and mental components of sexual functioning. How a surgical procedure influences postoperative sexual functioning depends on the:

- Reason for surgery, diagnosis, and prognosis related to sexual functioning
- Significance of loss of childbearing and fertility functions
- Knowledge of anatomy and physiology of sexual structures and functions
- Meaning, assumptions, and values related to sexual identity
- Type and rationale for premorbid sexual activity

The main difference between a health disruption resulting from chronic illness and surgical or accidental trauma is the psychologic preparation and the irreversible effect on nerves, blood vessels, and hormonal supply.

Most of the drugs reported to affect sexual functioning directly (see Table 14–1) act on specific neurotransmitters. There is evidence that the primary neurohormone in mobilizing sexual behavior is dopamine, while serotonin is the major inhibitor. Therefore, medications that block dopamine receptor sites and drugs that deplete dopamine interfere with central control of sexual function, while drugs that depress serotonin concentrations in the brain are expected to stimulate sexual function.

Many sexual responses are mediated through the parasympathetic nervous system; therefore, parasympatholytic or cholinergic blocking drugs may cause impotence in men and problems with vaginal lubrication in women. Orgasm and ejaculation are primarily functions of the sympathetic, adrenergic, and nervous system, so drugs such as anticholinergics may interfere with potency and orgasm.

Ganglionic blocking drugs, such as antispasmodics, impair both sympathetic and parasympathetic nervous system function. Drugs that stimulate or depress the CNS can affect sexuality, particularly the antianxiety agents and narcotics and many of the substances used socially such as caffeine, alcohol, cocaine, marijuana, and amphetamines. With few exceptions, most therapeutically useful drugs have some adverse effect on sexual function.

TABLE 14–1. **Drugs That Alter Sexual Behavior**

Drugs (Classification)	Probable Effects
Antihypertensives	Produce vasodilation and decreased cardiac output; depress CNS.
	Cause impotence in men and decrease vaginal lubrication in women.
Antidepressants	Anticholinergic side effects can cause impotence, premature ejaculation, delayed orgasm.
	Decrease depression.
Antihistamines	Anticholinergic side effects can cause impotence, premature ejaculation, delayed orgasm.
Antispasmodics	Smooth muscle relaxation can cause impotence.
Sedatives and tranquilizers	Depress CNS.
	Produce tranquilization and relaxation.
	Depress libido.
Oral contraceptives	Remove fear of pregnancy.
Alcohol	In small amounts, may increase libido.
	In large amounts, impairs neural reflexes involved in erection and ejaculation.
	Chronic use may cause impotence.
Opioid narcotics	Central sedation causes impotence in chronic users.
Cancer chemotherapy agents	Possible temporary or permanent testicular and ovarian failure causing impotence, lack of desire.
Estrogen	Suppresses sexual function in men.
Diuretics	Chronic use may cause impotence.

Lifespan Issues

CHILDHOOD

Gender identity is usually firmly established by the age of 18 months. In rare cases in which gender was misassigned at birth due to physical abnormality or where accidental damage was suffered, it is considered almost impossible to reassign a child to the opposite sex after age 2.

ADOLESCENCE

During adolescence sexual preference and active sexual behavior become more evident. A major concern at this time is sex education regarding sexually transmitted diseases, birth control, and the development of satisfying, long-term relationships with same-sex and opposite-sex friends.

ELDERLY

There are many myths and stereotypes about sexuality and the elderly. The most important factor in sexual activity in older adults is the availability of a healthy relationship between two healthy partners. The most significant health issues affecting sexuality for the elderly are fear of heart attack, poststroke dependency, fatigue related to chronic obstructive pulmonary disease, erectile dysfunction related to diabetes and impotence related to treatment for prostatic cancer in men, inadequate lubrication in women, and arthritis causing movement limitations. Surgeries more common in the elderly, such as prostatectomies, mastectomies, hysterectomies, and ostomies, also affect the older adult's sexuality. Institutionalization is a problem particular to the elderly, as the staff at such facilities may not understand or be sensitive to the sexual needs of their residents.

Possible Nurses' Reactions

- May be shy or insecure about the sexual aspects of their professional role even though they are sanctioned to touch others in an intimate and personal manner and to ask personal questions, including questions about sexual matters, related to their patients' health.
- May experience anxiety, even revulsion, when dealing with sexual questions or behaviors while caring for their patients.
- May deny their own or their patients' sexuality by avoiding any verbal or behavioral interaction regarding sexual

function, for instance, avoiding subject of sex, responding to sexually oriented questions in a vague manner, or
using euphemistic expressions like "private parts" or
"down below" when referring to genitalia.
* May use hospital rules to sidestep patients' sexual concerns. For example, they may assign male staff to male
patients when sexual behaviors or concerns develop.
* May not recognize or may actually encourage patients'
becoming emotionally involved with them.
* May experience pity for patients who are unable to perform some sexual acts following injury, such as spinal
cord injury. May feel insulted, denigrated, or angered by
some patient behaviors, such as flirting, pinching, and
exposing body parts.
* May feel uncomfortable dealing with sexual dysfunction
in patients.
* May have a mistaken belief that the seriously ill do not
have sexual needs or desires and may show a lack of
tolerance and empathy for a patient's sexual concerns
during illness.

Assessment

See Table 14–2, Guidelines for a Sexual Interview.

Behavior and/or Appearance

* Reluctance to answer questions related to sexual functioning
* Concern over changes in sexual performance, body
image
* Withdrawn, isolated, embarrassed
* Inappropriate sexual acting out, such as pinching or teasing the nurse, exposing genitalia, or wearing seductive
clothing
* May verbalize changes in functioning due to illness, injury, or surgery

Mood and/or Emotions

* Fear about future limitations on sexual performance or
attractiveness

TABLE 14–2. **Guidelines for a Sexual Interview**

These questions serve as a guideline. Adjustments in the focus and depth of the assessment depend on the nature of the patient's problem and the nurse's level of comfort discussing sexual concerns.

1. Does the patient's current physical condition affect his or her level of sexual function?
2. Does the patient have concerns about body image or self-esteem related to illness, injury, or surgery?
3. What does the patient know about potential or expected changes in sexual function related to the illness, injury, surgery, or medications?
4. What significance does the physical change or limitations have on the patient's perceptions and understanding of sexual function?
5. What are the patient's previous sexual patterns?
6. What does the patient's spouse or significant other understand and believe about the patient's sexual function and the impact of the illness, injury, surgery, or medications?
7. What are the patient's outlook and prognosis regarding sexual function?
8. What is the patient's level of comfort and willingness to discuss sexual function with health professional, spouse, or others?
9. Would the patient or significant other benefit from more education, counseling, or therapy?

- Fear, anxiety, or guilt about sexual abilities or loss of function resulting from illness, injury, or surgery
- Presence of stressors affecting sexual functioning, such as job problems, financial worries, religious conflict, value conflict with family or partner, separated or divorced partner
- Discomfort over lack of privacy, frequent physical exams, or invasive procedures
- Depression over lack of sexual satisfaction or loss of relationships

Thoughts, Beliefs, and Perceptions

- Lack of knowledge or incorrect information about sexual functioning

- Change in self-concept or body image due to illness, injury, or surgery
- Denies or misinterprets partner's reactions to sexual functioning
- Denies any concerns about sexual functioning but acts in a sexually inappropriate manner with staff or others

Relationships and Interactions

- Sexual dissatisfaction or decreased sexual desire
- Altered relationship with significant other
- Partner unavailable, unwilling, or abusive
- Poor past sexual relationships, absent or negative sexual teaching

Physical Responses

- Painful intercourse
- Inability to complete intercourse, early ejaculation, impotence in men
- Menopausal changes in women due to age, surgery, and medications (such as chemotherapy) causing vaginal dryness and lack of interest

Pertinent History

- Physical diseases or injuries affecting sexual functioning
- History of depression
- Sexual abuse and/or history of rape
- Alcohol or other substance abuse
- Previous sexual dysfunction, such as impotence, painful intercourse, premature ejaculation, or lack of lubrication in women

Collaborative Management

Pharmacologic

Any patient experiencing sexual dysfunction needs a thorough assessment of all medications being taken. Then alternative drug choices as well as changes in doses and timing can be tried.

There is a limited role for medications to enhance sexual

functioning. Hormonal therapy may be appropriate treatment in some cases. For example, postmenopausal women may benefit from estrogen replacement therapy to reduce discomfort during intercourse. Antidepressants can contribute to sexual dysfunction in some, but in others they have been known to increase desire and reduce depression. Any medications that would increase patient comfort such as analgesics may also be helpful to reduce pain during sexual contact.

Sex Therapy

A patient may need to seek out individual, couples, or group therapy to treat sexual dysfunction. Many mental health professionals have training specifically for sexual dysfunction. In addition, the patient may wish to seek out a professional who has obtained certification as a sex therapist from a national organization.

Nursing Management

SEXUAL DYSFUNCTION EVIDENCED BY IMPOTENCE, PREMATURE EJACULATION, VAGINISMUS, DYSPAREUNIA, OR OTHER CHANGES IN SEXUAL BEHAVIOR RELATED TO ILLNESS.

Patient Outcomes

- Relates valid, accurate information regarding sexual anatomy and function
- Able to verbalize correct information about previously believed myths and misinformation about sexual matters
- Identifies alternate sexual expressions that are pleasurable
- Discusses sexual functioning using correct information
- Resumes previous sexual activity
- Considers further evaluation and treatment when appropriate

Patient and Partner Outcomes

- Participate in treatment or practices that mediate problem or facilitate and enhance current sexual functioning

Interventions

- Create an atmosphere of understanding, openness, and acceptance between patient and nurse.
- Eliminate or reduce causes for patient to feel embarrassed while discussing sexual functioning.
- Provide privacy, and be nonjudgmental and supportive.
- Begin with other subjects, such as physical or family questions, then move into questions on biologic aspects of sexuality, such as menarche and age of onset of sexual development, before discussing sexual behaviors or fears. Focus on general knowledge and expectations before moving to specific individual concerns.
- Determine patient's knowledge and attitudes about sexuality and sexual function.
- Focus on patient's knowledge of anatomy and functioning of body parts that may be affected by disease, injury, or surgery.
- Pay attention to attitudes and words used by patient.
- Identify any misinformation, myths, or beliefs that may affect patient's adjustment to changes in sexual functioning. Validate correct information, and correct erroneous information.
- Accept person's feelings and concerns; explore cultural, social, religious, and parental influences on current beliefs.
- Provide new information appropriate to patient's maturational or educational level; include spouse or partner, as appropriate.
- Discuss with patient and partner the various etiologies for specific diagnoses; explain cause of problem, if known; provide information about its treatment and prognosis.
- Encourage couple to talk over the effect of dysfunction on their relationship.
- Discuss alternate methods of sexual gratification with patient or partner.
- Refer to a urologist or other specialist for further evaluation regarding surgical procedures for penile implants, or vaginal reconstruction when appropriate.
- Refer for further evaluation, counseling, or therapy, if indicated.

SEXUAL DYSFUNCTION EVIDENCED BY IMPOTENCE, PREMATURE EJACULATION, VAGINISMUS, DYSPAREUNIA OR OTHER DISSATISFYING CHANGES IN SEXUAL BEHAVIOR RELATED TO INABILITY TO ADAPT TO LIFE STRESSORS, E.G., DIVORCE, DEATH, LOSS OF JOB, DEPRESSION.

Patient Outcomes

- Identifies stressors affecting sexual function
- Identifies constructive coping patterns and sexual practices
- Resumes previous sexual activity

Interventions

- Assess for factors causing patient's ineffective coping and their influence on sexual function.
- Assist the patient to understand and discuss the relationship between life stressors and poor sexual functioning.
- Help him or her determine which stressors can be changed and which patient has no control over.
- Discuss the modifications of or changes in ways of dealing with stressors. Assist in problem solving for alternatives.
- Help the patient identify alternative methods to reduce sexual energy when partner is unavailable or unwilling, such as the role of regular physical exercise, alternative sexual practices (self-stimulation, increased social activities if spouse or partner is absent or deceased). Provide educational materials, as needed.
- Refer patient or partner for further counseling or therapy, as indicated, such as consider referrals to marriage counselor, sex therapist, social services as indicated by patient's specific problems.

ALTERED SEXUALITY PATTERNS EVIDENCED BY ACTUAL OR ANTICIPATED NEGATIVE CHANGES IN SEXUAL CHANGES AND/OR IDENTITY RELATED TO CHANGES IN OR LOSS OF BODY PART OR PHYSIOLOGIC LIMITATIONS.

Patient Outcomes

- Shows increased acceptance of change in or loss of body part

- Identifies practices that assist in restoration of sexual function despite change in or loss of body part
- Identifies practices that conserve energy and oxygen requirements for sexual activity
- Engages in satisfying sexual activity
- Discusses change in or loss of body part and its influence on sexual functioning

Patient and Partner Outcomes

- Identifies mutual concerns
- Shows increased acceptance of change or loss
- Identifies and uses practices that assist in satisfying sexual functioning

Interventions

- Determine the level of acceptance or adaptation of the patient or partner to the changed or lost body part or function. Note patient's reactions, such as anger, depression, or denial. Explain normal feelings about loss, grief and change.
- Convey an attitude of acceptance. Be sensitive to the patient's cues that a concern exists, and encourage any attempts to discuss the problem or fear.
- Respect the patient's need for privacy.
- Facilitate the partner's and family's understanding of patient's condition and concerns:
  - Encourage need to share by listening and answering questions.
  - Include spouse or partner in counseling and teaching as they express readiness. Also include them in discussions about fear of future losses, fear of rejection by loved ones, and fear of physically hurting partner.
- Help the patient realize that body changes and losses are acceptable to others by spending time with the patient, appropriate touching, and teaching about care during regular nursing care.
- Ask about strengths of relationship with partner, and encourage discussion of alternate sexual activities.
- Do not assume that patient knows about how the illness or injury impacts sexuality. Many patients will not ask

questions or give any indication at all about their concerns.

- Check to see whether the patient understands medical terminology by asking for feedback on what he or she comprehends. Use pictures and verbal explanations when providing information or giving instructions.
- Provide information over short, repeated visits so that patient has time to think over what you have discussed and to formulate questions for later clarification.
- Check which medications the patient is taking, and inform the patient about any adverse effects on sexual function.
- Encourage the patient to resume sexual activity as close to previous pattern as physically possible. Teach specific information applicable to individual physical condition:
  - For the patient with an ostomy, provide information on ways to control drainage odor.
  - Refer to enterostomal nurse specialist for assistance with appliances. Refer to other specialists, as needed.
  - For the patient with cardiac or respiratory disease, teach techniques for conserving oxygen and reducing cardiac workload.
  - Identify what symptoms indicate sexual activity should be terminated.
  - Provide information on specific techniques if patient is unable to move legs due to arthritis or spinal cord injury.
  - Take pain medication before sexual activity for pain due to arthritis, cancer pain, and so on.
- Promote the use of alternative methods of sensory and perceptual stimulation, such as body massage.
- Refer the patient and partner to further educational material, self-help support organizations, and therapy, as needed. Many self-help groups offer support related to sexual concerns, such as United Ostomy Association, Arthritis Foundation, American Cancer Society, organizations for the handicapped, and Reach for Recovery.

ALTERATION IN SEXUAL BEHAVIOR PATTERNS EVIDENCED BY INAPPROPRIATE SEXUAL BEHAVIOR IN THE MEDICAL SETTING RELATED TO INEFFECTIVE COPING.

Patient Outcomes

- Decreases or eliminates sexual acting-out behavior
- Shows willingness to discuss meaning of behavior and its impact on others
- Uses other behaviors for maintaining sexual identity
- Finds more appropriate ways to meet sexual needs in medical setting

Interventions

- Assess meaning of sexual behavior as release of sexual needs or anxiety, aggression, fear of loss of identity, re-action to change in or loss of body part, or need for closeness.
- Identify when inappropriate behaviors occur, what happened prior to acting out.
- Discuss behaviors with patient, and attempt to understand meaning to patient.
- Give feedback about staff reactions to behaviors. Assist patient to understand impact on other patients and staff. Point out which behaviors are most disturbing.
- Set clear limits with patient about what specific behavior is inappropriate.
- Discuss more appropriate ways for patient to meet sexual needs, such as exercise, reading, or spending private time with partner.
- Ensure that the patient knows that sexual acting out is not needed to maintain nurse's interest or concern as a person.
- Provide time to talk with or give physical care to patient when sexual behaviors are not occurring.
- Provide opportunity for the patient to express feelings about sexual identity and the impact of illness, injury, or surgery on body image and self-concept.
- Discuss and negotiate ways to provide privacy during long-term hospitalization.
- Provide structured activity or active games. If appropriate, ask volunteers to arrange for activities outside the current environment.
- Conduct care plan conference to discuss problem and appropriate interventions. When embarrassed or frustrated by sexually acting-out patient, get backup from

other staff, consultants, or administrator who can assist in setting limits and determining care plan goals.

ALTERNATE NURSING DIAGNOSES

Disturbance in self-concept
Impaired social interaction
Ineffective individual coping
Knowledge deficit
Social isolation

WHEN TO CALL FOR HELP

✔ Onset of sexually "acting-out" behaviors inappropriate to medical setting
✔ Increased staff complaints or conflict over management of patient behavior
✔ Increased staff anxiety over dealing with sexually inappropriate behavior
✔ Increased sexually inappropriate behavior in other patients
✔ Patient's sexual behavior interfering with treatment
✔ Staff inability to provide needed information or counseling to patient

Patient and Family Education

- Review with the patient and sexual partner, if requested, any effects of medications that may affect sexual function. Reenforce need to report these to physician so alternatives can be found.
- Teach probable causes and treatment for sexual dysfunction if patient and partner request this information.
- Provide information on birth control, and prevention of sexually transmitted diseases, as appropriate.

Charting Tips

- Use objective, nonjudgmental terms to describe the patient's sexual behavior.
- Document the patient's sexual concerns even if you do not feel comfortable providing information or education.

- Document the selected interventions for dealing with inappropriate sexual behavior on the patient care plan for consistency.
- Document the patient's understanding of cause and treatment of sexual dysfunction. Include responses of family members if they are involved in patient education and treatment.

Discharge Planning

- Consult with physician and inform patient and partner about appropriate resources related to sexual dysfunction.
- Provide referrals to appropriate support groups.
- Inform other healthcare professionals of patient's inappropriate sexual behavior if patient is being transferred to another facility.
- Inform patient and partner about expected changes in sexual behavior or dysfunction as disease progresses or patient is rehabilitated.
- Provide referral information for further sexual counseling or therapy, if needed.

Nursing Outcomes

- Staff caring for the patient selects interventions appropriate for patient's specific sexual dysfunction.
- Staff who are uncomfortable with talking about sexual dysfunction with patients arrange for other staff to intervene.
- Accurate and supportive information is provided as patient and partner exhibit readiness and willingness to receive teaching.
- Staff responds to patient's demands and behavior with understanding, support, and limit setting, as needed.

Suggested Learning Activities

- Attend a class on interviewing for sexual history.
- Share past experiences of dealing with patients with inappropriate sexual behaviors.
- Review the nursing literature on the sexual concerns of

the patient population you see most often. Do you include these concerns in your assessment of the patient?
- Obtain information from organizations who develop educational materials for patients in the population you see most such as the American Cancer Society or the Ostomy Association.

15

PROBLEMS WITH PAIN

The Patient in Pain

LEARNING OBJECTIVES

▼ Differentiate between acute, recurrent, and chronic nonmalignant and malignant pain.
▼ Examine the reasons for underassessment and undertreatment of pain.
▼ Describe important factors to be considered when assessing pain.
▼ Discuss age-related issues in pain management.
▼ Describe the role and routes of administration of opioid and nonopioid analgesics in pain management.
▼ Discuss the importance of alternative (nonpharmacologic) methods of pain relief.

Pain is what the person experiencing it says it is, exists when and where he or she says it does. The patient is the authority about his own pain (McCaffery, 1968).

Pain is a universal human experience occurring in all age groups and is the most frequent reason that people seek health care. However, no data exist that accurately reveal the true incidence of either acute or chronic pain. The frequency, and perhaps, the severity of pain may even be

---

Glossary

Pain—An unpleasant sensory and emotional experience arising from actual or potential tissue damage caused by noxious stimuli. Almost all pain has both physical and mental components.

Acute pain—Pain that lasts from seconds to usually less than 6 months after the noxious stimuli.

Chronic pain—Lasts for 3 to 6 months or more after the noxious stimuli. Types of chronic pain include *recurrent acute pain*, which has a potential for recurrence over a prolonged period but in between episodes, the patient is pain free; *chronic acute pain*, which lasts months or years but has a high probability of ending; and *chronic, benign pain*, which occurs almost daily and has existed for 6 or more months.

Pain tolerance—Duration and intensity of pain that an individual is willing to tolerate at any one time. Pain tolerance changes within an individual from one pain experience to another (see Table 15–1).

Placebo—Any measure that works because of its implicit or explicit therapeutic intent rather than its chemical or physical properties.

Drug tolerance—A *physiologic response* of the body, not under the person's control, in which the drug loses its effectiveness after repeated use. Occurs in almost all patients using narcotics more than 7 to 10 days.

Addiction—A *psychologic process* that involves the repeated use of a drug or drugs for psychologic reasons.

TABLE 15–1. **Factors Influencing Pain Tolerance**

May Increase or Decrease Tolerance	Generally Decreases Pain Tolerance
• Past experiences with painful stimuli • Knowledge about cause of pain, its treatment, and probable outcome • Personal meaning of pain • Knowledge and experience in coping with pain and willingness to try new techniques • Stress, fatigue, and energy levels • Secondary gains from the way others treat person when he or she has pain • Available resources • Positive or negative interactions with healthcare providers • Cultural background: Some cultures encourage the expression of even mild discomfort, whereas others expect stoic, quiet tolerance of even very severe pain	• Disbelief on the part of others • Lack of knowledge about pain and pain-relief measures • Fears about addiction or loss of control over pain • Poor experiences with past pain-relief efforts • Increasing or long-term disability • Fatigue or monotony

increasing as progress in medical science increases survival from birth through old age.

Studies do, however, consistently show that pain is underassessed and undertreated by healthcare professionals. The classic study by Marks and Sachar (1973) reported that 73 percent of hospitalized medical patients experienced moderate to severe pain despite receiving parenteral narcotic analgesics. Recent research indicates that nurses and physicians continue to undertreat pain in patients because they do not understand pain management principles, they fear causing the patients' dependence on narcotics, and they possess poor knowledge of narcotics, adjuvant therapies, and the components of pain assessment. In 1992, the Agency for Healthcare Policy and Research established federal guidelines on pain management assessment and intervention to address the problem.

Pain is a multidimensional and complex phenomenon, requiring effective assessment and management. Many disciplines are involved in pain management in a variety of clinical settings. Optimal pain management depends on cooperation among the different members of the healthcare team throughout the patient's course of treatment. The nurse usually has the most significant influence on how well the patient's pain is relieved because of being the one who has the most frequent contact with the patient. Consequently, the nurse is in a unique position to identify the patient who has pain, to appropriately assess the pain and its impact on the patient and family; to initiate action to alleviate pain using available resources; and to evaluate the effectiveness of those actions.

Patients vary greatly in their response to pain and its interventions as well as in their personal preferences and expectations regarding pain relief. Therefore, rigid prescriptions for the management of pain are inappropriate. An effective pain management program will incorporate the following requirements and principles:

1. Pain intensity and relief must be assessed and reassessed at regular intervals in a consistent manner (see Fig. 15–1, Initial Pain Assessment Tool).
2. Patient preferences must be respected when selecting methods of pain management.
3. Each institution must develop an organized program to evaluate the effectiveness of pain assessment and management.
4. Establishing positive relationships between patients and healthcare professionals is an important part of successful pain control. Patients should be informed that information about options to control pain is available and they are welcome to discuss their concerns and preferences with the healthcare team.
5. Unrelieved pain has severe negative physical and psychologic consequences. Aggressive pain prevention

INITIAL PAIN ASSESSMENT TOOL

Patient's Name _____   Age _____   Date _____

Diagnosis _____   Physician _____   Room _____

Nurse _____

I. LOCATION: Patient or nurse mark drawing.

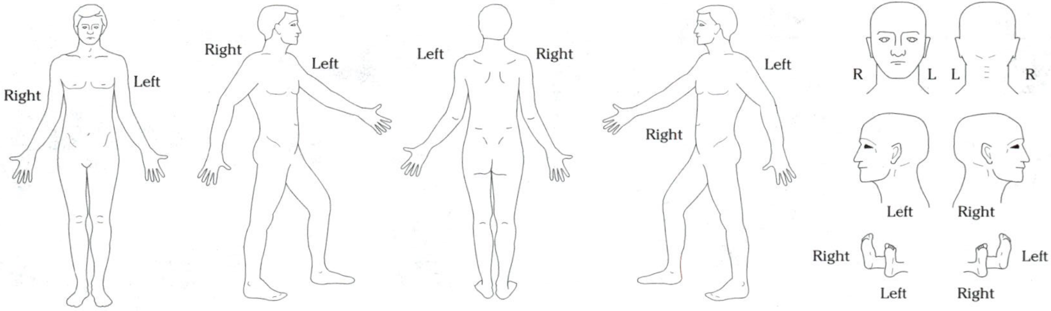

FIG 15-1

II. INTENSITY: Patient rates the pain. Scale used _____

    Present: _____

    Worst pain gets: _____

    Best pain gets: _____

    Acceptable level of pain: _____

III. QUALITY: (Use patient's own words, e.g. prick, ache, burn, throb, pull, sharp) _____

IV. ONSET, DURATION VARIATIONS, RHYTHMS: _____

V. MANNER OF EXPRESSING PAIN: _____

VI. WHAT RELIEVES THE PAIN? _____

VII. WHAT CAUSES OR INCREASES THE PAIN? _____

VIII. EFFECTS OF PAIN: (Note decreased function, decreased quality of life.)

    Accompanying symptoms (e.g., nausea) _____

    Sleep _____

    Appetite _____

    Physical activity _____

    Relationship with others (e.g., irritability) _____

    Emotions (e.g. anger, suicidal, crying) _____

    Concentration _____

    Other _____

IX. OTHER COMMENTS: _____

X. PLAN: _____

FIG 15-1 (cont.)

and control can yield both short-term and long-term benefits. Although complete elimination of some pain may not be practical or even desirable, techniques are now available to set reduced pain as a realistic goal.

6. Prevention is better than treatment. Pain that is established is too difficult to control.

Etiology

The exact mechanism of transmission and perception of pain is not known; however, neurophysiologic, psychologic, and sociologic research has contributed to the formation of pain theories.

The *gate control theory*, originally proposed in 1965 by Melzack and Wall, suggests that pain occurs when smaller-diameter type A nerve fibers and very small diameter type C fibers are stimulated. These afferent, or sensory, fibers penetrate the dorsal horn of the spinal cord and end in the substantia gelatinosa. When the sensory stimulation reaches a certain critical point, the "gate" opens and allows nearby transmission cells to project the pain message to the brain. In contrast, the large-diameter type A sensory fibers inhibit pain transmission. When these fibers are stimulated, fast-conducting afferent fibers oppose the smaller fibers' input and activate the substantia gelatinosa "gate" to close, thus blocking nerve transmission.

This theory explains why external methods of pain control work. For example, stimulating the large-diameter type A fibers by massage, applying heat or cold, acupuncture, transcutaneous electric nerve stimulation (TENS) can override sensory input in the smaller-diameter type A fibers and block pain transmission at the gate. Cognitive techniques, such as distraction, biofeedback, relaxation, and guided imagery, operate through the efferent fibers, closing the gate.

In the 1970s, the body's own internally secreted narcoticlike substances, called *endorphins*, were identified. Research found that the brain triggers the release of endorphins, which lock into the narcotic receptors at nerve endings in the brain and spinal cord to block the transmission of pain signals, preventing the impulse from reaching consciousness. This research has helped to explain why pain perception and the need for analgesia can vary greatly from one person to another. Endorphins are depleted with prolonged pain, recurrent stress, and the prolonged use of morphine or alcohol. Endorphin levels are increased during brief pain episodes, brief stress, physical exercise and sexual activity, massive trauma, some types of acupuncture, some types of transcutaneous nerve stimulation, and possibly with placebos.

One of the newest theories is called the *multiple opioid receptor theory*. This theory recognizes how not all narcotics work the same way and some cannot be switched back and forth without adverse consequences. There are at least three types of opioid receptor sites in the spinal column. Each type binds somewhat differently with different types of narcotics. For example narcotics like Stadol or Nubain (agonist-antagonist drugs) antagonize the effects of other narcotics like morphine and can contribute to withdrawal rather than pain relief. Knowledge of this theory enhances appropriate selection of analgesics.

Social and cultural factors also affect the pain response by influencing how the individual interprets pain and how he or she responds emotionally. Through family, social, and cultural values and attitudes, the patient learns which types of pain responses are appropriate within his or her group. Of course, family and social influences change as a child matures. By the time adulthood is reached, the individual may have modified or even rejected many family values or taken on the values of another subgroup. If the patient's values conflict with his or her family's, additional stress and anxiety may be felt. This may explain why certain patients act differently when family members are present.

Other factors influencing pain behaviors may include the body part involved, the patient's socioeconomic status and religious beliefs, and experience with folk medicine or alternative therapies. A patient's language and vocabulary affect how pain is described. Don't be too quick to assume you understand what the patient is trying to say, especially if his or her native language and ethnic background are different from yours.

Related Clinical Concerns

The physiologic and psychologic risks associated with untreated pain are greatest in frail patients with other illnesses, such as heart or lung disease, those undergoing major surgical procedures, and the very young or very old. Untreated pain can contribute to complications as the patient is unable to cough or deep breathe or gets inadequate rest or nutrition. In patients with psychiatric diagnoses such as depression, schizophrenia, dementia, malingering and hypochondriasis, pain may be the chief presenting complaint. Treating the underlying psychiatric disorder should lead to reductions in pain. Those with alcohol or drug withdrawal syndromes need special consideration in their pain management especially if they also have other medical problems. Patients with chronic benign pain are by far the most difficult to treat effectively over long periods of time and usually require a multidisciplinary pain team approach.

Each individual experiences and expresses pain in a unique manner, depending on age, sex, culture, and previous pain experience. All pain is real to the person experiencing it, regardless of its physical or psychologic etiology. Each person's ability to tolerate pain is also unique. Depending on the situation, pain tolerance can vary even in the same individual. Anxiety or depression can decrease pain tolerance. Most people with severe or prolonged pain also have emotional changes related to their pain.

About one-third of all patients with a diagnosed physical cause for their pain respond to placebos. Nurses should be aware that a positive response, meaning that the patient gets relief after taking the placebo, cannot be used to prove the pain is psychologically induced. Sometimes just listening to the patient, acknowledging the pain and giving a medication can enhance pain relief.

The benefits of adequate pain management are easier mobilization, shorter hospital stays, increased productive rehabilitation, and earlier return to previous work or lifestyle; or if the patient is terminal, increased comfort and peace of mind.

Lifespan Issues

CHILDHOOD

Research indicates that younger children, including neonates, may experience some pain more intensely than older children. For those children who cannot communicate verbally about their pain, one needs to assess pain by observing physiologic changes, nonverbal behavior, and vocalizations, such as crying or groaning. Consult parents or guardians about how the child expresses pain at home. Knowledge of the child's age and developmental level gives insight into how pain may be expressed.

If painful procedures are needed, be sure they are performed outside the child's room or the playroom so his or her bed, room, and the playroom continue to be safe places. If the child is verbal, try to use his or her words for pain when asking about the discomfort. Use one of the assessment tools for children (see Fig. 15–2, Pain Assessment Tools for Children).

Most dosage recommendations for narcotic analgesics in children are not supported by double-blind studies and underdosing is especially common. Initial recommended doses must be viewed as educated guesses and should be adjusted either up or down according to the individual child's response.

Toddlers and older children may obtain pain relief from cutaneous stimulation like massage and TENS and distraction similar to adults. Adolescents may report more pain than younger children, especially if the pain is chronic.

ELDERLY

Pain is not an inevitable part of aging; however, the elderly are at greater risk for many disorders that may result in pain such as arthritis, cardiovascular disease, osteoporosis, falls, hip fractures, and cancer. Elderly patients may deny pain more frequently than other age groups because they fear the consequences of admitting pain, such as longer hospitalization or more tests or they have the mistaken belief that pain is normal for their age. Special efforts must be taken to adequately assess pain, especially in the confused elderly.

Polypharmacy is of special concern in the elderly. Because of the physiologic changes that occur with aging, drug half-life and clearance times are increased in the elderly and that can lead to increased and unexpected side affects and toxicity making pain control more difficult in this group. Unrelieved pain may also contribute to confu-

Vertical Visual Analog Scale

```
——— 10  Worst pain
 +   9
 +   8
 +   7
 +   6
 +   5
 +   4
 +   3
 +   2
 +   1
——— 0  No pain
```

Have the child mark on the scale how he rates his pain.

Use the same scale for re-evaluation to chart pain relief progress.

Wong/Baker Faces Rating Scale

0

2

4

1

3

5

1. Explain to the child that each face is for a person who feels happy because he has no pain (hurt, or whatever word the child uses) or feels sad because he has some or a lot of pain.

2. Point to the appropriate face and state, "This face is…"

   0—"very happy because he doesn't hurt at all."

   1—"hurts just a little bit."

   2—"hurts a little more."

   3—"hurts even more."

   4—"hurts a whole lot."

   5—"hurts as much as you can imagine, although you don't have to be crying to feel this bad."

3. Ask the child to choose the face that best describes how he feels. Be specific about which pain (e.g., "shot" or incision) and what time (e.g., now? Earlier before lunch?).

FIG. 15-2

sion and dementia. Adjuvant analgesics must be used with caution in the elderly as sedation, confusion, and constipation may be compounded by the sedative and anticholinergic effects of many of these drugs. Low starting doses are recommended. Long-acting analgesics may be more prone to lend to side effects.

Possible Nurses' Reactions

- May rely more on physiologic changes or signs such as vital signs, body movement, facial gestures, and other nonverbal behavior than on patients' own verbal reports to assess patient's pain.
- May become immune to patient's expressions of pain.
- May have difficulty accurately assessing the patient's pain. Varying opinions among staff members over interpretation of behaviors suggesting pain and selected pain control modalities can lead to very divisive conflicts among staff members.
- May feel extremely frustrated over what can be done to help their patient.
- May fear causing a patient's addiction if the patient requires narcotics for an extended period of time.
- May think the need for greater pain control is more acceptable for certain types of pain, such as cancer pain.
- May believe that the patient will always accurately report pain when they have it.
- May become frustrated over what to do when the patient denies having pain to the physician but continues to request pain medication from staff.
- May feel manipulated by patients whom staff believe are faking pain for the purpose of obtaining more medication.

Assessment

ACUTE PAIN

Behavior and/or Appearance

- Reports pain as being sharp, highly localized with possible radiation. Onset may be sudden or slow. Intensity ranges from mild to severe.

- Guarded positioning.
- Tense or grimacing facial expression.
- Rubbing, pulling at, or splinting or protecting painful area.
- Fatigued, lethargic.
- Crying or moaning.
- Restless.

Mood and/or Emotions

- Fearful, anticipating more pain
- Angry, irritable, frustrated
- Depressed, hopeless, withdrawn
- Feeling out of control or helpless about pain if relief is inadequate

Thoughts, Beliefs, and Perceptions

- Wide variations in beliefs about pain, its causes, and methods for relief
- May be confused and unable to concentrate
- Lack of information or has misinformation about pain control methods
- Decreased motivation to participate in activities of daily living
- Unwillingness to try alternative pain-relief methods
- Lack of trust in caregivers if pain not believed

Relationships and Interactions

- Patient may withdraw socially or have angry outbursts related to pain.
- Secondary gains may influence pain behaviors. For instance, family members may cater to patient's needs more attentively if he or she is in pain.
- Caregivers may avoid the patient because of previous experiences with the patient when he or she was in pain due to feelings of helplessness.

Physical Responses

- Increased blood pressure, pulse, respirations
- Diaphoresis
- Tremors
- Redness and swelling around painful area

Pertinent History

- Previous pain experiences
- Effect of pain on work, sleep, eating, elimination, and sexual patterns
- Previous and current use of narcotics or other analgesics
- Drug or alcohol dependency
- Litigation pending after injury or an accident
- Medical problems, surgeries, and injuries

CHRONIC PAIN

Behavior and/or Appearance

- Presence of pain for more than 6 months
- Difficulty maintaining job or other activities
- Frustration, fatigue
- Changes in skin color over painful area
- Changes in muscle tone and reflexes

Mood and/or Emotions

- Depression
- Social isolation and withdrawal
- Hopelessness
- Suicidal ideations
- Angry and bitter
- Preoccupied with pain
- Fear that caregiver will give up on patient and pain problem
- Fear that pain is intractable and will always affect family, work, social life, finances, and mood

Thoughts, Beliefs, and Perceptions

- Perceives others do not believe that he or she is in pain
- Fears losing control over the pain and that the medication will lose effectiveness or be withdrawn before pain resolves
- Has misinformation about effectiveness or alternative pain-relief methods
- Lacks trust in caregivers who do not acknowledge or treat his or her pain
- Family experiences fear and frustration about the patient's using pain for secondary gains

Relationships and Interactions

- Family or work relationships may have changed since pain became chronic
- Patient's dependency increases with pain
- Patient withdraws from usual activities and friends
- Patient experiences decreased social activities and reduced satisfaction with relationships and diminished sexual interest

Physical Responses

- Anorexia or weight gain
- Impaired mobility
- Insomnia
- Intermittent pain relief with rest; pain recurring with increased stress or certain activities

Pertinent History

- Pain of more than 6 months' duration
- Changes in mood, sleep, appetite, and activity patterns
- Constipation related to prolonged use of narcotics
- Litigation pending after injury
- Prolonged use of medication without effective pain relief
- Physical dependency on pain medications, other drugs, or alcohol since pain became chronic
- Financial problems due to cost of medical care
- Possible multiple medical complaints with little satisfaction over treatment
- Seeking out numerous doctors for treatment

Collaborative Management

Pharmacologic

Several types of drugs are available to treat pain. Selection is based on the cause of the pain, its intensity and duration, and the patient's response. Mild intermittent pain may be treated with salicylate analgesics or nonsteroidal anti-inflammatory agents. More severe acute pain may need opioid analgesics. Determining the most effective medication requires careful assessment of the cause of the patient's pain and his or her perception of the pain and underlying condition. Factors that influence the effectiveness of medication include:

- Route of administration
- Amount and frequency of dosage
- Anticipated onset and duration of action
- Method of drug's action (central versus peripheral)
- Previous experience with medication

The patient experiencing pain needs to be constantly reevaluated to ensure that he or she receives maximal relief with the least potent drug. For instance, a surgical patient may require intravenous or intramuscular opioid analgesics immediately after surgery. As healing occurs, the drug can be titrated to a less invasive administration method and a lower dose while still maintaining adequate pain control. An equianalgesic list (see Table 15–2, Opioid Analgesics Commonly Used for Severe Pain) gives the dose and route of administration of one drug that produces approximately the same degree of analgesia as the dose and route of administration of another drug. There are many differences among individual patients, so these lists serve only as guidelines to the relative equivalences of various analgesics. Dose and time intervals must be titrated for each patient.

Patients on one or more other medications need to be evaluated for possible drug interactions. Drug pharmacokinetics may change because of alterations in cardiac, renal, and liver function, respiratory rate, and gastrointestinal absorption. Fever, sepsis, burns, and shock will also affect drug effectiveness.

Patients with psychiatric conditions taking antianxiety agents or psychoactive drugs must also be evaluated for possible drug interactions, in particular, the added sedative effects of opioids and many of the psychotropic drugs. Clinicians should be aware that patients in these categories may not respond as expected to pain medication.

Nursing Management

ACUTE PAIN EVIDENCED BY REPORT OF MODERATE PAIN, CHANGES IN AUTONOMIC NERVOUS SYSTEM (INCREASED HEART RATE AND

TABLE 15-2. Opioid Analgesics Commonly Used for Severe Pain

| Name | Equianalgesic Dose, mg | | Starting Oral Dose | | Comments | Precautions and Contraindications |
	Oral	Parenteral*	Adults, mg	Children, mg/kg		
Morphine	30†	10	15–30	0.3	Standard of comparison for opioid analgesics; sustained-release preparations (MS Contin, Oramorph, SR) release drug over 8–12 h.	For all opioids, caution in patients with impaired ventilation, bronchial asthma, increased intracranial pressure, liver failure.
Hydromorphone (Dilaudid)	7.5	1.5	4–8	0.06	Slightly shorter duration than morphine.	
Oxycodone	30	—	15–30	0.3		
Methadone (Dolophine)	20	10	5–10	0.2	Good oral potency; long plasma half-life (24–36 h).	Accumulates with repetitive dosing, causing excessive sedation (on days 2–5).
Levorphanol (Levo-Dromo-man)	4	2	2–4	0.04	Long plasma half-life (12–16 h).	Accumulates on days 2–3.

Drug				Comments
Fentanyl	—	0.1	—	Transdermal fentanyl (Duragesic) 25–50 mcg/h roughly equivalent to 30 mg sustained-release morphine q 8h.	Because of skin reservoir of drug, 12-h delay in onset and offset of transdermal patch; fever increases rate of absorption.
Oxymorphone (Numorphan)	—	1	—	5 mg rectal suppository = 5 mg morphine IM.	Like IM morphine.
Meperidine (Demerol)	300	75	Not recommended	Slightly shorter acting than morphine.	Normeperidine (toxic metabolite) accumulates with repetitive dosing, causing CNS excitation; avoid in patients with impaired renal function or who are receiving monoamine oxidase inhibitors; irritating to tissues with repeated IM injection.
Opioid agonist-antagonists					
Nalbuphine (Nubain)	—	10	—	Not available orally; not scheduled under Controlled Substances Act.	Incidence of psychotomimetic effects lower than with pentazocine; may precipitate withdrawal in opioid-dependent patients.

TABLE 15–2. **Opioid Analgesics Commonly Used for Severe Pain** *(Continued)*

Opioid agonist-antagonists						
Butorphanol (Stadol)	—	2	—	—	Like nalbuphine.	Like nalbuphine.
Dezocine (Dalgan)	—	10	—	—	Like nalbuphine.	May precipitate withdrawal in opioid-dependent patients; SC injection irritating.
Buprenorphine (Buprenex)	—	0.4	—	—	Not available orally; sublingual preparation not yet in U.S.; less abuse liability than morphine; does not produce psychotomimetic effects.	May precipitate withdrawal in opioid-dependent patients; not readily reversed by naloxone; avoid in labor.

Note: Equianalgesic doses are equivalent to 10 mg of IM morphine (i.e., morphine 10 mg IM = merperidine 75 mg IM = oxycodone 30 mg PO).

*These are standard IM doses for acute pain in adults and also may be used to convert doses for IV infusions and repeated small IV boluses. For single IV boluses, use half the IM dose. IV doses for children >6 mo = parenteral equianalgesic dose X weight (kg)/100.

†Some experts argue that 60 mg of oral morphine is the more accurate equivalent dose and suggest caution in converting patients from high doses of oral morphine to other drugs if the 30-mg equivalent is used.

Source: Adapted from American Pain Society: Principles of Analgesic Use in the Treatment of Acute Pain and Cancer, Skokie, IL, 1992.

BLOOD PRESSURE), AND REDUCED ABILITY TO PERFORM ADLs RELATED TO SURGERY, INJURY, OR ILLNESS.

Patient Outcomes

- Reports decreased pain levels
- Identifies previously successful pain-relief techniques to use now to decrease pain
- Identifies and minimizes factors that precipitate or aggravate pain
- Participates in assessment of pain and effectiveness of pain-relief methods
- Demonstrates increased mobility and activity

Interventions

- Perform a thorough pain assessment. Ask patient to rate pain on a consistent scale such as zero to ten with zero being no pain and ten being the worst possible pain. Be sure to determine the patient's perception of his or her pain, previous effective pain methods used, and any misperceptions they have about effective pain-relief methods.
- To reduce the patient's anxiety, explain the causes of pain, if known.
- Teach the patient and family about factors that may increase or decrease pain. Try to minimize factors that increase pain perception.
- Teach about any necessary painful procedures before they occur to reduce stress over anticipating the procedure. Patient teaching should include:
  - Basic description of the procedure or test, its purpose, and equipment to be used
  - A description of any sensations likely to be experienced
  - Anticipated duration of procedure and discomfort
  - Measures that can be used to reduce discomfort
- Provide accurate information about analgesics to reduce fear or misconceptions about addiction, tolerance, and physical dependence. Recognize that the patient or family may become anxious when medications are changed. Discuss any changes in medication, dose, or frequency with physician, and plan how to inform the patient about the pain control goals and parameters.

- Provide relief measures at regular intervals rather than on an as-needed basis, even when the pain is still tolerable. Do not expect patient to wait until pain is unbearable to administer the next dose:
  - Determine whether and when to give PRN medications.
  - Choose the appropriate analgesic when more than one is ordered.
  - Evaluate the effectiveness of administering medications at regular intervals.
  - Monitor response to administered medications, and report promptly any adverse reactions and when they are ineffective.
  - Suggest appropriate changes based on knowledge of the patient and previous response to pain-relief measures.
- Check with patient 30 minutes after administering a pain medication to assess its effectiveness. Include patient in rating level of pain before and after medication or other pain-relief method used. Use the same pain rating scale each time you assess the patient to ensure accurate evaluation.
- Encourage patient's participation in using alternative pain-relief methods such as relaxation exercises or use of heat or cold. Instruct the patient about rigid body position that can increase pain and techniques to reduce muscle tension:
  - Select a time when patient is relatively comfortable and able to concentrate so that teaching will be more effective.
  - Use pillows or other supports to splint and support body parts to reduce muscle tension.
- Discuss effects of stress, monotony, fatigue, and distraction on pain perception.
- Provide for privacy for pain expressions if the patient desires.
- Try to limit the number of caregivers interacting with patient and making decisions about pain management.
- Provide opportunities for rest and therapeutic use of distraction, such as visits or watching television, between uncomfortable treatments.
- If patient has a current or past history of drug or alcohol abuse, he or she still needs strong opioids to treat an

acute pain problem. Putting this patient on an around the clock dosing schedule of analgesics is usually recommened to avoid euphoria. Other suggestions include long-acting analgesics and making a contract with the patient about what medications can be given.

- Consult with other staff or with the physician about increased medication at bedtime and before painful procedures to keep pain at tolerable levels throughout the day and to maximize patient's participation in required activities.
- Institute measures to reduce any adverse effects of narcotics. For instance, administer stool softeners to combat constipation, antiemetics for nausea, and mouthwashes for dry mouth.
- Assist the patient to cope with the consequences of pain by encouraging discussion of fears, anger, and frustrations; acknowledge difficulty of situation; and praise and reinforce any efforts to handle pain.
- Consult with pharmacist and physician about alternative narcotic and analgesic combinations.
- Consider using aspirin or acetaminophen simultaneously with narcotics for maximal effect. Also consider use of nonsteroidal anti-inflammatory drugs (NSAIDs) for peripheral pain.

CHRONIC BENIGN PAIN EVIDENCED BY ONGOING EPISODES OF PAIN, DIFFICULTY PERFORMING USUAL ACTIVITIES, AND OTHER EFFECTS OF CHRONIC PAIN, SUCH AS SLEEP DISTURBANCE OR POOR NUTRITION RELATED TO ILLNESS, SURGERY, OR INJURY MORE THAN 3 TO 6 MONTHS AGO.

Patient Outcomes

- Acknowledges pain and accurately describes its intensity
- Participates in assessment of pain
- Able to discuss previously used effective pain-relief methods
- Uses one or more alternative measures to manage pain
- Increases participation in activities
- Decreases use of pain behaviors for secondary gain
- Decreases dependence on narcotics for pain relief

Interventions

- Assess patient's previous and current pain behaviors.
- Encourage the patient to learn and use noninvasive pain-relief methods, such as muscle relaxation, deep breathing, guided imagery, distraction, TENS, and application of heat or cold.
- Incorporate family or caregivers in alternative pain-relief measures.
- Use analgesic medications in conjunction with alternative pain-relief measure to effectively control pain.
- Discuss with physician or pharmacist plan for weaning patient off narcotics and onto nonnarcotics. Titrate intravenous or intramuscular pain medications, and switch to oral doses, as soon as possible, while ensuring adequate pain control.
- Teach patient and family that oral medication, when prescribed in appropriate dose and frequency can be as effective as parenteral.
- Administer a loading dose and then maintain a therapeutic drug level of oral medications when first switching to gain the patient's confidence in new treatment.
- Ask patient to participate in evaluation of pain-relief methods by keeping his or her own pain diary.
- Assist family or caregiver to recognize and decrease pain behaviors for secondary gain.
- Promote optimal mobility and meaningful activity in patient.
- Assess patient's nutrition and elimination functions related to use of medications and decreased mobility or activity.
- Assess patient's sleep pattern, levels of depression, or other psychologic reactions to prolonged pain. Consider use of adjuvant treatments, as indicated.
- Provide the patient and family with the opportunity to discuss fears, anger, and frustration in a private setting. Acknowledge the difficulty of the situation and any of their efforts to help the patient cope.
- As indicated, refer the patient for evaluation at a multidisciplinary pain clinic if problems are not improved before discharge.

ALTERNATE NURSING DIAGNOSES

Alterations in thought processes
Anxiety
Disturbance in self-concept
Fear
Ineffective individual coping
Powerlessness
Sleep pattern disturbance
Spiritual distress

Patient and Family Education

- Provide information about all pain-relief methods available to the patient. Keep the patient and family informed about changes in treatment plan.
- Teach relaxation techniques (see Appendix C).
- Allow the patient to make choices about relief methods used. Involve him or her in assessment of pain; teach how to use pain flow sheet or keep a pain diary, and select appropriate alternative pain-relief measures based on activities and effectiveness of relief methods.
- Initiate teaching with the patient, family, or caregiver related to pain-relief methods to be used after discharge. Review with them the ordered discharge medications, potential adverse effects and how to manage them, what to report to physician, and effective alternative pain-relief measures.

Charting Tips

- Include the selected pain rating scale in assessment and evaluation documentation.
- Use objective, nonjudgmental terms to describe pain behavior and responses to pain-relief measures. When possible, use the patient's own words when describing the pain.
- Document patient's responsiveness to all pain-relief measures used.
- Document any factors or activities that the patient or

family identify that increase or decrease pain tolerance or effectiveness of pain-relief methods.

WHEN TO CALL FOR HELP

✔ Pain-relief measures are ineffective.
✔ Pain levels increase.
✔ Patient or family is unwilling to learn about alternative methods of pain relief.
✔ Psychiatric problems are interfering with patient's use of prescribed pain-relief methods.
✔ There is increased frustration from dealing with the patient's or family's pain behaviors.
✔ Analgesics ordered are ineffective and physician refuses to make changes.
✔ Patient continues or increases use of pain behaviors for secondary gain.
✔ There are concerns over patient's or family's ability to manage pain after discharge.

Discharge Planning

- Review with the patient, family, or caregiver the patient's progress with pain management since admission.
- If being discharged with prescriptions for opioids, give patient referrals for local pharmacies that carry these medications.
- Allow sufficient time for the patient to adjust to the change from parenteral to oral administration of pain medications and to practice alternative pain-relief measures before discharge.
- Consult with the physician if patient's pain is not controlled before discharge or if pain is expected to continue for some time thereafter.
- Instruct the patient, family, or caregiver on how to use a pain flow sheet or maintain a pain diary at home.
- Suggest that the patient be referred to an appropriate pain treatment center where multidisciplinary treatment is offered.

Nursing Outcomes

- Staff responds to the patient's pain management needs with support and understanding.
- Staff caring for the patient frequently reassesses the patient's pain status using a reliable and consistent pain rating scale.
- Staff is knowledgeable about selecting equianalgesic medications administered by less invasive routes while still ensuring adequate pain control.
- Staff is knowledgeable about teaching alternative pain-relief measures.
- Nurse contacts physician to discuss alternative interventions if patient's pain is uncontrolled.

Suggested Learning Activities

- Attend pain management classes.
- Learn to teach new pain-relief methods.
- Evaluate use of a pain rating scale in your clinical setting.
- Learn to use an equianalgesic list for changing or substituting narcotic with nonnarcotic medications.
- Share personal experience with pain. Discuss how you coped with it.

16

PROBLEMS WITH NUTRITION

The Patient With Anorexia Nervosa or Bulimia

LEARNING OBJECTIVES

▼ *Describe the similarities and differences between anorexia nervosa and bulimia.*
▼ *Formulate nursing diagnoses and interventions for patients with anorexia nervosa and/or bulimia.*
▼ *Identify common nurses' reactions to the patient with anorexia nervosa and/or bulimia.*
▼ *Describe the complications of anorexia nervosa and bulimia.*

Dieting is a national obsession especially with women. Many sources indicate over 50 percent of American women are on a diet at any one time (Fontaine, 1991). Numerous fitness clubs are filled with individuals trying to attain the idealized thin, muscular body. It seems that it has become accepted behavior to be obsessed with body weight and shape. Self-esteem and happiness in young girls are often linked to weight and body shape even before adolescence. Adolescent girls may be rewarded for dieting with either increased social acceptance or praise from parents. When this social influence is combined with the right biologic, developmental, and family dynamics influences, it could be the beginning of an eating disorder. Eating disorders have little to do with simply not eating enough or overeating.

Anorexia nervosa and bulimia (sometimes called "bulimia nervosa") most commonly occur in young women, and the incidence of these disorders is on the rise. Patients with an eating disorder may be treated in psychiatric facilities but are often admitted to an acute care hospi-

---

Glossary

Eating disorders—Gross disturbances in the patterns of ingesting food.

Anorexia nervosa—A potentially life-threatening eating disorder characterized by self-starvation in a relentless pursuit of thinness, an intense fear of becoming fat, and delusional disturbance of body image.

Bulimia (bulimia nervosa)—An eating disorder characterized by consuming large quantities of food in a short time, terminating in abdominal pain, sleep, social interruption or self-induced vomiting.

Binge—Rapid consumption of large amounts of food in a short period of time (usually less than 2 hours).

Purge—Planned or unplanned episode to undo damage of binge including self-induced vomiting, laxative use, or diuretic use.

Compulsive overeating—Consuming large volumes of food without purging.

tal for treatment of complications or for initial diagnosis when ruling out other conditions. There are many similarities between these two eating disorders, and long-term anorexics may develop bulimia in later life (see Table 16–1).

The term *anorexia* is really a misnomer because this condition has very little to do with appetite. It has more to do with the person's morbid fear of obesity causing obsessive fear of losing control of one's intake. In fact, the

TABLE 16–1. **Comparing Anorexia Nervosa and Bulimia**

	Anorexia Nervosa	**Bulimia**
Epidemiology	• Over 95% female • Younger adolescent onset • Fairly rare	• 85% female • Young adult onset more likely • 2–3 times more frequent than anorexia
Appearance	• Emaciated • Below normal weight	• Normal or overweight • Weight fluctuations
Family	• Rigid, perfectionistic • Overprotection	• More overt conflict
Behavior	• Introverted • Socially isolated • High achiever • Excessive exercise	• Impulsive • More histrionic, acting out
Signs	• Cachexia • Hair loss • Amenorrhea • Dry skin • Pedal edema	• Dehydration • Chronic hoarseness • Chipmunk facies (parotid gland enlargement)
Prognosis	• 5–18% mortality rate • Frequent lifelong problems with food • Bulimia • Depression	• Death is rarer • Lifelong problems with food

person often is hungry and views the discomfort of hunger as a reminder of the deprivation needed to inflict on himself or herself. Only in the late stages is appetite actually lost. The distorted body image causes the patient to view himself or herself as fat even though appearing emaciated. No amount of weight loss relieves the anxiety causing this deadly cycle to continue, eventually causing electrolyte imbalance, arrhythmias, and cardiomyopathy. Complications can continue years later even after successful treatment.

The death rate from anorexia nervosa ranges from 5 to 18 percent (DSM-N, 1994). Purging, which promotes electrolyte imbalance and arrhythmias, combined with compulsive exercise make up a most lethal combination. Successful treatment is measured by weight gain, return of menstruation, and reduced number of compulsive behaviors.

Bulimia was officially designated as a psychiatric disorder in 1980 and is harder to diagnose than anorexia. As with anorexia, bulimia is mainly a condition of younger females; however, some studies show that up to 15 percent are male (DSM-IV, 1994). Males tend to be older at onset. Both men and women often demonstrate difficulties with impulse control associated with higher incidence of drug abuse and acting-out behavior like petty crime.

Unlike the patient with anorexia, the patient with bulimia uses food as a temporary relief of stress, causing the patient to binge. The resulting sense of shame and disgust causes the patient to purge. The cycle of binging and purging may begin as a way to lose weight but can become a compulsive behavior as the person eats large quantities when under stress and then feels uncomfortable as well as remorseful and then attempts to purge the body of the ingested food. Bulimia is associated with less life-threatening complications but can lead to chronic conditions including sore throat, dental erosion, and/or parotid gland enlargement.

Etiology

Most patients report a premorbid history of dieting and attempts to control their weight. What makes it progress to anorexia nervosa and/or bulimia is unclear, but most likely genetic, biologic, psychologic, and family factors are all involved. There are many similarities in etiologic theories between these two conditions. These disorders are also significantly associated with depression.

Anorexia nervosa may have *genetic* influences since there is an increased incidence among daughters and sisters of anorexics. The *biologic* influence may be multifactoral. Research suggests that there is an interrelationship between multiple neurotransmitters that regulate appetite, body size, and fat distribution. Dysfunction of the hypothalamus has also been implicated. Because the symptoms usually begin in adolescence, hormonal changes may be an important contributor.

Psychoanalytic theory suggests that the core of anorexia can be a child's fear of maturing and unconsciously avoiding developmental tasks. By not eating, the person forestalls sexual development and maintains the role as child in the family. Other dynamics include perfectionistic tendencies developed through demanding, overachieving parents. Anorexia gets out of control as the person tries to achieve the perfect image. Many family therapists believe anorexia symptoms represent a dysfunctional family situation as the patient tries to present a "perfect good girl" image, trying to meet the family's distorted view of perfection. Also the eating disorder gives the patient a sense of control that counteracts feelings of loss of control, anxiety, and need to avoid conflict. Some reports indicate a mother's preoccupation with weight and food becomes a source of conflict between mother and child, this becoming a means of control for the child. An overwhelming sense of worthlessness in the child may also be responsible.

Specific theories on the causation of bulimia are limited. *Biologic* views look at low levels of the neurotransmitters norepinephrine and serotonin associated with bulimia. Low serotonin is known to increase the need for intake of carbohydrates. Low levels are also associated with depression.

Family dynamics in bulimia are often characterized by a high degree of conflict, marital discord, and acting out. This may contribute to the patient's developing increased anxiety with intimate relationships and fear of abandonment and conflict surrounding parental authority. Low self-esteem contributes to feelings of inadequacy and a deep-rooted sense of shame and guilt. Some studies have noted an increased incidence of family members with a history of alcoholism and/or presence of physical or sexual abuse.

Related Clinical Concerns

Anorexic and bulimic patients may have a history of being overweight when young. Anorexics have been noted to weigh more at birth. Bulimics may have a history of anorexia when younger as well as a tendency for obesity within the family.

Lifespan Issues

CHILDHOOD TO ADOLESCENCE

Anorexia and bulimia remain a condition of adolescence and young adulthood. Children as young as 8 years old often admit to preoccupation with diet and atypical eating habits. A sense of self-consciousness and insecurity with their body is a normal part of growth and development; however, children whose self-esteem becomes more closely tied to satisfaction with their body size tend to become more prone to eating disorders. This is often influenced by how adult caregivers perceive and respond to them. Children who are overweight may experience increased criticism and demands made upon them leading to low self-esteem. In adolescence, awareness of cultural ideals becomes even stronger. Adolescents may notice that thin teens may have more friends or dates.

Possible Nurses' Reactions

- May feel shocked or disgusted by patient's behavior or appearance.
- May resent the patient because of the belief that the disorder is self-inflicted. This may make it difficult to express empathy, which in turn may make the patient feel rejected.

- The nurse may feel helpless to change the patient's behavior, leading to anger, frustration, criticism.
- The nurse may inadvertently re-create family power struggles with patient by trying to make the patient eat by nagging, cajoling, arguing, or even tricking. This will inhibit a trusting nurse-patient relationship.
- The nurse may feel overwhelmed with the patient's problems, leading to feelings of hopelessness or to the setting of rigid limits to feel more in control of the patient's behavior.
- Many nurses become embroiled in power struggles with these patients, which may trigger angry responses in the nurses.

Assessment

ANOREXIA NERVOSA

Behavior and/or Appearance

- Emaciated.
- Tends to cover up body with large clothing in attempt to hide appearance, though some may exhibit thinness with a sense of pride.
- Avoids being weighed. May try to manipulate weight by putting weights in pocket.
- High achiever in school and work.
- Ritualistic behavior surrounding food (such as eating every third bean).
- Spends time with food-oriented activities, such as cooking or shopping for others.
- At mealtimes, tries to hide not eating by:
  - cutting up food to give appearance of less food present
  - moving food around plate
  - hiding pieces of food in pockets or under plate
- Exercising obsessively (possibly in secret).
- May excessively use laxatives or foods with a laxative effect.

Mood and/or Emotions

- High anxiety associated with mealtimes, weight gain, being weighed, and especially any control issue

- When under stress, may feel need to starve self more
- Feelings of sadness and low self-esteem
- May feel need to punish self for feelings of pleasure
- Denies feelings of sadness or anger and will often appear pleasant and compliant

Thoughts, Beliefs, and Perceptions

- Distorted attitude toward appearance, weight, and food that overrides hunger and reason
- Distorted body image: Sees self as fat despite others saying that the opposite is true
- Perfectionistic, compulsive, rigid
- Sees self as helpless and dependent; has great difficulty making decisions
- Possible mental status changes from malnutrition such as memory lapses, poor attention span, poor judgment, and bizarre behavior
- Denies seriousness of low body weight

Relationships and Interactions

- Introverted; avoids intimacy and sexual activity
- Secretive
- Fears trusting others; needs to be in control

Physical Responses

- Extreme weight loss; weight less than 85 percent of expected for age and height
- Cachexia
- Fatigue
- Amenorrhea
- Hair loss; presence of lanugo (fine body hair covering)
- Low pulse rate, low blood pressure, low body temperature
- Chronic constipation
- Dry skin
- Altered lab values including: Low hemoglobin and hematocrit (or high if dehydrated), hypokalemic (especially if using laxatives or diuretics), high BUN and serum creatinine
- Insomnia

- Consuming large volumes of fluid to distend stomach, which may lead to hyponatremia
- Pedal edema related to malnutrition
- Late stages, may exhibit arrhythmias and congestive heart failure
- Pathologic fractures due to bone loss from estrogen deficiency and ovarian dysfunction

Pertinent History

- Involved in activities where small size is important such as ballet or gymnastics
- Uses food-oriented coping mechanisms to deal with stress such as stopping eating or excessive eating
- Family history of depression, eating disorders

BULIMIA

Behavior and/or Appearance

- Weight is normal, slightly overweight and/or fluctuating
- Routinely goes into the bathroom shortly after meals
- Patient eats normally or sparingly when with others, and binges in private. Purging behaviors may follow, including self-induced vomiting, laxative or diuretic misuse, fasting, or excessive exercise
- Patient may appear normal without obvious problems
- Patient functions normally
- Patient's behavior is sometimes histrionic or impulsive Patient tends to act out

Mood and/or Emotions

- Binge triggered by some emotional stress; initially some relief of anxiety during the binge but tension slowly increases as feelings of remorse and guilt build
- Purge in response to feelings of remorse and guilt
- Anxiety over one's appearance and weight
- Anxiety around mealtimes as fears loss of control
- Feelings of anxiety, depression, self-disgust

Thoughts, Beliefs, and Perceptions

- Perfectionistic
- Preoccupied with appearance, weight

- Self-critical
- Very aware that own behavior is abnormal
- Feels powerless over binge-purge cycle
- Believes unable to change
- Suicidal thoughts

Relationships and Interactions

- Overt conflict within the family
- Goes to great lengths to keep binge-purge behavior a secret from others
- Generally social and gregarious with a strong need to be accepted by others
- Sexually active

Physical Responses

- If binging: Abdominal pain, malaise, fluctuating blood sugars.
- If vomiting: Chronic hoarseness, parotid gland enlargement causing chipmunk facies, dental caries, loss of enamel on teeth, skin changes over dome of the hand. Use of Ipecac to induce vomiting can induce cardiac symptoms including palpitations, chest pain.
- If abusing laxatives: Abdominal pain, diarrhea.
- Other symptoms may include dehydration, hypokalemia, cardiac arrhythmias.

Pertinent History

- Anorexia nervosa as a teenager
- Drug and/or alcohol abuse (especially cocaine as a way to control appetite)
- Involvement in activities where weight must be kept down such as modeling, ballet, athletics

Collaborative Management

Pharmacologic

Medications have had some success in treating eating disorders. Antidepressants, particularly fluoxetine (Prozac), have been used in those patients with clinical depression. They may reduce the incidence of bulimic behavior as well. Some antidepressants also cause weight gain as a side effect. Doses of antipsychotic medications may be used in patients who are extremely obsessive-compulsive. Cyclopheptadine (Periactin) has been used with some success in anorexics to gain weight while exerting an antidepressant effect. It is an appetite stimulant, antihistamine, and serotonin antagonist. Antianxiety medications have also been useful. Bulimics have also been treated with lithium and phenytoin (Dilantin).

Dietary

Dietary regimen for the anorexic patient generally involves a slow, steady weight gain of not more than 2 pounds per week. Too rapid weight gain can put undue stress on the heart and precipitate complications. Management by a clinical dietitian or nutrition support team is essential. These patients need careful assessment as to their nutritional needs. In severely ill patients, malnutrition must be treated before any improvement from psychotherapy can be expected. For life-threatening situations, aggressive nutrition interventions will be required. This may include enteral feedings with nasogastric or gastrostomy tubes or total parenteral nutrition. Some patients do well with these aggressive measures as they feel relief that they do not need to make decisions about food. Others may react with more resentment and feel an increased loss of control, causing the patient to take more drastic measures to take control such as increasing exercise, using laxatives, or changing the drip rate or solution being infused. Bulimic patients need dietary education and supervision to control weight.

Psychiatric

Individual and group psychotherapy are essential in treating patients with bulimia and anorexia nervosa. Since both conditions also commonly exhibit troubled family relationships, family therapy is also needed. The treatment plan for anorexia nervosa may include a behavior modification program, as well. Patients are given rewards for any weight gains and increased restrictions for any weight loss or self-destructive behaviors. To increase the chance of success, patients should participate in developing the treatment plan. Written contracts that clearly explain the patient's behavioral expectations have been effective.

Bulimics may also benefit from keeping a diary of their food intake, feelings, and binge-purge behaviors. Patients who are hospitalized in the acute setting may benefit by evaluation by a psychiatrist.

Nursing Interventions

ALTERED NUTRITION: LESS THAN BODY REQUIRE-MENTS EVIDENCED BY WEIGHT LOSS, AVOIDANCE OF FOOD, EXCESSIVE EXERCISE, HIDING FOOD, SELF-INDUCED VOMITING RELATED TO SELF-STARVATION, BINGE-PURGE CYCLE.

Patient Outcomes

- Increased oral intake (anorexia nervosa)
- Weight gain at rate of no more than 2 pounds per week or per prescribed treatment plan (anorexia nervosa)
- Reduced incidence of strenuous exercise and/or purging (bulimia)

Interventions

- Recognize that patient may be very defensive about eating behavior and attempts to keep it secret. Mealtimes may be very stressful. Create environment of acceptance to encourage a trusting nurse-patient relationship.
- If personnel are available, stay with patient during meals to be sure food is actually eaten. Create a social atmosphere rather than a supervisory one.
- Give patient as much control as possible around eating behavior. Encourage him or her to select some foods. Set limits, however, on length of mealtimes. Lengthy mealtimes tend to increase anxiety and acting-out behaviors.
- Monitor food and fluid intake. Measure urine and fecal output. Assess skin turgor. Do this in matter-of-fact manner. Avoid power struggles or criticism. For example, note what patient has eaten without scowling or making demands. Recognize that telling a patient "You have to

eat more" will create tremendous anxiety and probably lead to defiance. For the patient at home, recognize that monitoring food intake and controlling binging may be more difficult and require a commitment from family members.

- Weigh patient regularly using same scale. Treatment plan may include setting a minimal safe weight range that must be maintained. This can remove the power struggle from mealtimes as patient knows what is expected.
- Set limits on dysfunctional behaviors such as strenuous exercise, and use of bathroom after eating.
- Set limits on time spent alone in the bathroom after meals. Also insist patient wait at least 30 minutes after eating before using bathroom.
- Present meals without threat, coercion, or criticism. Recognize that arguing about food will only increase the problem. In addition, avoid cajoling or tricking patient into taking more calories.
- If you suspect that patient is trying to sabotage treatment plan, talk openly with patient about your concerns. Be aware that patient may have a need to hide food to give impression that he or she is eating.
- Reinforce that patient can avoid more aggressive interventions, such as tube feedings, by meeting acceptable minimal weight standards, per treatment plan. For example, patient may need to gain 2 pounds a week. This can be a way for patient to maintain control as he or she can decide how they will accomplish it.
- Obtain specific information from a patient who purges including method of self-induced vomiting, laxative, or diuretic use.

BODY IMAGE DISTURBANCE EVIDENCED BY INACCURATE PERCEPTION OF APPEARANCE AND MORBID FEAR OF OBESITY RELATED TO DISTORTED THOUGHTS AND INABILITY TO PERCEIVE BODY SIZE AND PHYSICAL NEEDS REALISTICALLY.

Patient Outcomes

- Verbalizes more realistic perception of his or her body
- Refers to body in a more positive way

Interventions

- Encourage patient to express feelings especially about the way he or she thinks about or views himself or herself.
- Avoid overreacting to self-deprecating comments patient may make about his or her body. Recognize that these feelings and images are very real to patient. For example, the patient may dwell on having "fat" legs even though they may be very normal or even emaciated looking. Listen to patient, and explore how the fear of fat creates distress. For example, "I understand you see yourself as fat, however, I do not see you the same way." Avoid responding to patient's self-deprecating remarks by minimizing the patient's statements.
- Encourage discussion of positive personal traits especially regarding one's body image.
- Encourage patient to dress attractively and to use makeup and jewelry, as appropriate.
- Avoid insincere compliments about patient's appearance.

INEFFECTIVE INDIVIDUAL COPING EVIDENCED BY BINGING-PURGING BEHAVIOR, OBSESSIVE BEHAVIOR AROUND FOOD RELATED TO DISTURBANCE IN IMPULSE CONTROL.

Patient Outcomes

- Verbalizes feelings to others while in care of the nurse
- Demonstrates reduced number of behaviors that sabotage treatment plan
- Demonstrates more adaptive coping mechanisms while in care of the nurse
- Participates in decision making

Interventions

- If patient is panicked over personal feelings or behavior, remain calm, and help patient focus on abilities to remain in control. For example, patient may feel panicked over a weight gain and want to exercise or purge. Help patient focus on short-term goals that he or she can achieve.

Identify one area over which the patient has some control. Reinforce coping abilities.

- Communicate support and empathy to patient. Be non-judgmental to encourage sharing of feelings and coping mechanisms. Demonstrate acceptance by use of support and concern to help the patient feel lovable and accepted.

- Recognize the importance of developing a trusting relationship with patient. One or two staff members who attempt to develop a therapeutic alliance with patient can be particularly helpful. Recognize that patient may be very angry about entering treatment program. Developing a trusting relationship will take time. Show acceptance by use of touch, and if appropriate, talking about interests. Avoid just focusing on food.

- Be consistent in treatment plan. All staff members need to be aware of how to handle sabotaging of plan, such as hoarding food or self-induced vomiting.

- Listen for signs of perfectionistic thinking, and explore ways to challenge unrealistic expectations. Recognize that patient may have very rigid, fixed beliefs.

- Encourage patient to make small decisions. This tends to empower the patient and assists in feeling a sense of control and accomplishment.

- Assess for depression, suicidal risk, and substance abuse, and intervene as appropriate.

- Be aware of the family's role in patient's behavioral responses. Patient may need help in seeing himself or herself as a capable person outside the family unit.

ALTERNATE NURSING DIAGNOSES

Altered thought process
Anxiety
Compromised family coping
Fluid volume deficit
Ineffective denial
Knowledge deficit
Powerlessness
Risk for self-injury
Sexual dysfunction

WHEN TO CALL FOR HELP

✔ Patient expresses suicide thoughts or makes a suicide attempt.
✔ There is evidence of psychotic thinking, hallucinations, or severe obsessive-compulsive behavior including repetitive obsessive thinking.
✔ There are signs and symptoms of severe malnutrition or serious complications including cardiac symptoms, hypokalemia, or renal impairment.
✔ Patient uses other addictive behavior including drug abuse.
✔ Staff is in conflict over treatment plan.

Patient and Family Education

- Provide information on the long-term effects on the body of anorexia nervosa and bulimia.
- Involve family in what symptoms to identify and report. Review with them how to deal with self-destructive behaviors so as not to reinforce them.
- Provide information on the 12 Step program for dealing with addictions if appropriate. This is helpful for some people.
- Review nutritional information and recommended dietary program.
- Teach stress management and relaxation techniques to reduce anxiety especially at mealtimes or when feeling need to binge-purge.
- Educate patient and family on the need to continue long-term treatment.
- For patients who use self-induced vomiting, encourage adequate dental care.
- Reinforce need for close medical supervision.
- Teach central line care and tube feeding administration, as appropriate.
- Provide education on health effects of laxative and diuretic abuse.

Charting Tips

- Document intake and output.
- Describe behavior at mealtimes, purging behaviors.
- Describe interactions with family.
- Describe patient's verbalization about his or her body image.
- Document all self-destructive behavior.
- Document assessment of potential complications, for example, cardiac status.

Discharge Planning

- Psychiatric follow-up is essential, including family therapy. Referrals need to be made for appropriate treatment.
- Refer for adequate nutritional support follow-up if appropriate, including management of enteral feedings and central line care. If patient is being followed by a home health agency, encourage referral to dietitian. Home health agency social work referral may also be helpful to encourage compliance to psychiatric care, for family support, and for behavioral management.
- Refer patient and family to support groups if available.
- Refer patient to dental care follow-up if patient is vomiting.
- Refer patient to Overeaters Anonymous if appropriate.

Nursing Outcomes

- Demonstrates acceptance of patient's behavior
- Demonstrates consistency in treatment plan
- Avoids power struggles with patient

Suggested Learning Activities

- Arrange for inservice by eating disorder specialists to discuss dynamics and management of eating disorders.
- Obtain information on conditions from the National Association of Anorexia Nervosa and Associated Disorders, Box 271, Highland Park, IL 60035, or the American An-

orexia and Bulimia Association, 133 Cedar Lane, Teaneck, NJ 07666.
- Read and discuss the books *The Golden Cage* by H. Bruch or *The Best Little Girl in the World* by S. Levenkron. Popular movies and videos may also be available.
- Contact local chapter of Overeaters Anonymous.

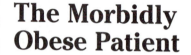

The Morbidly Obese Patient

LEARNING OBJECTIVES

▼ *Differentiate obesity from morbid obesity.*
▼ *Identify potential lifestyle restrictions and prejudices faced by the morbidly obese.*
▼ *Describe effective interventions to enhance self-esteem for these patients.*
▼ *Identify common emotional reactions of nurses to the morbidly obese patient.*

The cultural ideal of the thin body has no greater dichotomy than the image of the morbidly obese. Though aesthetic preferences for body size and shape vary from culture to culture, today the thin, fit body is idealized for women and men in America. Prejudice against the obese has a significant impact on anyone with a serious weight problem, but the morbidly obese often face outright discrimination.

The morbidly obese are often viewed in society as undesirable. They may be abused by strangers and treated with contempt by family members. Even healthcare professionals may view them as being emotionally disturbed even though there is no increased incidence of psychopathology in the morbidly obese. Others may view these individuals as lazy, unkempt, and lacking in self-control.

Glossary

Morbid obesity—A condition in which an individual is 100 pounds or 100 percent over his or her ideal body weight.

Obesity—Having an excess of adipose tissue and being at least 15 percent over ideal body weight.

Ideal body weight—Standards based on actuarial tables.

Developmental obesity—Obesity that began in childhood or adolescence and is more often associated with problems of self-concept.

Reactive obesity—Obesity that starts later in life and is the result of maladaptive coping styles at times of stress such as death or leaving home.

Chronic obesity—Lifelong overweight condition with few fluctuations.

Pickwickian syndrome—Individuals of extreme overweight where demands of the body size on a small chest wall lead to cardiovascular-respiratory changes including hypoxemia, cyanosis, reduced vital capacity, carbon dioxide retention, and pulmonary edema. Also known as *obesity hypoventilation syndrome*.

Many experts promote viewing these individuals as having a chronic illness rather than a cosmetic problem.

The morbidly obese face discrimination particularly in the workplace because they are viewed as less healthy, less diligent, and/or less intelligent than their thinner peers. Certainly with this kind of reaction, it is no wonder that these people often experience poor self-esteem, feelings of isolation and helplessness, and loss of control.

Morbid obesity crosses all ages and races though it is much more common in lower socioeconomic groups. Obesity is equally distributed between men and women. At least 20 percent of the population is obese, while only 0.1 percent of the population is morbidly obese (Lomax, 1989). Potential health problems include a wide range of chronic conditions including hypertension, cardiac problems, diabetes, respiratory insufficiency, and joint and back disorders. Mortality rates are 1200 percent higher than in the nonobese population with similar age and health status (Lomax, 1989). Nutrition deficiencies are also extremely common because the obese person may lack a well-balanced diet or experience protein deficiencies related to crash dieting.

Morbidly obese individuals often have subjected themselves to many weight-loss strategies only to regain the weight, which increases the stress on the body. Some studies suggest that individuals whose obesity has persisted for more than 5 years have very limited success with treatment.

Obesity is a complex issue, and any weight-loss program needs to include a multidisciplinary approach. Successful weight-loss programs need to include medically supervised diet and exercise programs and emotional and social support. When these measures have been unsuccessful, some people pursue surgical intervention possibly including maxillomandibular fixation (jaw wiring), intragastric balloon (inflated balloon in stomach to reduce space available for food), jejunoileal bypass (removal of a portion of jejunum to reduce absorption of food), gastric bypass (proximal segment of stomach is transacted to reduce volume), and gastric stapling (staples along lesser curvature of stomach to reduce its volume). All of these surgeries have serious complications and need to be combined with behavior modification, support, and education.

Etiology

Extreme obesity is a complex problem, and the etiology is probably multifactoral. Most often it begins early in life.

The *biologic* view considers that early onset is related to childhood development of large-size adipose or fat cells. The cellular hypertrophy results from increased food intake and decreased energy expenditure. Other factors may include impaired hunger-satiety mechanism in the hypothalamus and endocrine disorders leading to slower metabolism or changes in insulin or cortisol production. The set point theory focuses on the body as being programmed to maintain a certain level of fat stores. This could explain why some people gain weight so easily. *Genetic* studies have found that 60 percent of obese subjects have at least one or both obese parents (Galzis and Kempe, 1989). Recently, a defective gene has been identified that contributes to abnormal secretion of "satiety factors"; if present, the brain does not receive signals of being full.

Psychoanalytic theory views obesity as an expression of an intrapsychic conflict that occurred during the oral stage of psychosexual development. Unmet needs and stress in an infant can lead to overeating to decrease anxiety, express hostility, and compensate for lack of love. Unmet oral needs may contribute to behavior such as being demanding and impatient. Weight can provide a shield against intimacy. This can explain how individuals who lose large amounts of weight without adequate psychologic support may experience intense anxiety and feelings of vulnerability. *Learning theory* looks at how overeating occurs in response to tension, stress, or boredom. This can be a learned behavior from childhood as parents use food as a source of reward and attention.

Sociocultural factors must be included since food and eating are such important parts of our society. Social customs are often centered on food. Mealtimes may be an important part of family life and family traditions.

Related Clinical Concerns

Sedentary lifestyle, possibly related to a medical condition that limits mobility, is a significant factor in developing morbid obesity. In addition, treatment regimens for some conditions may increase the risk of severe obesity. Steroids can quickly contribute to increased adipose tissue development, and some antidepressants, antipsychotics, and estrogens can cause weight gain.

Lifespan Issues

CHILDHOOD

Obesity in childhood is linked to obesity in adulthood. Some contributing factors include more sedentary lifestyles with emphasis on television and computers, fast foods high in calories and fat, and reduction in sports programs in schools. Obese children are often seen by others as sloppy, less intelligent, lazy, and less likable. Obese children are often victims of teasing and social isolation, adding to poor self-image and causing these children to retreat to food as a coping mechanism. Poor self-image often remains throughout life regardless of the person's educational or vocational success. Childhood growth spurts may resolve some overweight tendencies while others go on to be morbidly obese.

ELDERLY

Past history of obesity is the major contributor to obesity in the elderly. Increased sedentary lifestyle due to failing health, medications, or poor nutrition due to low income, low energy, or depression also contribute.

Possible Nurses' Reactions

- May view patient as sloppy, lazy, weak, lacking impulse control, mentally ill
- May feel overwhelmed and hopeless with patient's problems
- May resent the demands placed on the staff with the heavy workload created by patient's size and need for special equipment

- May tend to focus on patient's size rather than view him or her as an individual with unique feelings
- May feel guilty for these negative feelings

Assessment

Behavior and/or Appearance

- Binge eating, secretive night eating, hoarding food
- Repeated dieting
- Dressing in large, oversized clothing
- Sedentary, may avoid chance to exercise
- May exhibit night eating syndrome with cycle of insomnia, increased hunger, eating large amounts, morning anorexia

Mood and/or Emotions

- Depression
- Difficulty being assertive
- Guilt, shame associated with overeating
- Strong emotions that trigger need to eat
- May feel hopeless, overwhelmed, out of control
- Unrealistic expectations, leading to disappointment

Thoughts, Beliefs, and Perceptions

- Food has many powerful meanings for patient such as comfort, love, and security
- Patient has a distorted body image
- Patient may see self as thinner, possibly indicating denial, or larger than true self
- Patient may respond to external cues and thoughts rather than hunger in deciding what and when to eat
- Weight loss may stimulate fears of success or intimacy on an unconscious level where he or she can no longer hide behind the weight

Relationships and Interactions

- May lack social skills
- May avoid social situations for fear of rejection
- May cover feelings of rejection with joking

Physical Responses

- Hypertension
- Diabetes
- Arthritis, trauma to joints and back
- High serum cholesterol
- Cardiac disease
- Malnutrition
- Fatigue
- Dyspnea on exertion
- Pickwickian syndrome: Includes sleep apnea, daytime somnolence related to carbon dioxide retention, and symptoms of congestive heart failure

Pertinent History

- Multiple attempts at weight loss
- Childhood obesity
- Chronic illness
- Parents with history of obesity and sedentary lifestyle

Collaborative Interventions

Pharmacologic

The drug traditionally used in weight-loss programs is amphetamine. It is included in many over-the-counter "diet pills" even though they have been of limited benefit in suppressing appetite. In addition, they frequently have adverse side effects including hypertension, stroke, and renal failure. Antidepressants, such as sertraline (Zoloft) and fluoxetine (Prozac), have a side effect of anorexia and have been used with success in long-term weight-loss programs. They also reduce irritability and depression.

Administering any medications to the morbidly obese requires extra caution as some may require dose adjustments. Some medications may need to be given in higher doses because of the increased body weight while other drugs, such as theophyllines, may need lower doses because metabolism of the drug is affected by the patient's lower protein or higher fat stores. Check with the pharmacist for specific information on the chosen drug. The route of administration can also affect absorption and distribution of the drug. Drugs administered intramuscularly may not be absorbed if the needle does not reach the muscle. If the medication is deposited in fat tissue, its absorption is slowed, and onset of action may be delayed. Intravenous administration may be the most effective route. Because IV access is often difficult, central line insertion may be the most efficient.

Dietary

Beginning and maintaining a weight-loss program with the morbidly obese requires close medical and dietary supervision. A complete nutrition assessment needs to be done. Patients with medical problems require very close supervision to maximize outcomes.

Nursing Management

SELF-ESTEEM DISTURBANCE EVIDENCED BY NEGATIVE SELF-IMAGE, FEELINGS OF POWERLESSNESS RELATED TO FEELINGS OF SELF-DEGRADATION AND RESPONSE OF OTHERS TO THE OBESITY.

Patient Outcomes

- Verbalizes positive traits about self
- Verbalizes concerns to nurse
- Demonstrates fewer self-critical remarks
- Participates in self-care
- Does not let self-consciousness about weight interfere with care needs

Interventions

- Avoid preaching or criticizing about need for weight loss as these approaches will only increase patient's negative feelings and sense of hopelessness and powerlessness.
- Provide privacy and treat with modesty. Be aware that the patient may be extremely sensitive to having body parts exposed.
- Have extra help available before turning or ambulating a patient to prevent falling and help the patient feel more secure.

- Have adequate-sized and reinforced equipment such as wheelchairs and beds to avoid embarrassment of squeezing patient in to accommodate your equipment. Check if patient has own custom wheelchair. Have family bring clothing from home if hospital gowns are inadequate.
- Recognize that the patient may feel very anxious at being stared at by strangers, particularly in a hospital situation. Prepare other departments for patient's appearance and needs.
- Listen for cues of how patient views self and appearance. If patient makes self-deprecating remarks, explore these feelings. Focus on positive traits other than body size. Patient does not need to be reminded of his or her large size.
- Give the patient the opportunity to share feelings. He or she needs to be viewed as an individual and encouraged to identify feelings.
- Explore use of makeup, hairstyle, and dress, as appropriate, to increase feelings of self-esteem.
- Encourage the patient's participation in treatment plan to avoid passivity. Provide encouragement to make decisions about all aspects of care. Work with patient to problem solve ways to maintain participation.
- Assess patient's support system and encourage his or her involvement.

ALTERED NUTRITION: MORE THAN BODY REQUIREMENTS EVIDENCED BY MORBID OBESITY RELATED TO EXCESSIVE INTAKE, EMOTIONAL FACTORS OR ALTERED HEALTH MAINTENANCE.

Patient Outcomes

- Begins to identify feelings or thoughts that contribute to overeating
- Demonstrates changes in eating patterns
- Identifies one short-term goal to attain
- Demonstrates non-food-related coping mechanisms

Interventions

- Assess the patient's condition and priorities of care before assuming treatment plan should include weight loss. Patient must be involved in deciding if weight loss is a

realistic objective at this time. Patient motivation is essential to the success of a weight-loss program.
- Obtain baseline weight. Identify scales adequate to handle patient's weight beforehand. Also, consider using two scales or, in the hospital setting, use a bed with adequate built-in scales.
- Assess the patient's eating patterns and typical daily intake. Provide a supportive environment so that patient can feel secure to be honest. Recognize that patient may feel need to minimize his or her intake.
- Assess the patient's knowledge level about eating patterns. Be alert to myths held about weight and weight loss by patient and family. For instance, he or she may say that the entire family is "fat" or "it's genetic."
- Assess skin and mobility. Patient may be prone to skin breakdown and complications related to poor mobility or hygiene.
- Identify coping mechanisms to deal with stress and anger that do not involve food such as taking a walk, deep breathing, or talking to a friend. Give patient feedback on alternative coping mechanisms and identify the link between stress and desire to eat.
- Focus on short-term goals to identify successes in weight loss or improved mobility. Help the patient identify nonfood rewards when goals are met.
- For the patient at home, help explain that removing easily accessible high fat/high calorie foods from the house will lessen temptation.
- Assess family involvement. Recognize that family can consciously or unconsciously sabotage weight-loss plans by exposing patient to old eating habits. Encourage the family to eat foods similar to those eaten by the patient for shared meals.

ALTERNATE NURSING DIAGNOSES

Activity intolerance
Altered health maintenance
Body image disturbance
Impaired gas exchange
Ineffective individual coping
Noncompliance

WHEN TO CALL FOR HELP

✔ Patient experiences serious complications from diabetes, hypertension, or heart disease.
✔ Patient expresses desire to start a potentially dangerous quick weight loss program.
✔ Patient exhibits signs of severe depression or self-destructive behaviors.
✔ There are signs of other addictive behavior, such as substance abuse.

Patient and Family Education

- Provide information on starting an exercise and weight-loss program.
- Strongly encourage the patient to maintain medical supervision for any weight-loss or exercise program.
- Provide information on behavior techniques for weight loss, such as eating slowly and serving smaller portions.
- Teach patient to become more aware of body signals of hunger and satiety.
- Teach appropriate exercises within patient's ability. Explain even minimal exercise, such as short walks several times a day, can help reduce weight and make the patient feel better.
- Teach patient how to monitor for possible complications such as diabetes and cardiac problems.
- Give family information on weight loss, nutrition, and ways to support patient.
- Consider focusing education on reducing medical complications and increasing activity rather than just weight loss.
- Teach coping mechanisms to reduce anxiety that do not involve food.
- Encourage patient to continue in psychosocial support program after weight loss is achieved to learn skills to deal with new image.

Charting Tips

- Document baseline weight, mobility, and skin condition.
- Document response to activity.

- Document eating patterns.
- Note coping mechanisms in response to stress.
- Note indications of motivation regarding treatment.

Discharge Planning

- Provide referral information to support groups such as Weight Watchers or Overeaters Anonymous as appropriate.
- Encourage nutritional and medical follow-up.
- Assess if patient needs assistance with transportation to medical care.
- Provide information to home health agency or other healthcare providers on patient's needs.

Nursing Outcomes

- Demonstrates acceptance of patient's behavior and/or appearance
- Demonstrates ability to treat patient as unique individual
- Provides care in safe, respectful manner

Suggested Learning Activities

- Obtain information and attend meetings at Overeaters Anonymous.
- Share information found in articles written for the obese in popular magazines.
- Arrange for weight-loss specialists to present an inservice.

17

PROBLEMS WITHIN THE FAMILY

Family Dysfunction

LEARNING OBJECTIVES

▼ *Differentiate between traits of functional and dysfunctional families.*
▼ *Discuss the role of systems theory related to the family.*
▼ *Describe the signs of caregiver role strain.*
▼ *Identify effective nursing interventions to help the family cope with the illness of one of its members.*

As the basic unit of society, the family is the most important influence on shaping whom we become. The traditional nuclear family, with two parents and children, has undergone tremendous changes in the last few decades, and some of those changes will impact generations to follow. According to the 1990 Census, only 26 percent of all U.S. families fit the description of a traditional nuclear family. Nearly half of all marriages end in divorce today (McNeil, 1992). Changing economic needs, changes in women's and men's roles, and a decreased tendency to accept unsatisfactory relationships have contributed to the increased divorce rate and significant changes in family structures. Single-parent households, step-families, and a variety of combinations of cohabiting individuals represent an increasing percentage of families.

Stresses caused by relationship adjustments can influence one's health status. Also, a change in the health of any member of the family can create family disorganization or even a crisis when roles, patterns, or routines must be restructured. Anger, guilt, and denial may all occur as the members try to adapt.

Glossary

Family—A small social system made up of people held together by strong reciprocal affections and loyalties and living in a permanent household that persists over time.

Family of origin—Family into which one is born or adopted.

Enmeshed family—Family organization in which boundaries between members are blurred and members are overconcerned and overinvolved in each other's lives, making acting on one's own impossible.

Dysfunctional family—A family that develops ways of interacting with one another that leads to impaired functioning both among the members and outside the family boundaries.

Disengaged family—A family with minimal involvement in each other's lives.

Even in those families who function satisfactorily, an illness may cause a tremendous crisis as the family shifts life patterns to meet the demands the illness has created. A family member may need to take on the added demands of being a caregiver to an ill person at the same time he or she is handling other major family responsibilities. Even the most healthy functioning family may enter a crisis period in response to a devastating illness or death. Relatives may need to move in, which changes the social structure of the family, or the family may need to outlay large amounts of money to provide extended care, affecting the family's future goals.

Because of the impact illness has on the family and the family members have on the patient's recovery, members need to be involved in the patient's treatment plan. Family response can represent a major source of stress to the nurse as family conflicts and dynamics are acted out. Family members' own fears, lack of sleep, conflicts with each other, as well as loss of emotional support can all contribute to their sense of isolation and possible mistrust of healthcare professionals.

Etiology

Bowen's *family system theory*, developed in the 1950s, views the family as a homeostatic system of relationships. A change in functioning of one member results in compensatory changes in the other members in an attempt to maintain equilibrium. For example, when a family member becomes ill, other members will adapt to fill the roles of the ill member while he or she is sick. The family system is always changing as it adapts to internal and external stimuli in its attempt to remain stable.

All families have unwritten, covertly expressed rules, such as conflict is wrong, and roles, such as "Dad makes the final decision." These covert roles are often more obvious as the family is coping with stress and often requires an enormous amount of adjustment when roles must be reversed. For example, if the father, who makes all the decisions, becomes ill, a normally dependent member may accept more of the decision-making responsibilities reversing the established roles. If past relationship problems do not support the changes, family members may exhibit un-healthy relationship behaviors, such as anger (possibly di-rected at the hospital staff) and guilt. The illness can also exacerbate any relationship problems among other family members.

In stressful situations, family members may exhibit be-haviors that seem to temporarily help the relationship while they focus on the current crisis reducing the anxiety and intensity of existing relationship problems. Some of these attempts at solutions can create more stress for a family member. At times, one member is identified as the "problem" and the rest of the family focuses attention on that member and his or her problem. This is called *scape-goating* and allows the family to avoid confronting the real conflicts within the family. For example, parents with mar-ital relationship problems may focus their attention on their child's behavior problems rather than their own.

Related Clinical Concerns

The family can play a key role in how a person responds to illness. Support and love from family may encourage a patient to concentrate on healing and strengthen his or her will to survive. In some families, however, the sick individ-ual may be viewed as dependent and unacceptable, reduc-ing his or her will to survive and remain a burden to the family.

Lifespan Issues

CHILDHOOD

The family represents the young child's whole world. The family gives the child a supportive environment in which a sense of trust and seeing oneself as a separate, competent person is developed. As the child grows, the world expands outside of the family, exposing him or her to new ideas, conflicts, and inconsistencies. Separation from this comfort can create an enormous amount of stress for the child and family.

Other outside factors may influence this separation anx-iety. As more and more children are being cared for by babysitters or in day care, adjustment to an environment outside the home may be less stressful. However, if the child has experienced a loss of a loved one, such as with death or divorce, separation may be even more stressful.

The great increase in the number of step-families has created new, complicated relationships. Children must adapt to new family members, yet maintain relationships with parents, siblings and others.

ELDERLY

With longer life expectancies, the elderly today are more likely to become incorporated into new families as they re-marry or cohabitate or maintain some type of group living situation. Adjusting to a new spouse's family at an advanced age can be a challenge as adult children may be ambivalent, or even extremely resentful, about their parent's new relationship. These new relationships can create some major relationship problems within the families and may result in very difficult situations when the parent becomes ill.

The need to care for sick elderly is also a source of family relationship problems. Today, as many families do not have one member who stays at home and has the ability to care for an ill parent, caregiving can become a tremendous burden, both physically and financially. The caregiver may be faced with overwhelming guilt and, possibly, anger. An ill parent may be viewed as an intrusion into a family already overwhelmed with caring for their children with both parents working. If an elderly person with a chronic illness is admitted to the hospital, it is essential to assess how well the family is coping with the situation and how well they are able to care for the elderly person. In the home, be aware of what family members are trying to verbalize. Sometimes, they would like more assistance but hesitate to ask for it because they are too afraid or feel guilty.

Possible Nurses' Reactions

- May anticipate problems with all families because such problems are so common
- May resent the disruption in routine that may result when family members want to be involved in patient care

- May feel uncomfortable in the presence of family members acting out their conflicts
- May resent the family's criticisms, which may be their attempt at maintaining control of the situation
- May relate patient's situation to personal family conflicts, possibly causing uncomfortable feelings
- May become overinvolved with a patient's family and experience the emotional highs and lows related to patient's progress and family response
- May incorrectly view a family as dysfunctional if their relationship styles differ from the nurse's past experience in a family
- May feel overwhelmed with dysfunctional family's problems

Assessment

Each family will exhibit unique behaviors related to the normal roles established within the family. Some of the common problem behaviors are listed below.

Behaviors and/or Appearance

- May exhibit behaviors that isolate others from family interactions
- Change in behavior patterns when in the presence of various family members
- May exhibit a defensive response to staff
- May consistently place blame on others
- May exhibit a lack of empathy toward the ill family member
- May be a lack of congruence between verbal and nonverbal communication
- Some family members may be open and realistic about diagnosis, treatment, and prognosis, and others may deny any problem, blame the staff for the problem, or avoid the patient altogether

Mood and Emotions

- May exhibit contradictory, confusing, or inappropriate affect to the situation
- May be unable to express or display feelings

- May avoid emotional situations

Thoughts, Beliefs, and Perceptions

- May indicate inaccurate or unrealistic beliefs about the patient's condition or prognosis or one's ability to provide adequate care
- May be operating on the basis of myths or inaccurate beliefs that impede care
- May think it is wrong to share concerns with others
- May focus on personal reactions to the patient rather than objectively viewing the patient's needs

Relationships and Interactions

- The roles among family members may be rigid.
- Individual family members may do anything to placate others to prevent an angry response or rejection.
- Family may have difficulty managing conflict.
- The family may be in a state of constant conflict.
- The family may pay undue attention to the ill family member.
- The family may appear to get along well when the history suggests that relationship problems have existed in the past.
- Family members may evade opportunities for communication.
- The family may avoid visiting or having contact with the patient.
- There may be inappropriate or miscommunication among family members. Communication may be unclear, nonspecific, or not direct.
- One family member may take the lead in defining the needs of the patient and family, or several members may jockey to assume the lead role.

Pertinent History

- History of child abuse, domestic violence, elder abuse, or family conflict
- History of psychiatric illness or substance abuse
- Recent losses or deaths in the family and past significant losses or trauma

Collaborative Management

Family Therapy

Family therapy can be an important treatment to assist the family under stress. Where problems such as emotional problems, abuse, marital conflict, and substance abuse are present, a therapist can assist the family in dealing with the current stressor and find more long-term solutions to their relationship or adjustment problems. Therapists may meet with all the family or limit meetings to a few key members. Young children can also be included.

Social Services

Social service agencies can investigate needed support services for families in distress on either a long- or short-term basis. They can direct the families to agencies that may provide additional finances or extra help, such as Meals on Wheels.

Nursing Management

ALTERATION IN FAMILY PROCESSES EVIDENCED BY INABILITY TO MEET DEMANDS OF ITS MEMBERS, AVOIDANCE OF MAKING DECISIONS, INAPPROPRIATE COMMUNICATION BETWEEN MEMBERS RELATED TO IMPACT OF ILL MEMBER ON FAMILY SYSTEM.

Patient and/or Family Outcomes

- Participates in treatment planning and care of ill family member
- Identifies resources available to assist family in coping
- Acknowledges diagnosis and prognosis of ill family member

Interventions

- Identify the family constellation, patterns of family interactions and who is considered to be the leader. Assess the ways that the family members interact with each other and the patient's response to family involvement.

Determine from patient whom he or she considers closest family and recognize that this could be close friends rather than relatives. Avoid making assumptions about whom the patient wants involved.

- With a large family, consider asking them to identify one member who will get the information on the patient's condition and take the responsibility to share it with the rest of the family. This avoids the need for multiple calls for information.

- As appropriate, ask the patient who he or she wants to be involved.

- Involve these family members in treatment plan. Inform them of what is happening according to patient wishes. Take the time to orient family to agency routines and visiting hours.

- Identify family support systems within the family.

- If family members exhibit disruptive behaviors, evaluate the underlying reasons. Talk with the patient and family to determine the cause.

- Analyze the family's ability to care for the patient and what they need to know when caring for the patient at home. Encourage family involvement in basic care needs if acceptable to patient. Involving the family in the care can help the patient accept his or her condition. For example, having the spouse care for a condition such as a colostomy can give the patient a sense that he or she is not disgusted by patient's body.

- If patient does not want family informed of his or her condition, talk with patient to identify reasons and fears. Not including the family may be a way of maintaining denial. Respect the patient's wishes, but continue to talk regarding the risk of social isolation. If patient is seriously ill, one person will need to be identified who knows his or her wishes.

- If family wants information withheld from the patient, discuss their fears. Point out that hiding the truth is not helpful to the patient. Dishonesty inhibits future trust and communication. Help family acknowledge their fears. However, recognize that certain cultures have strict rules concerning sharing bad news with loved ones, especially a parent. Avoid becoming angry with this situation and alienating the family. The family could distrust the healthcare team and block communication channels.

- Regularly assess the family's awareness of patient's condition and expectations for recovery and future treatment. Avoid use of medical jargon.
- If the family seems to avoid involvement in the patient's care or treatment plan, determine the reason. Consider giving them one task to do at a time to encourage their involvement without being overwhelmed.
- Encourage the family to verbalize their feelings about the illness. Respect their need for privacy to express emotions. Encourage family to leave patient's room to discuss areas of conflict. Use open-ended questions to promote sharing of feelings and concerns about problems with family interactions.
- Allow for flexibility in visiting, if possible. Recognize the need for family members to spend the night and for young children to be allowed to visit. As needed, set clear limits on disruptive behavior, and limit the number of visitors to reduce stress and fatigue on the patient. Encourage visitors to coordinate who will visit on certain days and times.
- As needed, organize a care conference with family members to discuss patient's care needs and any conflicts the family and staff may be having. Avoid having too many staff members in attendance as this could intimidate family. Focus on reassuring the family of the care and concern of the staff for the patient. Consider involving physician, social worker, or clinical nurse specialist to help intervene if conflicts continue.
- Acknowledge and facilitate family strengths. Promote self-esteem of individual family members by acknowledging their skills and influence on patient ("Your spouse really perks up when you visit").

CAREGIVER ROLE STRAIN EVIDENCED BY DIFFICULTY PERFORMING CAREGIVING ACTIVITIES, INABILITY TO MEET OTHER FAMILY RESPONSIBILITIES, DEPRESSION, AND ANGER RELATED TO MULTIPLE LOSSES AND BURDENS ASSOCIATED WITH CAREGIVING RESPONSIBILITIES.

Patient and/or Family Outcomes

- Expresses frustrations assertively
- Provides safe care to the patient

- Maintains personal needs along with caregiver needs
- Identifies resources available for assistance

Interventions

- Assess the caregiver's ability to meet the demands of the patient's care. Identify coping mechanisms and support systems available.
- Allow the caregiver the opportunity to share feelings and concerns away from the patient. Reinforce the need to express concerns and emotions. Give caregiver permission to express negative feelings, such as anger and resentment. Provide supportive, safe setting to do this. Reinforce that negative emotions are normal to reduce feelings of guilt.
- Encourage caregiver to be assertive in asking for assistance. Reinforce that others may not know what caregiver's needs are. This is especially important if the caregiver tends to demonstrate martyr behavior.
- Be aware of outside stressors on family members influencing their reactions. Fatigue and working long hours with an ill family member can contribute to ineffective coping mechanisms. Talk with them about possible resources to reduce stress including enlisting other family members to help, reducing expectations, and hiring outside help.
- Assess caregiver's expectations. Encourage caregiver to have realistic expectations of what he or she can do.
- Remind the family that past conflicts do not disappear even though someone is ill. When family members must spend long hours providing care, resentments can increase. Encourage the family to concentrate on dealing with the immediate stressor while taking steps to work on unresolved conflicts once the situation has resolved sufficiently.
- Encourage the caregiver to develop a routine to care for his or her own needs of sleep, eating, and socializing to effectively care for the patient. Enlisting other family members or hiring outside help can provide the needed break. If the caregiver is unable to get out, help him or her identify ways of maintaining contact with friends by regular phone calls and letter writing.

- At times families "promise" a loved one they will never put him or her in a nursing home so caregivers will hide their feelings. Talk openly about how these promises are sometimes made without realizing the full scope of the situation.
- Give the caregivers recognition for the good job they are doing.
- Be alert to caregivers' signs of increasing distress including depression, suicidal risk, hopelessness, and signs of potential physical and/or emotional abuse of the patient.

ALTERNATE NURSING DIAGNOSES

Anticipatory grieving
Ineffective family coping
Knowledge deficit
Noncompliance
Sexual dysfunction
Sleep pattern disturbance

WHEN TO CALL FOR HELP

✔ Indication of family not acting in the best interests of the patient such as taking patient out of hospital against medical advice or pushing inappropriate treatments.
✔ Any indication of abuse within the family must be reported per agency policy and state law.
✔ Indications that patient is not being cared for adequately include poor hygiene, decubitus ulcers, poor nutrition, or dehydration.
✔ Be alert for destructive behavior within the family such as substance abuse, attacking each other, or demoralizing patient.

Patient and Family Education

- Provide specific information about patient's illness and care needs such as pamphlets, videos, and other patient education materials. Make sure these materials match family members' reading level and language.

- Review with family what to expect from patient's illness and how this may impact communication and coping within the family. Let them know that family problems can either get worse or better during this time of stress.
- Reinforce the need for the family to maintain own self-care routines and to be aware of signs of stress that may lead them to being sick.
- Provide information on support groups and group education programs.
- Work with caregivers to develop routines that will make the care as easy as possible. For example, setting up the patient's room at home on the first floor of a two-story house will reduce the caregiver's need to go up and down stairs all day.
- Prepare family for possible course of the illness and anticipated changes in care.
- If the family is planning to hire help, provide suggestions on identifying and managing possible problems, such as the attendant not showing up for work on time or not caring for patient appropriately.

Charting Tips

- Describe which family members visit the patient and the interactions that occur.
- Document information on family structure, whom patient lives with, and care resources available.
- Document teaching given to family and include their response to any education given.
- Describe caregiver's ability to provide patient care.
- Document family awareness of the patient's condition and diagnosis.

Discharge Planning

- Involve family in the discharge plan early in the treatment.
- Provide specific referrals for additional help in the home or alternate care options.
- Provide specific information on appropriate support groups, such as for family members of Alzheimer's dis-

ease, stroke, or drug abuse. Also give information on hot-lines or other agencies that may be useful.
- Make sure social worker is involved, and consider social work evaluation in the home as well.
- Refer family to a family therapist, if appropriate.
- Identify appropriate equipment that will be needed in the home to provide care (for example, oxygen, hospital bed, wheelchair). Assist in making arrangements for delivery or refer to social service.
- Communicate with home health agency regarding family communication problems and conflicts that may impact care.
- Consider a home health referral after patient is discharged from the hospital to assess caregiver's ability to provide care.

Nursing Outcomes
- Staff will demonstrate appropriate assessments and interventions with families.
- Staff will provide adequate education to families and caregivers.
- Staff will demonstrate nonjudgmental care to families.

Suggested Learning Activities
- Arrange for an inservice from a family therapist to discuss role of family therapy.
- Obtain family therapy videotape if possible to observe the therapy process and observe family dynamics.
- Attend support groups that focus on a family's coping with a particular condition.
- Obtain information from the National Alliance for the Mentally Ill for caregivers of psychiatric patients (703) 524-7600 and the National Family Caregivers Association (301) 942-6430.

Family Violence

LEARNING OBJECTIVES

▼ *Identify suspicious signs of child abuse, domestic violence, and elder abuse.*
▼ *Discuss common traits of victims of any type of abuse.*
▼ *Discuss common traits of abusers.*
▼ *Identify common nurses' reactions to abuse.*

Family violence may be America's number one public health issue, yet many nurses caring for victims of family violence are often unaware that it is occurring within the family. Child abuse, domestic violence, and elder abuse can lead to lifelong emotional and physical problems for the victims and tears away at the very fabric of society as a whole.

Victims are often too fearful or ashamed to report

Glossary

Abuse—Willful infliction of physical injury or mental anguish and the deprivation by the caregiver of essential services.

Physical abuse—Deliberate violent actions that inflict pain and/or nonaccidental injury.

Sexual abuse—Occurs when the victimizer uses the victim for sexual gratification and the victim is unable to resist or consent. This includes rape and developmentally inappropriate sexual contact, incest, and using a child for prostitution or pornography.

Incest—Any type of exploitive sexual experience between relatives or surrogate relatives before a victim reaches 18 years of age.

Neglect—Deliberate deprivation of necessary and available resources, such as medical or dental care.

Psychologic abuse—Deliberate and willful destruction or significant impairment of a person's sense of competence by battering the victim's self-esteem and inhibiting normal psychosocial development.

Developmental neglect—Failure to provide emotional nurturing and stimulate physical and cognitive development.

Economic abuse—Using another's resources for one's own personal gain without permission.

Domestic violence (spousal abuse)—Intentionally inflicting or threatening physical injury or cruelty to one's partner.

abuse, become adept at hiding the signs, or use massive denial to convince themselves that the abuse is not that bad so that a violent family situation often goes unnoticed by outsiders. Healthcare professionals must be vigilant to the overt and covert signs of abuse. Every state mandates that suspected child abuse be reported and some states are enacting similar laws for domestic violence and elder abuse. The Joint Commission on Accreditation of Healthcare Organizations (JCAHO) also now requires that standards for identifying and providing services to victims of child abuse, domestic violence, and elder abuse be in place.

Child abuse includes physical and emotional abuse, neglect, and sexual abuse and occurs in all socioeconomic levels. Though statistics are difficult to attain, it is estimated that at least 1.5 million American children are abused each year by their parents or caretakers (Kashani, 1992), and homicide is the leading cause of death in children under age 4. Reported cases of child abuse have steadily increased over the last few years but there are many cases that are not reported.

Victims of child abuse are at an increased risk of becoming abusers as adults. Even though the child may hate the abusive situation, he or she never gets an opportunity to observe healthy parenting or to learn adaptive coping mechanisms to deal with frustration without violence. Other long-term effects include low self-esteem, high risk for substance abuse, tendency toward depression, difficulty trusting in close relationships, and violent lifestyle including crime.

Girls are the most frequent victims of sexual abuse. Long-term effects of sexual abuse include fear of intimacy, sexual problems, eating disorders, and an overwhelming sense of powerlessness. Victims may block out the memory of these incidents until later in life when a major event or trauma triggers memory recall. While false accusations of abuse have received much publicity in the past few years, any accusation must be investigated thoroughly.

Domestic violence most often refers to men abusing their female partners. This is an enormous societal problem. Like child abuse, it is found in all socioeconomic levels. It is the single largest cause of injury in women (Novello and Soto-Torres, 1992). Victims of abuse can endure physical, emotional, and sexual abuse. Abuse may increase if the woman becomes pregnant, if the abuser perceives competition from the baby. The battered woman syndrome refers to the common personality characteristics of these victims. These women are often economically dependent on their spouse or partner, exhibit very low self-esteem, and believe that they somehow deserve the abuse. Pediatrician offices may be the first to identify this victim because the woman often will not seek medical attention for herself but will take her children. In addition, many times when there is domestic violence in the home, the children are also victims of abuse or neglect. Fifteen percent of all homicide victims are spouses (Novello and Soto-Torres, 1992). The victim of the abuse may be the killer in retaliation for past abuse.

One of the most frequently misunderstood factors in domestic violence is why these women remain with the abusers. It is important to understand that these women often feel trapped and have little money, resources, or support, and fear being killed or losing or potential injury to their children. Permeating all these factors is the overwhelming sense of powerlessness.

Elder abuse includes physical, sexual, and emotional abuse, neglect, and the exploitation of the person's financial reserves by family, hired help, or strangers. This problem is greatly underreported and will continue to increase as the population grows older. One problem in reporting it is inconsistent laws defining elder abuse. Some states do not include neglect or psychologic abuse in their definition so it is essential to be aware of how elder abuse is defined in the state where you are working or reside. Because the abuser is often the victim's caregiver, including elderly spouse, victims rarely report the abuse. They fear reprisals or abandonment since they are dependent on the caregiver. Society's lack of interest in the elderly may add to the underreporting.

Etiology

There are similarities in all types of family violence (see Table 17–1). Family history of abuse remains the most common thread. Childhood exposure to abuse increases a gen-

TABLE 17–1. **Characteristics of Victims**

Type of Victim	Characteristics
Child All ages, with greatest risk under age 5 (including infants) and for fatalities under 2 years of age	• Incest generally begins after 9 years old • Self-blame for family conflict • Low self-esteem • Fear of parent or caretaker • Cheating, lying, low achievement in school • Signs of depression, helplessness • One child sometimes singled out in family due to being labeled as "difficult," product of unwanted pregnancy, reminds the parents of someone they dislike or even themselves, prematurity (inhibited parent-child bonding)
Spouse	• Low self-esteem • Self-blame for batterer's actions • Sense of helplessness to escape abuse • Isolation from family and friends • Views self as subservient to partner • Economic dependence on abuser
Elder	• Over 75 years old • Mentally and/or physically impaired • Isolated from others

eral sense of low self-esteem and reduced ability to deal with frustration as well as lack of role models to learn to interact in a healthy relationship. Another similarity is the presence of a vulnerable victim.

Various theories examine what causes a person to abuse another. *Psychologic* theory suggests that abuse provides the abuser with a sense of power and prestige that boosts one's self-image. The abuser hates the vulnerable powerless feelings within himself or herself and is able to block them out by creating (transferring) these denegrated feelings in others.

Sociocultural views examine the role of violence in our society. With easy access to weapons and the frequent exposure to violence from the media, potential abusers can identify violence as a socially acceptable coping mechanism. Another contributing factor is that abusers are often isolated with limited resources for assistance and very often have problems with drug and alcohol abuse.

Additional traits that contribute to child abuse include a parent who sees himself or herself in the child, child not meeting parent's expectations, and the parent's viewing the child as being there to satisfy the parent's needs. At times, a parent has no tolerance for normal child behaviors, such as crying, because of the past experience of being unable to express these needs in childhood. So the child's normal behavior reminds the parent of his or her own unmet childhood needs and unresolved anger toward his or her own parents. There is also a very high correlation with drug and alcohol abuse in this parent. The other parent is usually aware of the abuse but remains unable or unwilling to intervene. That parent may unconsciously deny the existence of abuse and is often a victim of spousal abuse. Step-parents may also be abusers as hostility for the new mate or previous spouse is projected on the child. Incest in the family may be related to sexual problems between husband and wife.

Domestic violence tends to escalate when the abuser is intoxicated. He often displays tremendous jealousy and fears losing his wife. At the same time he may blame his wife for his own problems. Inflicting injury on the woman gives the abuser a temporary sense of power and esteem. Other factors contributing to domestic violence include the victim's lack of financial support, belief that the children need both parents, and lack of a social support system.

As noted earlier, elder abusers are often caregivers. These abusers often have limited coping mechanisms, limited support, and are emotionally and financially dependent on the elderly person. Most often they live with the elderly victim. At times, family members can become abusers as resentment about the elder's dependency increases as well as retribution for perceived parent failures when younger.

Walker (1979) identified the *cycle theory of family violence*. This theory includes the following stages:

1. *Tension building stage:* Minor incidents of pushing, shoving, and verbal abuse occur.
2. *Acute battering stage:* Built-up tension is released by the abuser on the victim, leading to more brutal and uncontrollable abuse. Afterwards, the abuser often does not remember the intensity of the incident. The victim is often able to remember the incident in detail without the emotion.
3. *Honeymoon stage:* The abusers sense of remorse leads to a period of apology and attempts to make up for the abuse by presents, special treats, and affection. The victim is finally receiving the love and attention she or he so wants and desperately desires to believe there will be no further abuse. This may allow the victim to forgive the abuser and even drop legal proceedings or plans to report the abuse. Unfortunately, this stage is usually short-lived, and without intervention, becomes even briefer over time. The intensity and frequency of the cycle and severity of injuries tend to increase over time.

Related Clinical Concerns

Neurologic impairment and substance abuse can trigger the abuse cycle by disinhibiting impulse control in the abuser. Illness may be a risk factor to becoming a victim. Resentments may build from caregiving responsibilities when the potential victim is dependent on the potential abuser. In addition, more violence may be inflicted on the developmentally challenged child.

Possible Nurses' Reactions

- The most common reaction is anger and disgust directed at the abuser. These strong negative feelings can cloud the nurse's assessment and judgment and interfere with selecting appropriate interventions for the abuser.
- The nurse may feel great sympathy for the victims.
- The nurse may also feel anger toward the battered woman who displays powerlessness. May blame her for staying with the abuser or being helpless and become angry if she does not take advice offered.
- The nurse may feel overwhelmed with the family prob-

lems and helpless to change it, especially if possible victim denies abuse.
- The nurse may feel intense sadness and distress, which could lead to the wish to save or "rescue" the victim. The nurse may act out these feelings by making promises to the victim that in reality cannot be met or could create an unsafe situation for both of them. This could isolate the victim even more.
- Because abuse may be so upsetting, the nurse may deny evidence or refuse to believe it, especially sexual abuse.
- The nurse may fear reporting abuse because of fear of getting involved, possible legal implications, or reprisals from abusers. The nurse may not want to be responsible for displacing the victim from the family. (Note most states have Good Samaritan clauses in abuse laws that protect healthcare professionals from liability in reporting.)
- The nurse may be intimidated by abuser.
- The nurse may identify with the victim or abuser if he or she has had personal experience with abuse.

Assessment

CHILD ABUSE

CHILD BEHAVIORS
- History of injury inconsistent with child's developmental level (for example, baby turning on hot water)
- Failure to thrive; dull or inactive demeanor
- Signs of malnutrition, poor hygiene, or lack of health care
- Fears discussing how injuries occurred
- Lack of reaction to frightening events (for example, being given an injection) as child has learned to hide fear
- Unusual injuries such as cigarette burns, rope burns, spiral fractures from twisting injury, or bite marks
- May demonstrate magical thinking that doctor or nurse will know family secret
- Fear of returning home
- Apprehension when hearing a child cry because thinks another child is being hurt
- Antisocial behavior, such as lying and stealing

- Wearing inappropriate clothing that covers bruises
- Bruises or bleeding in external genitalia
- Torn, bloody underclothing
- Pain on urination or frequent urinary tract infections
- Abnormal discharge or odor in genital area, indications of sexually transmitted diseases
- Pregnancy in young child or adolescent
- Sudden onset of sexually related behavior, such as excessive masturbation, age inappropriate sex play, or overseductive behavior
- Child being given a variety of gifts or privileges
- Change in behavior including depression, anxiety, regression, running away from home, substance abuse, or decline in school performance

PARENTAL BEHAVIORS
- Exaggerated or absent reaction to child's injury
- Failure to show empathy for child
- Inconsistent explanations of injuries
- Care sought for child's minor complaints but not for more obvious illness
- Demands to take child home if pressured for answers or refuses hospitalization
- Explanations do not match injuries; attempts to blame the child
- Nonabusing parent may refuse to acknowledge even obvious abuse (see Table 17–2).

DOMESTIC VIOLENCE

VICTIM
- Injuries to head, abdomen, breasts, genitalia
- Injuries while pregnant
- Patterns left by item used to cause injury such as rope or teeth
- Frequent urinary tract infections
- Mother of abused child
- History of rape
- Lack of care for own chronic illness
- Demonstrates guilt for seeking treatment
- Use of alcohol or tranquilizers to cover hurt

TABLE 17–2. **General Warning Signs of Abuse**

> - Delay in seeking treatment for injuries, minimizing injuries
> - History of being accident prone
> - Pattern of injuries not accidental looking, for example, identical burns on bottom of feet, identical injuries on both sides of head
> - Multiple injuries in varying stages of healing
> - Conflicting stories from victim and abuser about cause of injury
> - Inconsistency between history and injury
> - Unusual, even bizarre explanation for injuries
> - Repeated visits to emergency rooms or clinics
> - Previous report of abuse
> - Patient reporting abuse
> - Patient fearful of caregiver or partner
> - Visits variety of doctors, emergency rooms for treatment

- Indicates acceptance of violence as a way to maintain her family
- Socially isolated with limited financial resources and family support
- Implies a sense of deserving abuse
- Stress-related complaints of headaches, insomnia, nervousness
- Wearing clothes and makeup to cover up bruises
- Denies abuse or gives explanations that do not match injury

ABUSER
- Minimizes injuries even when they become life threatening
- Speaks for victim or doesn't let her speak
- Controlling, angry
- Does not want victim to be alone with healthcare providers
- Tends to isolate victim by eliminating her social support system
- Insists on taking patient back home even if inappropriate
- Criticizes or humiliates the victim in front of others
- Access to guns, other weapons

TABLE 17–3. **Interviewing an Abuser or Abuse Victim**

Do	Don't
Conduct the interview in private.	Conduct the interview with a group of interviewers.
Be direct, honest, and professional.	Try to prove abuse by accusations and demands.
Be understanding.	Display horror, anger, shock, or disapproval of the abuser or the situation.
Be attentive.	
Inform the patient before making the referral to child or adult protective services and explain the process.	Place blame or make judgments about the abuser or the victim.
Assess for risk of danger and help reduce that risk before discharge.	Allow the victim to feel "at fault" or "in trouble."
	Probe or press for answers the victim is not willing to give.
For Children	
Tell the child that the interview is confidential.	Force the child to remove clothing.
Use age-specific language.	
Ask the child to clarify his or her meaning or words you do not understand.	
Tell the child whether any future action will be required.	

Source: Reproduced with permission. Smith-Dijulio, K, and Holzapfel, SK: Families in crisis: Family violence. In Varcarolis, EM (ed): Foundations of Psychiatric-Mental Health Nursing. WB Saunders, Philadelphia, 1994.

- Rationalizes his actions ("she deserved it") (see Table 17–3)

ELDER ABUSE

VICTIM

- Evidence of malnutrition, dehydration, poor hygiene, decubitus, not receiving needed medical care
- Unusual injuries such as twisting fractures, cigarette

burns on face or back, perforated eardrums from being slapped
- Evidence of sexually transmitted diseases, unusual genital injuries
- Deterioration in mental status including confusion and depression
- Sudden lack of funds in someone who previously had resources
- Frail, dependent, possible mental impairment requiring care from family member or hired help
- Extreme dependency, attachment to new caregiver
- Evidence of inappropriate use of restraints

ABUSER
- Often lives with victim, lacks resources to live elsewhere
- Refusal to allow diagnostic tests, hospitalization
- Much younger than patient
- Cashes victim's social security and/or pension checks
- Sudden, intense involvement with patient with little input from other family members
- Evidence of drug or alcohol abuse
- Expects dependent elder to meet his or her needs
- Caregiver overwhelmed with patient's care needs, demonstrates frustration and resentment, isolated with limited assistance
- Elderly spouse with dementia
- Coerces senior to change will to his or her benefit
- Shows no guilt or rationalizes actions

Collaborative Management

Psychotherapy

Individual and/or group psychotherapy are often used to treat both victims and abusers. For the victim, individual therapy may focus on the damage done to self-esteem and facing and resolving intense emotions toward the abuser, as well as toward others who may have tolerated the abuse (often the other parent in child abuse). The victim should be removed from living with the abuser before entering treatment to reduce the fear of retaliation. In spousal abuse, therapists often recommend the couple separate for a period of time before starting treatment.

Repressed, traumatic events of the past, such as childhood sexual abuse, may be uncovered during therapy. This repressed abuse could be influencing the patient's current life without his or her knowledge. However, this is very controversial since repressed memories have been found to be inaccurate. Group therapy may also allow the victim to learn from other victims and develop assertive skills.

More intensive psychotherapy or psychiatric treatment may be required for the abuser if psychopathology is suspected.

Because family violence is a symptom of family dysfunction, family therapy is often part of the overall treatment plan. When children are in the home where abuse has occurred, they must be part of the healing process. In addition, support group programs are available for both victims and abusers.

Nursing Management

INEFFECTIVE FAMILY COPING: DISABLING EVIDENCED BY CHILD ABUSE RELATED TO HISTORY OF ABUSE IN THE FAMILY, LACK OF RESOURCES, ISOLATION.

Child Outcomes

* Remains free from injury or neglect
* Seeks comfort and assistance from nurse

Parent Outcomes

* Seeks assistance for abusive behavior
* Demonstrates nurturing behavior toward child
* Refrains from abusive behavior

Interventions

* Establish a trusting relationship with child and parents. Avoid threatening behavior or criticizing parents in front of child.

- Observe parent-child interaction closely, especially when they are under stress. Observe caring and feeding behavior. In the home, observe sleeping arrangements and environmental conditions.
- Recognize that the child very often will not betray his or her parents. Even in the worst situations, the child may fear losing the only security he or she knows and consequently, will deny any problems.
- Involve the child in treatment plan to increase his or her sense of control.
- Demonstrate support, acceptance, and affection of the child. Reinforce child's self esteem by positive feedback and recognition.
- If child needs discipline, discuss punishment, and clarify that no physical abuse will be used. Consider referral for psychiatric or play therapy evaluation to better understand what is being expressed.
- Encourage play. Be aware that child may be better able to express feelings through play.
- Reinforce parent's strengths, and acknowledge importance of continuing medical care for the child.
- Reinforce positive parenting behavior. Role model caregiving behaviors for them.
- Avoid hostility toward the parents. At the same time maintain the child's safety. If child is at risk for being taken inappropriately by parents, have staff remain in attendance with security nearby and inform the parents of your reasons for doing so.
- Be aware of agency policy, and state laws on reporting suspected child abuse. Contact supervisor and/or social worker to implement appropriate reporting. Participate in collecting evidence, as indicated, and ensure that proper procedures are followed.
- Be sure that supervisors, physicians, and social services are informed when a suspected abuse is reported.

INEFFECTIVE FAMILY COPING: DISABLING EVIDENCED BY SPOUSAL VIOLENCE RELATED TO VULNERABLE VICTIM, ABUSER WITH HISTORY OF ABUSE IN HIS FAMILY, ISOLATED, LIMITED RESOURCES, INTENSE JEALOUSY.

Victim Outcomes

- Acknowledges the abuse
- Identifies options to escape abuser
- Remains in treatment even if pressured to not obtain care

Abuser Outcomes

- Seeks assistance for abusive behavior
- Refrains from harming others

Interventions

- Establish a trusting relationship with the abused woman. Avoid displaying shock or disgust at her story. Encourage her to share her fears and concerns. Ask specific questions to avoid a vague response.
- Assess the victim's safety. If there is a risk, implement agency security policies, as appropriate. If in the hospital, phone calls and visitors can be restricted. For patients at home, determine need to involve the police and information on legal restraining orders. If there are children in the home, determine their risk of injury. Be aware of state and agency policies for reporting domestic violence.
- Reinforce victim's self-esteem. Identify positive traits and coping mechanisms that she has been using. Encourage her to talk about accomplishments and goals.
- Encourage victim's participation in treatment plan. Help her take control of some areas of her life and make some decisions.
- If possible, identify available support systems and determine their awareness of family's problems. Encourage patient to involve some people in her life. Encourage her to maintain regular social contacts.
- Encourage her to realistically evaluate her partner and situation. Do not reinforce denial or avoidance.
- Be aware that during the "Honeymoon Stage" the victim may not be willing to discuss abuse. Describe the cycle of abuse to the victim. Give the victim written information on resources to use at another time.
- Encourage problem solving. Challenge her to identify realistic options, and reinforce all efforts to be assertive.

- Encourage her to talk about events that led up to the abusive event. Dispel any myths of guilt or responsibility for causing or deserving the abuse.
- Be sure that supervisors, physicians, and social services are informed when a suspected abuse is reported.

INEFFECTIVE FAMILY COPING: DISABLING EVIDENCED BY ELDER ABUSE RELATED TO MULTIPLE STRESSORS ASSOCIATED WITH ELDER CARE.

Elder Outcomes

- Identifies resources available for assistance
- Remains safe and without injury
- Continues to receive adequate health care

Caregiver Outcomes

- Identifies resources available for assistance in patient care
- Demonstrates more effective coping mechanisms
- Provides safe care to the elderly patient

Interventions

- Assess the elderly patient's condition and determine the role of caregiver in providing adequate care. Patients with decubitus ulcers, dehydration, lacerations, and bruises need to be evaluated; however, be aware that these may occur unrelated to abuse or neglect.
- If abuse is suspected, talk with patient and caregiver separately. With the patient, listen to his or her description of the caregiver and any complaints he or she may have. Then, verify the information, if possible, with the caregiver, other family members, or healthcare providers. Establish a trusting relationship with the caregiver by acknowledging positive accomplishments, as well as the stress of caregiving.
- If signs of abuse occur in a long-term care facility, observe patient care routines and the care of other patients. Note the use of restraints and the quality of hygiene provided. If patient is being left alone while restrained, ac-

tion must be taken immediately to stop this unsafe practice.

* Recognize that patients with altered mental status may falsely accuse caregivers of abuse. However, every accusation must be evaluated.
* Encourage the patient to be as independent as possible by remaining involved with family and friends, having his or her own telephone, and having neighbors check his or her status regularly. Appropriate independence will also promote self-esteem and self-reliance. Even in the highly dependent patient, it is important to maintain the individual's sense of control.
* Encourage problem-solving skills in patient and caregiver. Promote their abilities to find alternate solutions under stress.
* If patient is in an unsafe environment, implement agency policies and state laws as appropriate to determine reporting mechanism and action. If patient refuses to leave environment, determine patient's ability to make decisions. Involve physician, and/or social worker, as needed. Consider psychiatric evaluation. Involve family and friends if needed to encourage patient action.
* Determine caregiver's stress level, and determine if additional resources are available and would defuse the situation.
* Be sure that supervisors, physicians, and social services are informed when a suspected abuse is reported.

ALTERNATE NURSING DIAGNOSES

Altered family processes
Altered parenting
Caregiver role strain
High risk for violence
Knowledge deficit
Noncompliance
Posttrauma response
Powerlessness
Rape trauma syndrome

Patient and Family Education

* Teach effective parenting skills, including appropriate discipline. Abusive parents need skills in disciplining

children without violence and often need to learn acceptable outlets for their frustration.

- Incorporate assertive skills to teach potential victims, including young children, to speak up when rights are violated and learn to say no.
- Teach family members the signs of abuse and how to report it.
- Teach a victim of domestic violence to identify a plan in advance to leave her home, when needed. This plan should include having a place to go, setting aside money, and implementing security measures for herself and her children.
- When children must be removed from their home, prepare them for the emotional grief response that may occur when they are separated from their parents. No matter how bad the home was, children will still grieve. Be sure they understand that they are not being punished.
- Suspected abusers need information on alternative ways to resolve conflicts. If appropriate, refer them to counselors who specialize in abuse who can educate them on the role of substance abuse and violence.
- Review with victims and abusers the need to involve family and friends for assistance.

Charting Tips

- If abuse is suspected, carefully document, possibly with photos, any evidence of wounds, injuries, or poor hygiene. Follow institutional protocols carefully if called upon to participate in evidence collection.
- Document the nature of interactions between victim and abuser.
- Note victim's reaction to the abuser especially when discharging patient.
- Document victim's report of abuse.
- Document interventions made including reporting abuse and maintaining patient safety.

WHEN TO CALL FOR HELP

✔ Aggressive, belligerent behavior escalates to violence.

✔ Presence of abuser leads patient to fear of violence or of being kidnapped.
✔ Abuser is intoxicated.
✔ Abuser intimidates patient or staff.
✔ Victim leaves healthcare agency to return to unsafe environment.

Discharge Planning

* Provide written information on appropriate resources including: parenting support groups such as Parents Anonymous; parenting education programs; shelters; safe-houses; 24-hour local crisis hotlines for abuse or National Child Abuse Hotline (800-422-4453); and National Organization for Victim Assistance (800-TRY-NOVA). If abuse is suspected and patient denies it, provide the information, and encourage patient to keep it in a safe place.
* Provide information on legal referrals and security measures. If police are involved, reinforce information they give to patient.
* As appropriate, refer patient for counseling or family therapy.
* Refer for home health follow-up to assess home environment. Inform all referring agencies of concerns over abuse. Vocational counseling information may be helpful to the domestic violence victim.
* Anticipate caregiver needs in the home, and provide adequate support and equipment.
* Discuss day-care options for children or elderly.

Nursing Outcomes

* Staff demonstrates nonjudgmental approach in working with victim and abuser.
* Staff report all suspected abuse per agency policy and state law.
* Staff provides safe environment for the victim.
* Staff follows agency policies on reporting abuse.

Suggested Learning Activities

* Arrange for inservice by abuse specialists and counsellors.

- Consider attending Parents Anonymous support group or other support groups for victims or abusers where possible.
- Arrange to spend time with local child or elder abuse teams at social service or law enforcement agencies.
- Contact American Association of Retired Persons (AARP) for information on elder abuse.
    - Contact abuse hotlines.
    - Visit local women's shelters or foster child placements if possible.

18

PROBLEMS WITH SPIRITUAL DISTRESS

The Patient With Spiritual Distress

LEARNING OBJECTIVES

▼ *Define spiritual distress.*
▼ *Identify some life event and physical changes that may precipitate spiritual distress.*
▼ *Differentiate between religion and spirituality.*
▼ *Identify effective interventions for dealing with an individual experiencing spiritual distress.*
▼ *Describe common nurses' reactions to patients' spiritual distress.*

All people have a spiritual dimension regardless of whether they participate in formal religious practices. Spiritual distress is an existential crisis in which the beliefs or values around which the person has organized his or her life are threatened. Parents' belief system may be shaken when they learn that their child has an incurable illness or will not recover from an accident. For individuals, it can be learning of a life-threatening illness. When faced with these situations, you may hear an individual say "Life will never be the same" or "How can we go on living?" The very foundation of their life as they know it is threatened. They may no longer feel safe and able to go about their everyday activities. Some may question their belief in God.

Spiritual distress may manifest itself in many different ways. Individuals are a complexity of biologic, psychologic, sociocultural, and spiritual parts, all interacting and affecting all other aspects of the individual's life. When caring for someone in this time of specialization, it is important to keep in mind that an insult to one's spiritual

---

Glossary

Spirituality—Beliefs of individuals which permeate all areas of their life and influence attitudes, beliefs, values, and health.

Spiritual distress—A disturbance in the belief or value system that is a personal source of strength and hope; may be accompanied by an inability to carry out religious practices, possibly creating even more stress because the individual cannot use spirituality to cope with stress.

Chaplain—Clergy who has a formal relationship with a particular health organization.

Spiritual leaders—Officers and persons who provide spiritual support, including chaplains, priests, ministers, rabbis, monks, pastors, elders, deacons, mullahs, or hajjis.

Religion—A system of beliefs, worship, or conduct. Generally refers to formal, institutionalized practices.

dimension can affect every other dimension of the individual and influence the patient's experience of illness.

Spiritual distress occurs when a person believes that life no longer has meaning or purpose or experiences a sense of hopelessness. Like many other entities that can be viewed on a continuum, spiritual distress may be a temporal, transient phenomenon that is a response to a specific stressor or it may be a longer-reaching event prompting the individual to question or reexamine assumptions and priorities. In a few rare instances, extreme spiritual distress may indicate psychopathology.

In many ways, spiritual distress can be compared to the grief response. Grief of small losses may be short term, and with proper support, recovery will be rapid. Great losses affect the individual more profoundly and can be seen in changes in the person's mood, affect, energy level, interest in life, and somatic condition. In the most extreme pathologic grief, in which individuals are not recovering, their ability to carry out activities of daily living is greatly reduced and may sometimes require psychiatric hospitalization.

Both grief and spiritual distress deal with loss. The major difference is that spiritual distress disrupts the meaning which governs a person's life. There may be a perceived or real deterioration or collapse in his or her relationship with a supreme divine being, or with persons who represent the supreme being.

The presence of stressors does not necessarily predict or cause spiritual distress. The Chinese character for crisis, which is a combination of the symbols for danger and opportunity, helps one to understand this. For some individuals, a stressor or crisis, such as a life-threatening illness or tragedy, can ultimately become the source of a tremendously positive experience. While they readily acknowledge that they would have never chosen such events, they ultimately view them not as traumatic events but as opportunities for growth. In some ways, it parallels a wilderness experience. The arduous physical demands allow an individual to transcend his or her immediate surroundings and experience a sense of empowerment resulting in being better equipped to handle the challenges of life.

Nurses may feel uncomfortable or experience conflict when providing spiritual support if the patient is religious and the nurse is not or if the patient's spirituality differs from his or her own. These are normal responses to the unknown. How one responds to a patient's spiritual needs will depend both on one's education and background. It is important, however, not to evaluate the patient's value system by personal standards.

Certain nursing settings, such as hospice, require incorporating a spiritual assessment. Nurses who work or have worked in this type of setting are often more comfortable responding to spiritual distress.

Etiology

Spiritual distress occurs when particular stressors or life events threaten the individual's belief system as well as impact biologic, psychologic, sociocultural, and spiritual aspects of life. These stressors may be unique to the individual, or they may be similar to reactions experienced by others after certain events. Crisis or loss may have a variety of causes including loss of a significant person, employment, position, or status; financial reversal; or major illness or loss of a body part, or a change in self image. In some cultures it may also result from shame. However, what is lost is not as important as the value that the individual ascribes to it.

Cognitive theory looks at the role of beliefs on feelings, and *psychodynamic* theory helps one understand the underlying process of spiritual distress. For instance, when a person believes that he or she could never be forgiven, a great deal of spiritual distress can be experienced even to the point of affecting physical health. One's belief in the ability to be forgiven may be associated with his or her perception of how others show approval. The individual may accept forgiveness from God or a higher power in the manner forgiveness was accepted from parents since the dynamics of one's relationship with God or a higher power is often similar to the relationship with his or her parents.

Psychologic theories look at the various dynamics that can result in spiritual distress. A person with a high degree of inner strength, or ego functioning, may experience less spiritual distress in response to a loss than one who has a lower level of ego functioning. How one normally adapts to crises and change will also influence the risk of spiritual distress. Persons who are inflexible may have more difficulty accepting major changes. Similarly, individuals prone to anxiety, in the face of major change, may feel overwhelmed and have difficulty dealing with it.

Crisis theory considers not only the normal changes in life and life event stressors but also looks at the impact of disaster or massive crisis for the individual. Faith or a belief system may help a person cope with a crisis, but if the crisis is of a high magnitude, the person may feel that his or her belief system is challenged or inadequate and may be of little help.

One of the hallmarks of a disaster or massive crisis, such as a devastating hurricane, earthquake, or crash of an airplane, is the enormous sense of the individual's loss of control and extreme feelings of vulnerability. There may be a sense of betrayal, and the events may be expressed as not being "right." The individual reveals a sense of how things "should" be, his or her expectation of the world. The sense of betrayal and anger may be expressed in spiritual terms— "How can God let this happen"—toward God or their higher power.

A sense of mastery over one's environment, highly prized in American culture, is threatened when a major crisis occurs. No longer feeling safe in usual activities, a feeling of unease can spread to other areas of life. Hypervigilence may be a result. Many disturbing responses can be seen as normal responses to abnormal events.

Related Clinical Concerns

Although identifiable traumatic events may precipitate spiritual distress, it is important to be aware of physiologic conditions that may exacerbate the situation.

While there is no clear relationship between specific disease entities and spiritual distress, a spiritual state can be influenced by biologic changes, such as changes in neurotransmitters, endocrine levels, or blood chemistry. Just as there are differences in coping mechanisms, there are differences in how the individual as an organism responds to illness. Even when an event appears to be a precipitant for spiritual distress, biologic factors could also be at work. A complete physical assessment and other supporting tests can help determine biologic factors.

Psychoactive substances can influence mood and consequently the way the individual perceives the situation and how well he or she functions in responding to it. Nurses need to be aware of the many prescription drugs that have similar effects, such beta-blockers, steroids, antihypertensives, immunosuppressants, and chemotherapy.

Certain diseases, such as multiple sclerosis and AIDS, not only cause significant physiologic changes but also have the potential to cause overwhelming spiritual distress because of the meaning of the illness and the possibility of dying.

Lifespan Issues

CHILDHOOD

Since the belief system of young children is not as developed as the adult, children may not be able to adequately verbalize their sense of spiritual distress. Instead, they may present with such physical symptoms as weight loss, failure to thrive, and reversing developmental milestones. Most frequently their stress is in response to loss of a parent or caretaker or major change affecting a parent or caretaker. The child can sense the distress of the parent. For example, a young child may not fully understand the impact of death, but he or she can sense, and be negatively affected by, the tremendous distress the loss of a child or spouse can have on his or her caretaker. The child often responds by being more clinging or dependent at times of crisis.

Signs of distress in older children may be more subtle. Some children experiencing depression may act out in different ways. Behavioral problems may be exacerbated. It is important to pay attention to subtle changes in a child, such as a lack of interest in usual pursuits, withdrawal or isolation, or a decrease in school performance. One of the most traumatic events for children is either loss of parents or siblings by death or divorce. Children may mistakenly believe that they personally caused the loss of the parent and may not comprehend other dynamics at work.

Children's spiritual and/or religious beliefs are strongly influenced by those of the parents. More questioning tends to occur as adolescence approaches.

ADOLESCENCE

Adolescents are generally more able to articulate distress, but they may be hesitant to confide in an adult. More aware of complexities of life and often having a strong personal moral code, they may be traumatized by idealized parental failings. Loss of parents, siblings, classmates, or acquaintances by death, divorce, or relocation can be tremendously stressful events for the adolescent. Youths whose sexual orientation differs from parental or societal expectation may either act out or experience their crisis in secret. Other traumatic events include sexual exploitation from peers or adults. Even though pregnancy during teen years is rising, it may be exceedingly traumatic for the individual. The teen must deal with the dilemma of pregnancy and the changes it will have on her life and confront disappointing parental expectations. The teen is also vulnerable to life's tragedies like death of a parent. This can lead to questioning spiritual beliefs and loss of hope.

Because adolescents are so impressionable and idealistic, they are very vulnerable to cults and religious conversions. The beginning recognition that life is not as ideal and perfect as they once believed may cause individuals to lose hope and question spiritual beliefs.

ELDERLY

This is a period that is characterized by extremes. Individuals are most distinct in their elder years. There is tremendous variety in functioning. Many individuals may experience death of spouse and friends as well as changes in residence. Some may rely more on their spiritual life as their acquaintances diminish and limitations grow.

Possible Nurses' Reactions

- May not feel comfortable or adequately prepared to help patients with spiritual concerns.

- May be influenced by his or her own background, beliefs, values, and experiences, which may differ from those of the patient.
- May react negatively, or judgmentally, or distance themselves from patients whose beliefs, practices, lifestyles, or cultures differ from their own.
- May focus attention on religious content rather than assessing other issues that may be the cause of anxiety.
- May attempt to change or argue with religious content of patient's beliefs.
- May feel powerless when unable to help patients with spiritual concerns. Nurses may distance themselves from these patients to cope with their own feelings of inadequacy.
- May not understand the meaning of the loss from the patient's spiritual perspective and may try to reassure the patient in ways that are not effective or meaningful.
- May resent clergy because of their closeness and ability to meet some patients' needs.
- Conversely, out of feelings of fear and inadequacy, may refer patients to the chaplain too quickly rather than attempt to deal with the concerns.
- May reassure patients based on their own knowledge of illnesses and fail to hear the patients' concerns.
- May discount the loss or crisis of a patient if in their view the patient "should" be able to deal with it.
- May feel judgmental about individuals, expressing spiritual concerns or practices especially if those concerns are unfamiliar to the nurse.
- May feel anxious when encountering unfamiliar practices.

Assessment

Behavior and/or Appearance

- Many religious items or literature at bedside
- Frequently quotes from the Bible or other spiritual literature
- May display exaggerated religious rituals or behavior such as reading the Bible excessively rather than talking
- May appear withdrawn and preoccupied with own beliefs

such as being unable to focus on conversations and events in immediate environment
- Makes constant reference to religious themes in conversation
- Asks frequent questions such as "Is this God's will?" "Why is God letting me suffer?"
- Lethargic; may exhibit a lack of interest in surroundings
- Overtly or passively suicidal
- Frequently questions others about their spiritual beliefs
- States spiritual beliefs are no longer comforting
- Behavior changes, such as increased alcohol use or acting out

Mood and/or Emotions

- Highly anxious
- Denial of emotions or concerns
- Expressions of bitterness or anger over perceived abandonment by God or belief that God is causing the suffering
- Appears depressed
- Expresses feelings of helplessness or hopelessness
- Lack of enjoyment and satisfaction in formerly pleasurable activities

Thoughts, Beliefs, and Perceptions

- Believes that nothing can help
- Exhibits global, all-or-nothing thinking
- Believes life is overwhelming and cannot continue living
- Questions long-held beliefs and may doubt his or her faith
- Believes he or she has committed unpardonable sins that cannot be forgiven
- Self-absorbed in own belief system
- Views self as guilty and in need of punishment
- Views self as spiritually superior to others
- Believes a higher power requires suffering and pain, and therefore patient refuses pain control measures
- Views self as having a great mission to accomplish
- Claims to hear voices of God, Moses, or other religious figures
- Holds omnipotent view of self—a specialness that rests in the inability to be forgiven by God or higher power

Relationships and Interactions

- Feels isolated and alone even in the presence of others
- Withdraws from others who do not share similar beliefs
- Change in relationship with family or friends who are involved with religious beliefs

TABLE 18–1. **Assessing for Spiritual Beliefs**

Initial Assessment
1. What is your source of strength and hope?
2. What is your religious affiliation, and how important is this in your life? Any recent changes?
3. Is there a minister or other appropriate religious leader available to you while in the hospital?
4. Are there any religious or spiritual practices that are important to you while in the hospital?
5. Are there any religious or spiritual articles that are important to you while in the hospital?
6. Is there any spiritual literature that is important to you while in the hospital?
Advanced Assessment
1. Has being sick or in the hospital made any difference in your feelings toward God or in your beliefs?
2. What has bothered you the most about being sick or in the hospital?
3. What helps you the most when you are afraid or in need of special help?
4. What religious or spiritual idea or concept is most important to you?
5. What did your family believe? What was meaningful and important to them?
6. What exposure, if any, did you have to religious or spiritual beliefs as a child? Has that changed? How?
7. Have your religious interests arisen gradually or out of a crisis?
8. Do you have special religious leaders? How do you view them?
9. What would help you maintain your spirituality?
10. Does prayer provide comfort for you? If you pray, about what do you pray? When do you pray?
11. What happens when you pray or meditate?

Physical Responses

- Reports increased discomforts
- Change in eating or sleeping patterns

Pertinent History

- Involvement in specific religious groups, cults, or in a variety of different religious groups (see Table 18–1)
- History of emotional disorders or emotionally charged prior situations, such as abortion or catastrophic events

Collaborative Management

Some healthcare agencies may have full-time chaplains on staff. Others may have volunteer chaplains or links to clergy in the community. Chaplains provide spiritual counseling and are often knowledgeable about community support resources that may be useful for the patient. Working with the social workers, they can help in making funeral arrangements or locating needed services or volunteers. Chaplains can help both patients and staff find ways to cope with the problem situation. However, not all patients hold clergy in high regard. Some can talk about spiritual concerns more effectively to a nurse. Others may view clergy negatively or with suspicion, depending on previous life experiences. Also, depending on the situation, the patient may prefer to share concerns with a clergy other than the one associated with where he or she worships.

Clergy are restricted on what information they can share with nursing staff and others. Similar to the professional privilege held by mental health professionals and lawyers, clergy are bound by professional ethics and law regarding what they may reveal that was told to them in confidence.

Nursing Management

SPIRITUAL DISTRESS EVIDENCED BY QUESTIONING BELIEFS, DESPAIR, OR INABILITY TO PRACTICE BELIEFS RELATED TO SUFFERING, ILLNESS OR HOSPITALIZATION.

Patient Outcomes

- Verbalizes "I feel better," "I feel relieved," "I feel at peace," or similar statements
- Demonstrates increased social interaction
- Reports feeling rested and comfortable
- Demonstrates reduced crying or other signs of distress

Interventions

- Empathize with patient's degree of pain or despair.
- Recognize that your own personal values and beliefs may not be effective for others. Be willing to set aside your own beliefs when analyzing the patient's spiritual needs.
- Become familiar with the patient's beliefs and practices.
- Use self-disclosure of own spiritual beliefs only to foster patient's therapeutic goals.
- Seek assistance of or referrals to hospital chaplain or other resources when uncomfortable or unable to meet the patient's spiritual needs.
- Promote use of prayer and scripture when appropriate if within patient's belief system (see Table 18–2).
- Become familiar with agency policy regarding praying with patients.
- Provide supportive, private environment to meet these spiritual needs.
- Substitute supportive response for prayer when the setting or timing is inappropriate.
- Work with patient and staff to adapt patient's schedule or activities to incorporate rituals whenever possible.
- Allow patient to ventilate thoughts and feelings. Explore what precipitated the feeling of loss. Help patient clarify any underlying feelings of guilt. Help the patient explore and evaluate whether the source is rational or distorted.
- Help patient explore previously held false assumptions and, as indicated, refer to spiritual passages affirming hope, if within the nurse's comfort and knowledge.
- Make referrals to appropriate support groups such as Bereaved Parents or Reach for Recovery.
- Allow family to participate in religious rituals such as ritual body care after death or baptism of a critically ill child.
- Be open to patient's expression of spiritual concerns.

TABLE 18–2. **Guidelines for Use of Prayer and Religious Literature**

1. Prayer combined with therapeutic use of self can be used to meet the patient's spiritual needs and show empathy. A therapeutic relationship must already be established with the patient before engaging in prayer, a more intimate form of communication.
2. Prayer can consist of simply sharing a few brief sentences to express an immediate need or can be taken from a formally written source.
3. The request for prayer and religious literature should be initiated by the patient. If you are not comfortable, discuss with colleagues other alternatives.
4. Ask the patient to define the specific needs for which he or she is requesting prayer.
5. Ask what passages the patient wants to read and how they are significant.
6. Validate expressed feelings such as pain, fear, anxiety, stress, helplessness, or anger at God.
7. Know that prayer can be an affirmation of God's presence and hope for the patient.
8. If reading from religious literature, select passages carefully. Consult with chaplain or other staff if in doubt. Some passages may be misinterpreted, be interpreted literally, or be beyond the level of this patient.

Avoid dismissing practices as inappropriate or pathologic.

SPIRITUAL DISTRESS EVIDENCED BY RELIGIOUS DELUSIONS OR OBSESSIONS RELATED TO IMPAIRED THOUGHT PROCESS.

Patient Outcomes

- Demonstrates improved reality orientation
- Verbalizes concerns and conflicts
- Verbalizes improved sense of well being
- Demonstrates appropriate social interactions

Interventions

- Become familiar with the norms of the patient's particular religious group to assess the patient's deviation from standard practice.

- Be aware that delusions may represent areas of personal conflict or concerns. For example, the Messiah complex may reveal that patient has a need to feel special, and dwelling on past sins may show that patient feels badly about self. Focus on feelings the patient is having rather than on content of delusion.
- Use great caution in reinforcing religious beliefs with psychotic patients as this may perpetuate reality distortions. Seek assistance from available mental health resources.
- Set limits on time spent talking about obsessions and performing ritualistic behavior with the patient. Make a contract regarding time you will listen. Be consistent.
- Encourage patient to discuss concerns other than religious issues. Bring patient back to recent specific experiences or events.
- Avoid arguing with the patient about the validity of his or her beliefs. Rather, acknowledge the feelings these beliefs may evoke such as fear or sadness.
- Recognize that reducing obsessional thoughts or compulsive behavior may result in increased anxiety or possibly even a panic reaction (see Chapter 7, Problems with Anxiety, for interventions). Discuss with the physician the need for evaluation by a mental health professional and appropriate medication.

HOPELESSNESS EVIDENCED BY DEPRESSION, APATHY, WITHDRAWAL, REJECTION OF SPIRITUAL BELIEFS RELATED TO LOSS, IMPENDING DEATH, INCURABLE DISEASE, LACK OF MEANING; SPIRITUAL CRISIS.

Patient Outcomes

- Verbalizes phrases like "I hadn't thought of it that way" or "I feel better"
- Demonstrates increased social interactions
- Able to identify one or more future goals

Interventions

- Encourage patient to share feelings and concerns and talk about what has triggered the sense of hopelessness.
- Maintain a concerned yet positive attitude around patient, but avoid an overly cheerful approach that may inhibit communication.

- Focus on short-term, concrete goals; identify specific things the patient can do now. For instance, focus on the pleasure of visiting with granddaughter today rather than the hope to be playing tennis next year. Make a plan with patient for achievable goals, such as sitting up in chair for 5 minutes longer today than yesterday. Often a patient may feel less hopeless and depressed if progress in one area can be achieved.
- Recognize that pain, fatigue, and other stressors will affect ability to maintain hope. Use interventions to deal with these stressors.
- Seek out chaplain to discuss patient's beliefs to help challenge hopelessness and support a more hopeful view.
- Recognize that with time to work through a loss or crisis, the patient may be able to focus on the future. Allow the patient the time to work through the grieving process.
- Be aware of your own anxiety around patient. Patient could sense your tension and think that his or her issues are unacceptable.

ALTERNATE NURSING DIAGNOSES

Altered thought processes
Anxiety
Grieving

WHEN TO CALL FOR HELP

✔ Patient is suicidal or homicidal.
✔ Religious practices severely interfere with health-care regimen.
✔ Patient becomes psychotic.

Patient and Family Education

- Educate patient and family on ways to incorporate religious practices into the treatment plan for the specific illness. For instance, the patient can adapt dietary restrictions and fasting requirements around specific beliefs.
- Educate the family on importance of patient's spiritual beliefs if the family is not supportive of them.

- Encourage family to not impose their beliefs on the patient if they are different.
- Encourage family to bring in Bibles or religious articles, as appropriate

Charting Tips

- Document patient's beliefs especially as they relate to patient's illness.
- Document conflicts between patient and family.
- Document patient's response to visit with clergy.

Discharge Planning

- Refer to clergy or agency chaplain, as appropriate.
- Encourage attendance at religious or health-related support groups, such as Reach for Recovery.
- Encourage participation in patient's own house of worship as indicated.

Nursing Outcomes

- Staff remain objective and nonjudgmental regarding patient practices and beliefs.
- Staff makes efforts to incorporate patient's beliefs and practices in treatment plan.

Suggested Learning Activities

- Arrange for in-service education with spiritual leaders from a variety of religions.
- Incorporate spiritual assessment as part of the nursing assessment tool.
- Explore practices and beliefs of faiths other than your own with special emphasis on healthcare beliefs and practices.
- Share with colleagues the role of spiritual beliefs and religious practices in your family's lives.

19

NURSING MANAGEMENT OF SPECIAL PROBLEMS

The Chronically Ill Patient

LEARNING OBJECTIVES

▼ *Describe some important tasks that a person needs to accomplish to adapt to chronic illness.*
▼ *List common nurses' reactions to the chronically ill.*
▼ *Describe appropriate interventions for chronically ill patients with self-care deficit, alteration in self-concept, and impaired social interactions.*

Even though more Americans are affected by chronic illness than acute illness, the U.S. healthcare system focuses more money and research on treating acute illness. According to the National Health Survey (1989), nearly 80 million Americans live with one or more chronic illnesses including arthritis, hypertension, diabetes mellitus, respiratory disease, and mental illness. In addition, heart disease, cancer, and stroke, which are the leading causes of death in adults, can cause major disability and have significant impact on long-term care. Though the highest incidence of chronic illness is in the over 65 population, all ages are affected.

Unlike acute illness, which is time limited, chronic illness is often permanent with no definite timetable to give the person a frame of reference to plan for the future. Most chronic illnesses require major adjustments in the individual's lifestyle. The periods of uncertainty, remissions and exacerbations, and in some cases, a slow, steady decline in health can significantly strain the coping mechanisms of the individual and his or her family. Whether the individual and family can continue to effectively cope with the anxiety this creates depends on how

---

Glossary

Chronic illness—A condition not cured by medical intervention and requiring periodic monitoring and supportive care to reduce the degree of illness and to maximize the person's functioning and responsibility for self-care.

Acute illness—A condition caused by a disease that produces symptoms and signs soon after exposure to the cause, that runs a short course, and from which there is usually a recovery or an abrupt termination in death.

Exacerbation—Resumption of pronounced symptoms from an illness.

Remission—The period during which the disease is controlled and symptoms are not obvious.

Disability—Any long- or short-term reduction of activity that results from an acute or chronic condition.

long the individual's normal routine can be maintained, how frequently medical crises require treatment, and how easily treatment can be incorporated into the individual's normal lifestyle. In addition, changes in family routines such as caregiver responsibilities, role changes, financial strain, and changes in socializing patterns and sexual relationships significantly influence the psychosocial response to chronic illness.

Etiology

Many psychologic theories address the process of adapting to a chronic illness. *Grief* theory is one of the most significant. During the grieving process, the individual can experience denial, anger, depression, and finally, acceptance.

Denial can occur at the time of diagnosis or during remissions and/or exacerbations as a protective mechanism against the distress and fear created by the disease. Anger occurs as the individual struggles with giving up dreams and hopes because of the illness. Anger can energize the person to try to gain control over the illness. There may be need to obsessively seek second or third opinions, call information hotlines, talk to others with the condition to gain information on new treatments, and go to extremes to implement lifestyle changes such as diet or giving up smoking. Depression occurs when the individual feels the pain of giving up his or her former healthy self. Experiencing fear, sadness, and discouragement and reminiscing about the past can occur as part of the grieving process. Acceptance occurs gradually and may come and go as the illness changes. If unable to come to some acceptance, each new limitation will feel like a fresh emotional injury and the person experiences ongoing demoralization.

Poor adaptation of chronic illness can cause noncompliance, dependency, loss of self-esteem, and depression. Noncompliance may be the result of denial, used to protect one's self from having to acknowledge the illness; anger, used to maintain control over the situation; or fear of dependency.

Most patients with chronic illness need to accept a dependent role at some point in their illness, even if it is for a short time with dependence on medication or equipment.

However, people who view themselves as weak and vulnerable may become dependent for longer amounts of time, possibly for the rest of their life.

In those individuals who have preexisting low self-esteem, physical or lifestyle changes such as becoming dependent on medical equipment can negatively affect body image and, ultimately, lowers self-esteem even further. These patients may reject others because they feel unlovable. As they become more isolated, they are at a higher risk for depression.

Clinical Concerns

Chronic illnesses can influence an individual's response to an acute illness and the potential for recovery. For example, persons with chronic pulmonary disease may have difficulty surviving major surgery. The presense of more than one chronic illness often adds to the demands made by even a relatively minor illness.

Lifespan Issues

CHILDHOOD

Up to 20 percent of children have a chronic illness, with the most common being asthma (Copeland, 1993). How the child responds to the illness depends on the child's developmental stage and the parent's response. Under stress the child may regress to a previous developmental stage. Denial, overprotectiveness, rejection, and overcompensating are examples of poor parental responses and can significantly influence the child's adaptation response. The child's illness can cause dysfunction within the family as frequent doctor's appointments, changing living arrangements, and financial stress cause disruption in family life and increase the child's anxiety. Siblings may experience jealousy and resentment for the increased attention to the ill child, embarrassment, shame, fear of becoming ill, guilt at causing the illness, or an extreme sense of overprotectiveness. These feelings are influenced by the parent's response. The sibling may also regress to a previous developmental stage during times of stress.

ADULTHOOD

Chronic illness can be a devastating blow in adulthood, a time when expectations are highest. Many illnesses can impede performance of an important role as breadwinner or parent.

ELDERLY

By age 65, 86 percent of the elderly have at least one chronic illness, and by age 80, 50 percent of men and 70 percent of women have two or more chronic conditions (Burke and Walsh, 1992). In addition to the common chronic illnesses, the elderly also are frequently afflicted with cataracts, osteoporosis, and hip fractures. Adapting to chronic illness depends on resources available to the person, including caregiver availability, financial resources, and living arrangements. Spouses or other supportive people may be chronically ill as well. Advancing chronic illnesses may force the elderly to move out of their home into unfamiliar surroundings, such as to a retirement home or nursing home. Also, treatment for multiple chronic illnesses can drain one's coping reserves, and the symptoms of one chronic illness such as reduced vision from cataracts impacts the management of another one such as being able to give oneself insulin.

Possible Nurses' Reactions

- May view caring for the chronically ill as depressing because of deteriorating patient health, negative psychologic responses from the patient, an overwhelming sense of helplessness, and fear of losing someone with whom the nurse has established a relationship.
- May have difficulty defining care goals as optimal maintenance rather than curative.
- May lack empathy and blame noncompliant patient as causing his or her own problems.

Assessment

Behavior and/or Appearance

- Obvious disability or change in appearance due to illness

- Unkempt, poor hygiene due to lack of energy and depression
- May require obvious assistive devices such as oxygen and a wheelchair

Mood and/or Emotions

- Depressed
- Angry
- May lack emotional reaction caused by denial
- Guilt over burden created by illness
- Fear and anxiety caused by uncertain future or physical discomfort

Thoughts, Beliefs, and Perceptions

- Powerless to control condition, complications, or side effects
- May generalize view of self as weak and ineffectual into all areas of life
- May think obsessively about his or her health or physical condition
- May view body as unattractive or damaged
- May be able to maintain self-esteem and sense of competence

Relationships and Interactions

- May need to become dependent on others for care, transportation, financial support
- May have difficulty in maintaining personal relationships because of lack of energy, physical discomfort, or embarrassment
- May need to change living arrangements to facilitate care causing the individual to develop new or changed relationships with others
- May experience changes in sexual relationships because of physical discomfort, loss of energy, or poor self-image
- May experience a sense of social isolation or rejection because friends and family may avoid patient if they are uncomfortable being around someone with a disability

Physical Responses

- These vary depending on specific illness.

- Symptoms must be reassessed frequently as they may or may not be related to the chronic illness.
- Ability to perform activities of daily living can be affected.

Pertinent History

- Past history of chronic illness, other conditions, or disabilities
- History of psychiatric disorders especially depression and substance abuse

Collaborative Management

Pharmacologic

Because patients with chronic illnesses are often on multiple medications, there is an increased risk of interactions between medications or between medications and food. Each new symptom needs to be assessed carefully to determine if the cause is from the illness or treatment. For example, confusion and lethargy could be a sign of deteriorating medical condition or the result of overmedication.

Nursing Management

IMPAIRED SOCIAL ISOLATION EVIDENCED BY INABILITY TO ESTABLISH AND/OR MAINTAIN STABLE, SUPPORTIVE RELATIONSHIPS RELATED TO LOSS OF BODY FUNCTION DUE TO CHRONIC ILLNESS.

Patient and Family Outcomes

- Patient identifies behaviors that deter socialization.
- Patient demonstrates behaviors that encourage socialization.
- Family provides support to patient.

Interventions

- Assess the patient's support system, living arrangements, and care needs. Identify areas where patient needs assistance in his or her care routine.
- Identify types of behavior that may impede socialization,

such as manipulative, dependent, hostile, depressed, or passive-aggressive. As needed, help the patient become aware of how these types of behaviors may discourage interactions with others. Explore ways to change these behaviors.

- Encourage patient to share worries and concerns with others, as appropriate. Also encourage patient to make an effort to provide support to family members as they learn to adjust. If the patient consistently focuses others' attention on his or her health problems, give the patient feedback on understanding others' responses.
- Encourage patient to accept help from others, as needed, while maintaining independence within the limitations of the illness.
- Patient may need assistance to express feelings and wishes to his or her caregiver in a nonthreatening way. Role play with patient. This promotes independence and self-esteem of patient and caregiver.
- Encourage patient and family to be aware of communication patterns when under stress, and explain how these may negatively impact their relationships.
- Allow family to share their concerns and frustrations with you about the patient. Explore with the patient ways to resolve these issues. Consider bringing patient and family together to discuss if both agree to participate.
- Encourage patient to participate in activities and interests that do not involve his or her illness.
- Encourage the patient to maintain contact with supportive people through phone calls, letter writing, computer, and tapes.
- Assist patient in identifying ways to establish new relationships.

SELF-CONCEPT DISTURBANCE EVIDENCED BY SELF-DESTRUCTIVE BEHAVIORS, UNWILLINGNESS TO FACE EFFECTS OF ILLNESS, EXCESSIVE DEPENDENCY, DEPRESSION RELATED TO ALTERATION IN BODY IMAGE FROM CHRONIC ILLNESS.

Patient Outcomes

- Remains as independent as possible within limitations of illness
- Demonstrates acceptance of his or her body by such be-

haviors as talking positively about self, taking care of own physical needs
- Implements adaptive coping mechanisms

Interventions

- Develop a trusting relationship with patient to encourage sharing feelings with you. Providing privacy and respect for patient's feelings and body will enhance that trust.
- Encourage patient to express feelings and thoughts about the illness and the way the illness has changed self image.
- Assess the effect of illness on the patient. Clarify misconceptions, myths about illness, treatment, and functional ability. For example, patient may believe the portable oxygen tank cannot be taken in the car so he or she no longer goes out with friends.
- Help the patient begin to accept self with the new limitations. Involve the patient in own care, gradually increasing those areas for which the patient can take responsibility. Encourage expressing feelings about the illness and body image. As appropriate, involve the family.
- Be aware of what others' behavior communicates to patient. For example, if patient's wife puts on disposable gloves every time she is with patient, she is nonverbally communicating her discomfort being around him. She needs to be encouraged to examine how this behavior effects him.
- Explore the patient's strengths and interests. Provide encouragement to focus on these, not just the illness. Explore ways to develop former interests that are within his or her functional abilities.
- Encourage participation in rehabilitation and education programs, as appropriate.

SELF-CONCEPT DISTURBANCE EVIDENCED BY NOT PARTICIPATING IN ACTIVITIES OF DAILY LIVING AND DEPRESSIVE BEHAVIOR RELATED TO PAIN OR IMPAIRED MOBILITY OR COGNITION FROM CHRONIC ILLNESS.

Patient and Family Outcomes

- Demonstrates participation in care within limitations of illness
- Performs activities of daily living within limitations of illness

Interventions

- Assess patient's ability to perform activities of daily living and the patient's ability to maintain medical regimen for chronic illness care.
- Provide needed education and resources to enhance performing these activities to encourage independence.
- Involve family and caregivers in identifying ways to promote independence. Teach them ways to help patient without taking over completely.
- In areas where patient must be dependent on others, promote patient participation in decision making and timing of care to promote some control.
- To successfully promote independence in an activity, you may need to break down each activity into small segments and then focus on one segment at a time.
- Explore the patient's feelings regarding activities he or she is no longer able to perform. Encourage the grieving response to express feelings and encourage acceptance. Then explore activities of interest within the patient's functional abilities.

ALTERNATE NURSING DIAGNOSES

Grieving, anticipatory or dysfunctional
Ineffective individual coping
Noncompliance
Powerlessness

WHEN TO CALL FOR HELP

✔ There are indications that the patient is not being cared for adequately such as poor hygiene, decubitus ulcers, poor nutrition, or dehydration.
✔ Patient is not complying with treatment plan, which

> could lead to life-threatening complications—for ex-
> ample, the patient is not taking insulin or refusing
> dialysis
> ✔ Patient is demoralized by destructive behavior
> within his or her family, such as substance abuse.

Patient and Family Education

- Provide appropriate education for the individual's chronic illness and medical regimen.
- Provide information on prevention of complications or progression of the illness.
- Involve family and/or caregivers in this education.
- Teach assertive and problem-solving skills to patient who is dependent on others for much of his or her care to gain a sense of control over healthcare.
- Review with family the ways to promote independence and self-esteem in the patient.
- Teach relaxation techniques as a way to reduce anxiety (see Appendix C).
- Teach family the stages of grieving and ways to cope with these.

Charting Tips

- Document patient and family response to health teaching.
- Note caregiver responses to patient. Use specific examples rather than a subjective opinion of the response.
- Document patient's reaction to illness, prognosis, and body image changes.
- Document patient's participation in treatment plan.

Discharge Planning

- Involve patient and family in the discharge plan early in treatment.
- Provide specific referrals for additional help in the home or alternative care options as needed.
- Identify equipment patient will need in the home such as hospital bed and wheelchair to enhance independence and caregiving.

- Refer patient and family to support programs and self-help groups specific to patient's illness such as ostomy or stroke groups.
- Refer to counseling as needed.
- Consider home health referrals to assess caregiver's ability to provide care and patient's compliance in the home.
- Communicate with all referring agencies regarding identified problems.

Nursing Outcomes

- Staff will provide adequate education to patient and family.
- Staff will demonstrate appropriate assessment and interventions for the psychosocial needs of the chronically ill patient.
- Staff will demonstrate nonjudgmental care to patient and family.

Suggested Learning Activities

- Arrange for an inservice from a specialist on psychosocial needs for patients with particular chronic illnesses, such as sickle cell disease or asthma.
- Attend support groups and self-help programs for people with specific chronic illnesses.
- Obtain information from national organizations on specific chronic illnesses such as the Arthritis Foundation or the American Lung Association.

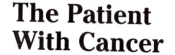

The Patient With Cancer

LEARNING OBJECTIVES

▼ Describe the psychosocial responses that occur most frequently in patients with cancer.
▼ Discuss the effects of specific cancer treatment modalities on psychosocial coping.
▼ Define appropriate nursing diagnoses related to the psychosocial care of the patient with cancer.
▼ Determine effective nursing interventions to promote coping and adaptation for the patient and family along the cancer continuum.

The diagnosis of cancer is a powerful, overwhelming, and life-changing event. To understand the psychosocial dimension of the cancer experience and the threats and challenges inherent in facing the disease, McGee (1990) has identified some important characteristics that influence the patient's responses to this illness. These include:

- Cancer is a unique experience for the individual.
- Cancer is a chronic illness.
- Cancer and cancer treatments are marked by uncertainty.
- Cancer results in a changed identity.
- Cancer affects the social system of the individual.

Each patient's emotional responses to facing the diag-

Glossary

Cancer—A group of neoplastic diseases characterized by the abnormal growth and proliferation of cells destructive to body organs and function.

Recurrence—Return of the disease after initial diagnosis and treatment. Recurrent disease signifies an inadequate response to therapy. Many cancer survivors express that the fear of recurrence continues to hang over their heads years after successful treatment, and this fear decreases their sense of personal control. Every illness may be interpreted as a return of the disease.

Remission—Absence of all clinical signs and symptoms of cancer.

Metastasis—Malignant lesions originating from the primary tumor but spread to anatomically different sites, for example, breast cancer that has spread to and infiltrated the bone.

Alopecia—Destruction of the hair follicles resulting in hair loss. Alopecia may result from chemotherapy or radiation. Hair loss from chemotherapy will be dependent upon the type of drug employed and will be temporary. Alopecia will occur from radiation therapy only if the head is in the field of radiation and most likely will be permanent depending upon the dose of radiation utilized.

nosis of cancer must be assessed within the context of the personal meaning of cancer, their developmental life stage, and their previous history of coping. Becoming aware of the unique personal meaning of cancer to the individual is the first step in assessing the impact of the diagnosis and treatment. Common threats posed by this disease include facing one's own mortality, changes in body image and self-concept, and challenges to role functions and relationships. The person's appraisal of the current harm and loss incurred by the illness and the threats to future equilibrium provide the keys for understanding that individual's response.

Advances in medical treatment have changed the course and treatment for cancer. Cancer is now viewed as a chronic illness, and long-term survival has emphasized the need to address psychosocial issues and quality of life. The cancer experience extends over a continuum of time and can be viewed as a developmental process demanding different psychosocial tasks at each stage. The emotional reactions to diagnosis may be similar or very different to those experienced during treatment, remission, or at the stage of recurrence. Underlying each stage is the uncertainty and ominous threat that cancer will return and overcome the individual. Coping with the reality of one's own mortality is a major task that extends into the stage of survivorship.

The cancer experience profoundly impacts the individual's identity. Facing the constant challenges of the disease and its treatments forces the individual to reassess priorities, life goals, and valued relationships. Cancer influences every facet of the patient's life: personal goals, family roles, employment, financial security, and social interactions. Most importantly, the internal resources that make up a person's "being" are constantly challenged. These resources include such facets as one's self-esteem, coping abilities, culture, sexuality, and spirituality. Cancer is a transitional point altering how the individual regards the future.

Finally, the individual's experience of cancer does not happen in a vacuum. It affects the entire social system of the individual, including family, friends, and coworkers. Because the family is the "unit of care," assessment must include the impact of cancer on family roles, homeostasis, and responses to the chronic illness. For instance, a mother diagnosed with breast cancer will face many challenges and so will her family. At the time she is diagnosed, she may be juggling a work schedule along with child and home care responsibilities. Treatment schedules and side effects will interfere with her roles as wife, mother, homemaker, and employee. Chronic fatigue has been cited as one of the major stresses related to cancer treatment due to its disrupting activities of daily living.

Family members will have a variety of responses to these new demands. The husband will need to take on additional roles, and the expectations of the children may change. At a time when the adolescent is attempting to become more independent from the family, a sick parent may require that he or she fulfill more responsibilities at home. For young children, a sick parent's experience may become internalized, and the young child may fear being at fault for what has occurred. It is important that all family members are included in the nursing care plan and that assessment includes the stresses and new role demands of all members.

Etiology

Cancer will make physical, psychologic, and social demands on the individual and family, and these will change depending on the patient's stage of illness. By identifying the specific psychosocial challenges that present at different stages of the illness continuum, Christ (1993) and Sales (1991) provide frameworks for understanding the emotional responses to these demands and the coping and adaptive abilities required of the patient and the family at each stage. The stages include diagnosis, treatment, remission, recurrence, and terminal. Each stage presents new and different challenges for the patient and family. Once these challenges and responses to them are understood, appropriate interventions can be selected to strengthen the adaptive tasks and provide professional support where needed.

The *diagnosis* of cancer is overwhelming and frightening for the patient and family. Confronted not only with the diagnosis but also with treatment decisions, this stage produces acute anxiety and distress. Personal meaning of cancer will influence how the individual responds during this stage, but shock and disbelief are common reactions. The crisis of diagnosis may be compounded if the patient feels guilty for choosing lifestyle behaviors he or she thinks contributed to the development of the illness.

In the *treatment* stage the patient is faced with side effects and the interruption of normal roles and relationships.

The adaptation or *remission* stage may resurge the patient's initial anxiety because active treatment is completed and fear of recurrence begins.

The patient's response to *recurrence* of disease will depend on many variables, including the patient's symptoms and physical status. Recurrence of disease may refute the hope that the cancer can be conquered or cured.

The stage of metastatic disease and *terminal* illness challenge both the patient and family because of overwhelming uncertainty, fear, and existential and spiritual concerns.

It is important to identify the patient's past coping mechanisms and the support systems currently available to him or her. The crisis of cancer may tax the patient's emotional reserves and present such overwhelming challenges that former coping mechanisms are inadequate. Anxiety can be viewed as adaptive and motivational if it does not overwhelm the patient. In addition, denial may also be a defense mechanism employed by patient's experiencing cancer. Denial allows the patient to incorporate the impact of the diagnosis in small increments, allowing time to reflect and solve problems without becoming engulfed and overwhelmed by the situation. Coping with reality-based issues presented by cancer needs to also be differentiated from coping with issues that are intrapsychic in origin. Concrete information regarding the disease, treatment options, and prognosis is most helpful in reassuring the patient and family. Social support systems such as friendships, work relationships, and community resources have also been found to buffer the impact of stress on the patient and family.

Identifying high-risk patients begins with an understanding that responses such as anger, fear, and sadness may be very appropriate in response to the diagnosis and treatment of cancer. These responses become maladaptive if they are prolonged and exaggerated. Significant prior psychiatric history such as chemical dependency, major depression, anxiety, or personality disorders may predict maladaptive responses to cancer and treatment. However, symptoms of clinical depression may also result from the effects of the disease or adverse effects of the treatment. Therefore, it is important to assess if these symptoms are a change from previous level of functioning, if they are persistent, or if they influence the patient's adjustment to cancer and treatment. Depression will have a negative impact on the patient's ability to cope, and these symptoms may also exacerbate physical illness or disease-related symptoms such as pain.

Valente, Saunders, and Cohen (1994) suggest that depression is one of the most commonly undetected psychiatric disorders associated with the diagnosis and treatment of cancer. The risk of major depression increases at diagnosis, treatment failure, or cancer recurrence. If major depression is untreated, it decreases the quality of life and increases the risk of suicide. Patients with cancer who are experiencing major depression will have an increased risk of suicide especially during terminal illness. Other factors that may increase the cancer patient's suicide risk are uncontrolled pain, intolerable fatigue, impaired cognition, and a poor prognosis. The nurse should also be aware of any irrational thinking, suicidal ideation, or lethal plans that the patient may have. A past history of prior suicide attempts, substance abuse, major depression, and/or poor social support are also important influencing factors. Delirium in the endstage patient is often undiagnosed and inadequately treated. It is associated with high morbidity and suffering.

Related Clinical Concerns

TREATMENT CONSIDERATIONS

Cancer treatment may include surgery, chemotherapy, radiation, immunotherapy, bone marrow and stem cell transplantation, or other investigational treatments. Each treatment modality has associated adverse effects that may influence psychosocial coping and adaptation. The patient may suffer loss of a body part or function following surgery.

Nausea, vomiting, fatigue, and alopecia will occur with chemotherapy and radiation. Intensive treatments such as bone marrow transplantation or extensive or exhausting research protocols can increase fears and uncertainty regarding outcomes.

PHYSIOLOGIC EFFECTS OF CANCER AND TREATMENT

Changes in physical function will occur from the treatments, disease progression, and the physiologic effects of the illness, and, ultimately, these changes will influence psychologic status. Loss of physical function will directly impact body image, self-concept, and sexuality. These changes in turn may cause the patient to experience feelings of sadness, powerlessness, grief, and loss. In addition, tumor growth may affect normal organ function such as in the case of brain metastases or bone metastases. Symptoms resulting from brain metastases, such as confusion and mental changes, can be mistaken for psychiatric disorders. Hypercalcemia resulting from bone metastases can also cause apathy, depression, restlessness, and confusion. Primary or metastatic tumors to the central nervous system, fluid and electrolyte imbalances, infection, and cerebral hypoxia can contribute to a state of impaired mental functioning. The patient experiencing pain from the cancer or treatment can exhibit anxiety, fear, restlessness, and depression. Inadequate pain management can lead to significant psychosocial impairment.

Lifespan Issues

CHILDHOOD

For the child experiencing cancer, the vital developmental tasks of trust, autonomy, and initiative may be threatened from repeated hospitalizations and treatments that cause separation from parents, missed school and socialization opportunities, physical dysfunction, fear, and anxiety. Cancer may cause the young child to become emotionally dependent, interfering with autonomy, and or unduly fearful, preventing initiative. Feelings of mistrust, shame, and doubt can remain if successful resolution is not possible due to illness.

ADOLESCENCE

If cancer strikes the adolescent, the tasks of achieving identity and independence will be disrupted. Just as the adolescent is forging his or her own self-concept and separation from parents, there is a need to become more dependent because of the illness. This may result in anger, resentment, and acting-out behaviors. The adolescent may withdraw from family and social interactions and be unable to share the vulnerability and confusion being experienced. Cancer may also cause the adolescent to feel alienated from peers and social activities due to changes in physical appearances, weakness, and long hospitalizations.

ADULTHOOD

The emotional, financial, and physical hardships endured by the young adult experiencing cancer threatens emotional and sexual intimacy. Developmental tasks of the young adult will be disrupted: autonomy from parents, attending college, focusing on one's career, or choosing a life partner. Sterility from cancer will threaten the ability to procreate and extend oneself into the next generation. The major goals of a young adult to forge a self-identity and plan for the future will be permanently affected by the crisis of cancer.

ELDERLY

For the elderly patient cancer may interfere with plans such as retirement, travel, and financial security. Dependency demanded by illness, loss of a partner, and other losses incurred by the aging process may overwhelm the individual. Grief and depression can thus interfere with achieving the final psychosocial task of ego integrity, and the elderly patient with cancer may experience despair and unresolved loss.

Possible Nurses' Reactions

- Emotional responses of the nurse will be framed within the nurse's own experiences in life, especially those experiences dealing with cancer, pain, crisis, and loss.
- May have fear and uncertainty caring for the patient if he

or she lacks sufficient knowledge of oncology, radiation, and chemotherapy.

- May avoid developing a therapeutic relationship with patient because of overwhelming feelings of powerlessness to control symptoms such as pain.
- May become overinvolved emotionally with patient, leading to enmeshment (feeling the patient's experience as her own).
- May be shocked by changes in the patient's appearance: alopecia, cachexia, amputation.
- May be judgmental by assessing patient's responses within the framework of own values and standards.
- May experience grief when supporting patient's grief and losses.
- May be unable to identify symptoms of burnout such as irritability, anxiety, insomnia, and detachment.

Assessment

Behavior and/or Appearance

- Inability to cope manifested by anxiety, irritability, or depression
- Dramatic changes in physical appearance due to alopecia, cachexia, amputation
- Unable to concentrate, follow directions, or make decisions
- Difficulty in carrying out tasks of daily living
- Disheveled appearance
- Dramatic behavior changes like giving up eating meat, stopping smoking
- Destructive behavior toward self or others
- Change in communication patterns

Mood and/or Emotions

- Inappropriate use of defense mechanisms such as denial, isolation, projection
- Inappropriate affect
- Shock and disbelief
- Unstable mood swings
- Anxiety and panic

- Uncontrolled anger
- Grief and depression, sad, tearful
- Hopelessness

Thoughts, Beliefs, and Perceptions

- Blaming self or others
- Feelings of failure
- Guilt regarding chosen lifestyles or behaviors linked to the development of the disease, such as smoking, or for impact of illness on family
- Questioning of self-worth
- Difficulty adjusting to the perceived meaning of the loss of a body part, such as a mastectomy
- Difficulty adjusting to the perceived meaning of lost roles
- Fears of dependency, pain, disfigurement, and death
- Feelings of powerlessness regarding disease and treatment
- Belief that cancer is a death sentence and that it brings severe pain and suffering

Relationships and Interactions

- Inability to express needs, expectations, or goals
- Difficulty communicating with healthcare providers
- Breakdown of normal family communication patterns
- Projects anger onto others
- Refuses to use appropriate resources
- Inappropriate dependency and resignation
- Social isolation

Physical Responses

- Multiple side effects of disease and treatment
- Low energy or fatigue resulting from anemia
- Increased risk of infection and septicemia resulting from leukopenia
- Increased risk of hemorrhage with thrombocytopenia
- Insomnia or hypersomnia
- Loss of appetite or overeating
- Flushing, sweating, and/or shortness of breath
- Palpitations

Pertinent History

• History of psychiatric disorders including substance abuse
• Concurrent illnesses and medications
• Unresolved losses

Collaborative Management

Pharmacologic

Patients experiencing mild to moderate anxiety and depression can be evaluated to determine if antidepressants would be helpful. For extreme fears, extreme anger, and moderate to severe depression, antidepressants, benzodiazepines, and occasionally antipsychotics may be helpful. It is important to recognize in these patients that multiple drug use can also cause anxiety, depression, and confusion, and that aspect should be evaluated before instituting additional pharmacologic treatment.

Chemotherapeutic agents that cross the blood-brain barrier, such as the nitrosureas or specific antimetabolites and vinca alkaloids, have been associated with neuropsychiatric disturbances such as delirium, hallucinations, lethargy, cognitive dysfunction, and depression. Depression is a direct side effect of some specific agents such as the vinca alkaloids, corticosteroids, interferon, and tamoxifen. Corticosteroids are used in many chemotherapy and radiation protocols and can cause adverse psychiatric symptoms ranging from sleep and mood disorders to personality changes and mania. Analgesics and antianxiety drugs can also contribute to lethargy and depression.

Nursing Management

INEFFECTIVE INDIVIDUAL COPING EVIDENCED BY BEHAVIORS SUCH AS DENIAL, ISOLATION, ANXIETY, AND DEPRESSION RELATED TO THE DIAGNOSIS AND TREATMENT OF CANCER.

Patient Outcomes

• Identifies stressors related to illness and treatment

- Communicates needs, concerns, and fears
- Absence of symptoms related to ineffective coping, such as acute anxiety
- Uses appropriate resources to support coping

Interventions

- Assess effective coping strategies based upon the patient's self-report of past coping mechanisms and those coping resources currently available to the patient. Assist patient in strengthening those behaviors that are effective and in recognizing those behaviors that are ineffective.
- Provide a safe and nonjudgmental environment for the patient to express feelings and fears. Use active listening skills and provide consistent care and support. Help patient to express concerns regarding the actual and potential losses incurred by the illness and the uncertainty regarding the outcomes of treatment.
- Assess the patient's readiness to learn the type and amount of information provided. Realize that using denial as a defense mechanism may be appropriate if it does not interfere with the patient's safety or compliance with necessary treatment. Be specific, clear, and honest in answering questions. Information may need to be repeated and reinforced as the patient's anxiety decreases.
- Facilitate communication between patient, family, and healthcare providers. Allow the patient to determine the amount of information to be shared. Encourage and assist patient in verbalizing needs, concerns, and expectations to others.
- Help the patient and family to identify immediate stressors and priorities in meeting the demands of illness and treatment. Focus on the patient's quality of life issues, and assist the patient in reframing life's goals within the context of cancer, such as sperm banking prior to chemotherapy. Promote adaptation by encouraging positive change and by reinforcing effective behaviors, such as healthy lifestyle behaviors.
- Ensure that patient's pain and other symptoms are controlled. This will contribute to improved coping.
- Use an interdisciplinary approach to care, and refer patient to appropriate resources. Work closely with the pa-

tient's physician, social worker, and clinical nurse specialist to provide a plan of care that is consistent and that ensures open communication. Identify other resources that may be important for the patient, for instance, the agency's chaplain.

- Assess for suicide risk. Identify symptoms of major depression and feelings of hopelessness. Provide adequate pain management. Identify any family or personal history of psychopathology that could increase the patient's risk. Refer the patient for psychiatric evaluation if appropriate.

SELF-ESTEEM DISTURBANCE EVIDENCED BY ANXIETY, MOOD DISTURBANCE, GRIEF, AND DEPRESSION RELATED TO THE DIAGNOSIS AND TREATMENT OF CANCER, LOST BODY PART(S) OR FUNCTION(S), ROLE DISTURBANCES, AND UNCERTAINTY ABOUT THE FUTURE.

Patient Outcomes

- Verbalizes meaning of lost body part(s) or function(s)
- Participates in self-care activities
- Reframes role performance and expectations
- Positively incorporates changed identity

Interventions

- Assess perceived or actual changes in body structure(s) or function(s) such as amputation, mastectomy, alopecia, and cachexia.
- Identify the personal meaning of the loss to the individual. Support normal grieving over lost body parts to aid resolution of the loss. Be aware, for example, that a hysterectomy is a threat to a woman's fertility, sexuality, and femininity.
- Encourage the patient to take responsibility for self-care, for instance, by monitoring mastectomy wound, and provide a safe environment for the patient to cry and verbalize feelings. Validate the patient's feelings, and give the patient permission to grieve.
- Evaluate the impact of cancer and treatment on the patient's sexuality. This not only includes the obvious threat of treatment on sexual performance, for instance, radical prostatectomy for prostate cancer, but also the

other components of one's sexual being. Provide the patient with a safe environment to verbalize fears and feelings regarding altered sexual health.

- Identify ineffective behaviors such as social isolation or avoidance of intimacy. Help patient to incorporate changed body image and changed self-concept by encouraging patient to verbalize feelings regarding the personal meaning of the losses and the meaning to significant others.
- Identify the impact of cancer and its treatment on the patient's role performance. Chronic fatigue, stress, nausea, and vomiting will ultimately interfere with the patient's ability to meet prior role demands. Assist the patient and family to communicate their needs and to support one another with the new demands.
- Refer the patient and family to community resources available to them, and assist them in planning daily activities during treatment so that they do not feel overwhelmed. Provide information on transportation to treatment if needed.
- Encourage the patient to be an active participant in decision making and to be as independent as possible in self-care to bolster self-esteem.
- Educate the patient regarding the disease and treatment and encourage the patient to be an active member of the healthcare team to diffuse feelings of powerlessness. Fear of the unknown and uncertainty regarding the future can contribute to overwhelming anxiety and depression. Assist patient to identify beliefs and myths that could negatively impact coping, such as new back pain means the cancer has spread.
- Assist the client and family to identify current stressors and coping strategies, allow independent self-care and autonomy, and enhance self-competency at each stage of the illness.
- Reinforce hope to prevent hopelessness leading to depression. Hope is tangible even in late stages of terminal disease. Hope for relief from pain or hope to spend quality time with loved ones can enhance the patient's self-esteem and quality of life.
- Identify the role of the patient's spirituality and religious beliefs to see what role they play in the patient's hope-

fulness or hopelessness. The patient may question former beliefs, ask "Why me?" or find comfort and solace in his or her own spirituality.

ALTERNATE NURSING DIAGNOSES

Anxiety
Body image disturbance
Coping, ineffective family
Denial, ineffective
Family processes
Grieving, dysfunctional
Knowledge deficit
Powerlessness

WHEN TO CALL FOR HELP

✔ Patient's unresolved grief leads to extreme anger, social isolation, or other behaviors
✔ Extreme anxiety and/or depression
✔ Patient pursuing unproven treatment methods that contribute to life-threatening complications
✔ Extreme anxiety in patient, evidenced by anger, inability to concentrate, and immobilization
✔ Patient expressing suicidal ideation
✔ Patient not complying with treatment plan, which may have life-threatening complications
✔ Emotional exhaustion or burnout in staff
✔ Escalating symptoms of depression in staff

Patient and Family Education

- Assess the patient's readiness to learn, and provide information accordingly so as not to emotionally overwhelm patient.
- Answer questions clearly and honestly.
- Educate the patient regarding pathophysiology of disease and rationale behind chosen treatment modalities.
- Instruct the patient regarding expected side effects of treatment.

- Teach the patient effective coping strategies to deal with stressors.
- Reinforce positive behaviors so that the patient learns effective strategies.
- Educate the patient and family on patient care needs and medical follow-up required for treatment.
- Prepare the family for possible treatment side effects and changes in condition and appearance.

Charting Tips

- Document the patient's understanding of diagnosis and treatment.
- Describe the patient's emotional, cognitive, and behavioral responses.
- Describe the patient's perception of stressors and effectiveness of coping strategies.
- Document the use of antianxiety or antidepressant medications and the patient's response.
- Describe the family's responses to the patient and cancer experience.

Discharge Planning

- Use an interdisciplinary approach to planning discharge—physicians, nurses, clinical nurse specialists, and social worker.
- Assess data regarding support systems, home environment, and outpatient care on a continual basis.
- Educate the patient and family regarding treatment protocol, expected side effects, and follow-up appointments.
- Identify the patient's needs, such as transportation to treatment and follow-up appointments.
- Ensure that patient has prescriptions and teaching regarding needed medications.
- Instruct the patient and family to inform the healthcare team of any new symptoms, adverse side effects, or significant changes in condition.
- Refer patient and family to home health care and appropriate community resources, such as the American Cancer Society.

- Refer the patient or family for individual or family counseling or support groups in the community if appropriate.
- Refer to psychiatric consult, if psychoactive medication is needed and to evelute confusion.
- Refer for hospice care if the patient is terminally ill.

Nursing Outcomes

- Recognizes own stressors of caring for patients experiencing cancer.
- Comes to terms with own fears regarding cancer and death.
- Provides nonjudgmental care to patient and family.
- Provides support and comfort to these patients whatever the stage of the illness.
- Seeks support from colleagues and other professionals when needed.

Suggested Learning Activities

- Visit community resources such as the American Cancer Society.
- Attend cancer educational programs, such as I Can Cope, or support group meetings, such as Make Today Count or Reach to Recovery.
- Arrange for inservice programs from mental health professionals who counsel patients with cancer.
- Contact professional cancer nursing organizations for information regarding care of the patient with cancer, such as the Oncology Nursing Society.

The Patient With AIDS

LEARNING OBJECTIVES

▼ *Identify one issue specific to children, women, homosexuals, and drug abusers with AIDS.*
▼ *List common nurses' reactions to HIV-positive patients.*
▼ *List common symptoms of AIDS dementia.*
▼ *Select appropriate nursing interventions for the AIDS patient with altered body image.*

The Centers for Diseases Control and Prevention (CDCP) reported over 500,000 cases of AIDS in the United States through 1994. Originally seen as a disease of male homosexuals, an increasing number of women, children, and IV drug users are now being affected. In 1994, the World Health Organization (WHO) noted for the first time that more than 50 percent of newly reported cases of AIDS worldwide are women. The majority of these individuals are young. Seventy-three percent of women and 65 percent of men with AIDS are under 40 years old. Up to 30 percent of infants born to women who are HIV-positive will be infected with the disease (CDCP, 1995).

AIDS generates a unique series of stressors for patients and their family and loved ones. The fear and stigma associated with this disease has caused incredible suffering. The diagnosis of AIDS initiates a roller coaster existence. Initially this patient faces unpredictable episodes of acute illness followed by periods of stability. Medications and

---

Glossary

Acquired immunodeficiency syndrome (AIDS)—An acquired defect in immune system functioning that reduces the affected person's resistance to certain types of infection, cancer, and progressive conditions. Diagnosis based on presence of opportunistic infections or rare forms of cancer as well as on CD4 lymphocyte count (T-helper cells) below 200.

Human immunodeficiency virus (HIV)—The etiologic agent that produces the widespread immunosuppression resulting in AIDS. Once exposed to the virus, the individual produces HIV antibodies and converts to HIV-positive status. This person is then at risk for developing a variety of infections and most likely AIDS.

Opportunistic infections—Infections caused by organisms in the environment that usually do no harm to a healthy human.

AIDS dementia—Cognitive changes due to direct invasion of HIV into the central nervous system. Also referred to as *HIV-associated cognitive and motor complex*.

doctors' visits become part of the regular routine. As it becomes more debilitating, fatigue and increasing discomforts must be faced. As the disease takes its toll, the weight loss often makes the diagnosis more identifiable to others. This can make it difficult to continue in social and employment settings. This is especially true for those who have hidden their disease from others.

The social stigma of having AIDS causes enormous problems for the individual and family. He or she may fear rejection because the chosen lifestyle is seen as unacceptable to others. Anticipating others' fear of contagion, or an overwhelming sense of guilt because the chosen lifestyle is creating such problems for loved ones. He or she may also experience severe economic devastation due to loss of job and lack of insurance. Social supports may be compromised because they may be infected with the virus as well. In addition, neuropsychiatric effects of AIDS result in depression, anger, excessive fear, and dementia.

Etiology

Psychosocial reactions to being at risk for AIDS (HIV-positive status) and being diagnosed with AIDS depend on a number of variables. At-risk individuals may defend against facing exposure to this disease by refusing to be tested or denying symptoms. Some may challenge their vulnerability by continuing high-risk behaviors. Others may become part of the "worried well," obsessively checking themselves for lesions, monitoring weights, or being tested frequently. This individual can develop severe anxiety to the point of emotional paralysis, particularly if that person has had problems with anxiety in the past.

The diagnosis of AIDS often forces families to face issues that have been hidden for years, such as homosexuality, bisexuality, drug use, or promiscuity. Those patients with a dual diagnosis of AIDS and substance abuse must deal with the devastating effects of both disorders, possibly overwhelming their coping skills and leading to inappropriate acting-out behavior, depression, and anger. In addition, using drugs such as cocaine and stimulants often adds to increased likelihood of participating in high-risk sexual behaviors.

The social stigma and poor prognosis combine to lengthen feelings of isolation and hopelessness and may lead to depression, suicide ideation, and anxiety symptoms. The risk for suicide is increased at the time of learning of HIV-positive status, the diagnosis of AIDS, and in later stages of the illness when pain and dementia overwhelm the individual's coping mechanisms. Those at higher risk include those with a history of depression, high levels of environmental stress, inadequate counseling before and after the HIV antibody test, and poor support networks (Frierson and Lippmann, 1988). Another factor may be that homosexuals and drug abusers are also known to have higher than average suicide rates.

AIDS dementia is one of the most feared yet most frequent complications because the patient loses control of many mental and emotional functions. Selnes (1990) notes 65 percent of AIDS patients are found to have anatomic evidence of dementia on autopsy. It is caused by invasion of the virus into the central nervous system. The loss of mental faculties represents a poor prognostic sign, and rapid deterioration often follows. This patient requires supervision over activities of daily living, adding to loss of control and independence. In addition to AIDS dementia, other causes of psychiatric complications include meningitis, cytomegalovirus (CMV) in the brain, toxoplasmosis, brain tumors, progressive multifocal leukoencephalopathy (PML), as well as metabolic imbalances.

Related Clinical Concerns

Aggressive treatment of AIDS will produce many side effects and complications including fatigue, alopecia, and anemia. The many opportunistic infections create complex symptoms including blindness, severe diarrhea, cachexia, pain, pneumonia, and cerebrovascular accidents. These will all complicate other coexisting diseases like asthma or diabetes.

Lifespan Issues

CHILDHOOD

In the past, HIV-positive infants tended to deteriorate very quickly because of their immature immune systems. However, today, early intervention with antiviral medications is resulting in much longer survival. Infected infants, children, and adolescents develop the same opportunistic infections as adults.

A child with AIDS usually represents a whole family at risk for infection as most often the child is infected from an HIV-positive mother who may have been infected by her male partner. So family members facing this devastating illness in the child may also be dealing with their own illness, as well as poverty and weak social supports.

A child with HIV-positive status or AIDS faces severe emotional distress, rejection, and possibly discrimination. This child may be ostracized by school officials and friends, and be particularly vulnerable to low self-esteem. To protect their child from emotional distress, parents may try not to reveal the diagnosis to the child or others. However, this rarely prevents problems and more often causes the child more anxiety and fear, sensing that some information is being withheld. The child should be given information appropriate to his or her developmental level and coping abilities.

A family may be facing multiple losses if more than the one child is infected. They often experience constant grief, depression, and exhaustion from caregiving. Siblings who are not infected may face guilt, fear, and confusion about what is happening to the family.

ADOLESCENCE

Because adolescents have little experience with serious illness and tend to be risk takers, they are more likely to exhibit denial. This puts them at higher risk for participating in high-risk behaviors like multiple sex partners or sharing needles that could put them at risk for AIDS or for spreading the virus to others.

ELDERLY

Up until now the impact of AIDS on the elderly population has been minimal. However, as the population ages and the disease spreads via heterosexual contact, this will change.

Possible Nurses' Reactions

- May identify with patient if the patient is about the same age or has a similar lifestyle, possibly leading to an overinvolvement with the patient or rejection.
- May be overwhelmed by the complexity of patient care.
- May become a surrogate family if the patient has limited support systems due to family rejection or death of significant other. This may lead to the need to face intense feelings of loss and discouragement, possibly causing exhaustion, numbness, or burnout.
- May resent the patient because he or she believes patient has caused own problems. This may make it difficult to express empathy and cause the patient to feel rejected.
- May be uncomfortable caring for patients with alternative lifestyles.
- May respond with anger and resentment at lack of resources available to this patient. May also feel anger toward the mother or lover who infected the patient.
- May fear accidental exposure to patient's blood.
- May fear caring for the patient due to fear of contagion.
- May deny potential risk of exposure and not use appropriate precautions.

Assessment

Behavior and/or Appearance

- Fatigue
- Weight loss
- Change in high-risk behaviors, e.g., stop IV drug use, abstain from sexual activity
- Signs of dementia (see Table 19–1)

Mood and/or Emotions

- Depression from illness, facing death

TABLE 19–1. **Signs of AIDS Dementia**

Early	Late
• Forgetfulness • Poor concentration • Apathy • Insomnia • Severe depression • Social withdrawal • Confusion • Regressed behavior • Changes in personality • Impaired abstract thinking	• Severe cognitive deficits • Mutism • Hypersomnolence • Psychosis • Loss of bowel and/or bladder control • Violent outbursts

- Anger
- Chronic grief from multiple losses from deaths of significant other, close friends
- Powerlessness
- Guilt, shame
- Denial

Thoughts, Beliefs, and Perceptions

- Hopelessness
- Poor judgement, confusion, inability to concentrate
- Low self-esteem
- Views self as a victim
- Change in body image

Relationships and Interactions

- May be estranged from parents or siblings because of lifestyle choices
- May have kept lifestyle choices or HIV-positive status a secret from family, limiting support network
- Support system may include more friends than family
- Significant others and friends may also be infected
- Patient may have been caregiver for others with AIDS
- Isolated due to others' fears of contagion
- Change in sexual relationships

Physical Responses

- Pain from neuropathies, tumors
- Multiple medications with many side effects
- Anemia
- Chronic diarrhea
- Impaired physical mobility
- Loss of vision
- Weight loss, problems with eating, poor nutrition

Pertinent History

- Substance abuse
- Psychiatric disorders
- Sexual promiscuity

Collaborative Interventions

Pharmacologic

Because these patients are on multiple medications, they are at particular risk for adverse effects. Many of the commonly used antiviral medications, such as zidovudine (AZT) and gancyclovir, can have adverse psychiatric effects, such as depression and mania. Amphotericin can cause delirium.

Detoxification and appropriate medication will need to be used for those patients with an existing substance abuse problem.

Because so many AIDS patients have psychiatric symptoms, antidepressants, antipsychotics, and antianxiety drugs are frequently used. HIV-positive patients taking antipsychotics are more vulnerable to extrapyramidal symptoms, and appropriate precautions must be taken.

Nursing Management

ALTERED THOUGHT PROCESSES EVIDENCED BY CONFUSION, INABILITY TO EVALUATE REALITY, OR DELUSIONS RELATED TO AIDS DEMENTIA OR OTHER AIDS-RELATED NEUROPSYCHIATRIC PROBLEMS.

Patient Outcomes

- Remains oriented to time, place, and person
- Remains safe and injury free
- Communicates clearly to others

Interventions

- Assess the patient's mental status frequently.
- If the patient has a history of substance abuse, determine if he or she is still actively using the drugs. The clinical symptoms could be associated with the abused substance rather than the illness.
- Orient patient regularly to date, time, place, and recent activities. Talk with patient about recent news events, such as the weather. Make sure a clock and a calendar are at the bedside. Encourage family and friends to bring personal items and photos.
- Avoid arguing with patient who is confused or agreeing with confused statements. Try to direct patient back to reality and attempt to gently correct inaccurate statements.
- Provide simple instructions. Encourage staff and family to structure patient's day. For example, give the patient a daily schedule of activities.
- When talking with the patient, reduce extraneous stimulation, such as television, to reduce distractions. If the patient is unable to concentrate, keep interactions brief. Consider using yes and no questions to reduce pressure on patient to answer.
- Evaluate potential safety hazards if patient exhibits poor judgment. If he or she is at risk to walk out of the hospital or home, make sure others are aware and provide adequate supervision.
- Consistent staff assignment will enhance patient trust. Recognize that patient may have limited short-term memory.
- Encourage verbalization of fears about changes in mental functioning.
- Be aware that patient may become agitated or violent because he or she is aware of losing his or her mental faculties. Intervene as appropriate to reduce risk of injury to patient and others.

- Address inappropriate behavior in quick and matter-of-fact manner.

BODY IMAGE DISTURBANCE EVIDENCED BY NEGATIVE COMMENTS ABOUT HIS OR HER BODY, LACK OF SELF-CARE, OR AVOIDANCE BY OTHERS RELATED TO WEIGHT LOSS AND/OR KAPOSI SARCOMA LESIONS.

Patient Outcomes

- Refers to self more positively
- Maintains social contacts with friends and/or family
- Demonstrates acceptance of appearance in his or her grooming and dress

Interventions

- Assess patient's reaction to changes in his or her appearance. Note how the patient talks about himself or herself and takes care of personal grooming.
- Encourage patient to talk about body changes being experienced and how they make him or her feel. Acknowledge the difficulty in accepting these changes rather than minimizing them. Patient will need to grieve over the loss of previous appearance by facing the changes and experiencing feelings of anger and sadness.
- Make sure the patient is aware of temporary changes such as hair loss from chemotherapy, and the permanent ones, such as severe weight loss.
- Encourage him or her to dress in ways that will minimize changes in appearance caused by weight loss. Encourage nutrition program and appetite stimulants, as appropriate. Encourage participation in support group programs to learn effective coping strategies from other AIDS patients.
- Use touch to show your acceptance of patient. Use gloves only when coming in contact with body fluids, observing universal precautions. Role model this behavior to family and friends. Provide education to others to reduce fears of physical contact with patient.
- Prepare the patient for possible reactions of others to patient's appearance. Encourage the development of per-

sonal strategies to respond to others who may appear uncomfortable or even reject the patient.

- Encourage the use of humor to cope, if appropriate.
- Encourage the patient to participate in some social activities. Suggest he or she start with only a few friends with whom he or she feels comfortable.

POWERLESSNESS EVIDENCED BY ANGER, FRUSTRATION, NON-COMPLIANCE, AND DEPRESSION RELATED TO PROGRESSIVE, DETERIORATING ILLNESS.

Patient Outcomes

- Verbalizes frustrations
- Makes decisions about his or her care and treatment
- Participates in treatment plan

Interventions

- Assist patient to identify sources of frustration.
- Encourage talking about feelings generated by changes in his or her condition and treatment regimen.
- Identify ways by which the patient can maintain independence. Set up the environment to promote self-care, where appropriate. Encourage participation in decisions about the treatment plan. Make sure patient has adequate knowledge to make these decisions.
- Negotiate the areas of care over which control can be maintained. Allow the patient some flexibility in his or her care and daily routine. Present options as choices rather than demands, and then honor those choices. The patient may need to accept that certain areas cannot be changed.
- Recognize and acknowledge patient's knowledge and abilities.
- Encourage patient to participate in own care and take responsibility for it. For example, patients at home can learn to set up hyperalimentation or flush central lines. This reduces the sense of dependence on others.
- Encourage exploration of new coping mechanisms to use to deal with new frustrations by reviewing the steps of the problem-solving process.

- Encourage completion of advance directive so patient's wishes are clear to others.

ALTERNATE NURSING DIAGNOSES

Anticipatory grieving
Anxiety
Caregiver role strain
Risk for suicide
Self-concept disturbance
Social isolation

WHEN TO CALL FOR HELP

✔ Suicidal threats or attempts
✔ Onset of aggressive, violent behavior
✔ Onset of psychotic behavior
✔ Extreme conflicts between family and significant others in decisions about patient's care
✔ Patient's noncompliance in critical areas of care
✔ Staff refusal to provide care for the patient
✔ Patient participating in high-risk behavior such as unprotected sex, not informing partners of his or her HIV-positive status

---

Patient and Family Education

- Patients need specific information on ways to prevent transmission of HIV including:
- safe sex practices
  - using a condom
  - abstaining from intercourse
  - avoiding high-risk sex acts that increase contact with blood or body fluids
  - informing any sex partners of HIV-positive status
- never sharing needles
- reminding others to avoid contact with patient's blood or body fluids. When providing education on sex practices, avoid using medical terminology that the patient may not understand. If uncomfortable doing this, seek

out other staff members who may have more experience. Use literature provided by many AIDS organizations to enhance this education.

- Patients, family, and caregivers need to understand modes of transmission and know precautions to take including appropriate use of disposable gloves and antiseptics and proper disposal of contaminated material.
- Educate the family that close physical contact, such as touching, or kissing are not modes of transmission.
- HIV-positive women need counseling on the use of birth control and the risks of pregnancy.
- Discuss completing an advance directive to document patient's wishes if he or she is no longer able to express them. This is especially important if patient does not want parents or siblings making decisions and would prefer friends or lovers to take on that role.
- If patient is a drug abuser, educate on coping mechanisms to avoid drug use especially under stress, such as call sponsor when stressed.
- Review with family and/or significant others the early signs of mental deterioration.
- Explain the difference between HIV-positive status and having AIDS. Educate the HIV positive on the signs of converting to AIDS.
- Educate on care of central lines, adverse effects of medication, and signs of secondary infections.
- Encourage any family and/or significant others to obtain HIV testing if they are fearful of exposure.
- Encourage healthy lifestyle for the patient as way to prevent deterioration and maintain immune system.
- For children with AIDS, recommend an education program for school officials and schoolchildren and their parents on the risks of exposure. AIDS support organizations may be able to provide these programs.

Charting Tips

- Document patient and family response to teaching.
- Describe family's and/or caregiver's response to patient.
- Describe any changes in mental status. Describe specific behaviors rather than a subjective opinion.
- Document the patient's coping mechanisms.

Discharge Planning

- Encourage the patient to contact local AIDS organizations for emotional and financial support and caregiver resources.
- Refer the patient to appropriate support groups and counseling.
- Assess the resources available to maintain the patient at home as long as possible, including caregivers and adequate equipment.
- Arrange for home health care and home infusion care, as needed.
- Refer the patient to hospice care (in the home or a facility), if appropriate.
- Refer the patient to the social worker to review financial concerns and insurance issues.
- Ensure that the family and significant others are aware of discharge plan.

Nursing Outcomes

- Staff will demonstrate adequate and concerned care to patient.
- Staff will demonstrate nonjudgmental care to patient or family or significant others.
- Treatment plan is carried out consistently.
- Staff demonstrates appropriate psychosocial assessments and interventions.

Suggested Learning Activities

- Contact local AIDS organizations to obtain information on services available within your community.
- Attend AIDS support groups for patients or families.
- Consider volunteering in AIDS support organizations.
- Obtain videos of recent films on AIDS including *And the Band Played On* or *Longtime Companion*.
- Become familiar with the national hotlines that provide a variety of information about AIDS including: National AIDS Hotline, which provides information on services and publications from the CDC (800-458-5231), and National HIV Consultation Service (800-933-3413).

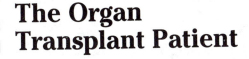

The Organ Transplant Patient

LEARNING OBJECTIVES

▼ *Identify aspects of the "emotional roller coaster" experienced by most transplant patients.*
▼ *Recognize the role of the nurse in caring for the transplant patient through each of the transplant stages.*
▼ *Select the most appropriate interventions for patients before, during, and after transplant.*
▼ *Identify possible nurses' reactions to issues related to transplant patients.*

Transplantation of tissues and organs has become an accepted, rather than experimental, treatment for tissue and organ disease and failure during the past 30 years. It is now possible to remove, replace, or substitute the heart, heart valves, lung, liver, kidney, pancreas, small intestine, adrenal cells, bone marrow, blood stem cells, cornea, skin, bones, joints, ligaments, tendons, and blood vessels. Improvements in medical diagnosis and patient

Glossary

Autografts—Transplanting tissue from one part of the body to another.

Allografts—Transplanting tissue from one member of a species to one of the same species.

Xenografts—Transplanting tissue from a member of one species to a member of another species.

Histocompatibility—The match between donor and recipient tissue as determined by immune response.

Immunosuppression—An alteration in normal protective responses, which brings about a state of unresponsiveness of the immune system.

Rejection—An immunologic response involving the recognition of HLA antigens on the donor tissue by recipient lymphocytes or antibodies and subsequent destruction of the antigen-bearing graft.

Hyperacute rejection—Occurs within hours of vascularization of the graft, caused by the presence of preformed circulating cytotoxic antibodies.

Acute rejection—Occurs within a week to 3 months of transplantation; it is a cellular immune response and can be treated with immunosuppressants.

Chronic rejection—Occurs after 3 months; mediated by both cellular and humoral antigen responses; leads to insidious, progressive loss of graft function.

Graft-versus-host disease (GVHD)—The principal limitation to histocompatible bone marrow transplantation; GVHD can be either acute or chronic.

Brain death—Specific criteria determined by state law to define brain death and establish who can determine that criteria have been met; organs and tissue may be donated after brain death has been determined if the patient and designated next of kin consent.

preparation and selection for transplant, as well as the availability of drugs that prevent rejection, have contributed to the high success rate of transplantation. There are more than 100 heart, 80 liver, and 200 kidney transplant programs in the United States today.

For those fortunate enough to receive organs, the transplant success rate is high: One-year survival rates are 92 percent for kidney transplants, 79 percent for heart, 76 percent for liver, 59 percent for heart and lung, and 89 percent for pancreas transplant. Most recipients return to normal activities and live for an average of 8 to 9 years after transplant.

More than 32,000 people in the United States are on a waiting list for organ transplant. The number has almost doubled over the last 5 years. Approximately seven people die each day because an organ cannot be found in time. About 12,000 to 15,000 medically appropriate potential organ donors are available each year. However, only one-third of these, or about 4500, actually donate organs. Organ donations have barely increased in the last 5 years. The number of transplants cannot keep up with the ever-increasing demand because of the shortage of donors. Potential donors are lost because patients have not considered organ donation before their hospitalization and because families deny consent or are not offered the option of donation when the patient becomes a potential donor. See Table 19–2, Laws Affecting Organ Procurement and Donation.

Generally Americans have a fairly high level of awareness about organ donation and the benefits of transplantation. Most Americans (89 percent) believe organ donation allows something positive to result from a death. More than half (59 percent) feel that organ donation helps families cope with their grief, and most Americans believe transplant recipients gain additional years of healthy life. About two-thirds of Americans report they are very or somewhat likely to want their organs donated after their death; but only about one-fourth have granted permission for organ donation by signing a donor card or indicating willingness to be a donor on their driver's license (see Table 19–3, Nursing Interventions to Assist Families of Potential Donors).

TABLE 19–2. **Laws Affecting Organ Procurement and Donation**

Law	Impact
1968 Uniform Anatomical Gift Act (UAGA)	Established legality of the organ and tissue donor care
1987 UAGA Revised	Defined rights and responsibilities of the donor and recipient
1978 Uniform Brain Death Act	Expanded traditional definition of death (cardiopulmonary) to include brain death
1980 Uniform Determination of Death Act	
1984 National Organ Transplant Act	Established the national Organ Procurement and Transplant Network (OPTN)
	Prohibited sale of human organs
1986 Omnibus Budget Reconciliation Act (OBRA)	Established hospital procedures that require a designated person to approach family members about donation at a time of a patient's death (Required Request)
1987 OBRA	Organ procurement organizations to be notified by hospitals regarding potential donors

There are many misconceptions, however, about organ donation. For example, almost 80 percent of Americans incorrectly believe that only a signed donor card is needed for organ donation. More than 40 percent do not realize that permission from the deceased person's next of kin is also required. About one-third believe that organs for transplant can be bought and sold on the black market (Gallup, 1993).

As transplantation is increasingly becoming an option for more patients, the technical aspects are more standardized, and outcomes are more predictable. The major limitation is the potential that tissue transplanted from another human being will be rejected if the recipient's im-

TABLE 19–3. **Nursing Interventions to Assist Families of Potential Donors**

- Make sure that brain death or death has been discussed with the family.
- Ensure family has had some time to grieve.
- Be aware of agency policies in identifying potential donors.
- Try to determine the beliefs of the potential donor such as has he or she ever mentioned donation or signed a donor card.
- Identify key family members to involve and provide a private place for discussion.
- Ascertain family's understanding about brain death and hope for recovery.
- Provide information slowly.
- Refer to potential donor by name.
- Provide accurate information on the need for informed consent, that other evaluations will be required, and that there is no cost to the family.
- Assure family understands that the donation will not interfere with funeral plans or having an open casket.
- Provide time for family to discuss request and make a decision without pressuring or inducing guilt.
- Seek input from transplant professionals throughout this process.

mune system recognizes the new tissue or organ as foreign. Histocompatibility testing is used to minimize graft foreignness and reduce donor-specific immune responses to the transplanted organ. Bone marrow has the greatest capacity to induce reactions, followed by skin, pancreas (Islets of Langerhans), heart, kidney, and liver. The ABO and HLA (human leukocyte antigen) systems have been identified as the major transplantation antigens in humans. These are the most commonly tested before transplantation.

The phenomenon of rejection is not a problem in genetically identical individuals. In all others, there may be some level of rejection caused by both donor and host factors. The major donor factor is the presence of HLA antigens on the donor tissue. The major host factor is prior sensitization against ABO and HLA antigens expressed on the graft. Rejection is classified as one of four types: hyperacute, accelerated, acute, and chronic. Anti-rejection drugs are used to minimize the effects of rejection.

The psychosocial aspects of transplantation are very challenging. Patients facing transplantation share many concerns regardless of the organ transplanted. Most are quite frightened when they realize that a vital organ is failing and that they will need a transplant to sustain life.

The transplant process has been described as a series of stages. These stages coincide with specific time periods and activities during the transplant process and are characterized by common stressors and emotional responses in both the recipients and their families. The stages of transplantation commonly described in the literature are: transplant proposed, evaluation, awaiting a donor, perioperative period, postoperative period, complications and possible loss of organ and death, discharge and postdischarge. The stages of transplant, common patient and family responses, and nursing diagnoses are listed in Table 19–4, Transplant Stages, Common Patient Responses, and Nursing Diagnoses.

Living donors as in kidney and bone marrow must face pain and some risk to help another. These donors often have high hopes that their tissue will save a loved one from death.

Etiology

The psychologic difficulties of patients who are undergoing a transplant experience have been widely documented in the literature. The response varies from very mild to severe. Coping with these problems may result in poor physical and psychologic adaptation to the new organ and post-transplant lifestyle. Common problems include anxiety and fear about the transplant and being a burden to the family and guilt that someone else has to be put at risk or die in order to receive an organ. Most patients experience some level of depression, behavioral problems, changes in body image, sexual dysfunction, and a sense of isolation due to infection precautions during some phase of the transplant process.

They may also experience hopelessness and helpless-

TABLE 19–4. **Transplant Stages, Common Patient Responses, and Nursing Diagnoses**

Transplant Stage	Common Responses	Nursing Diagnoses
Transplant proposed	Fear of death Lack of knowledge Grief over loss of organ	Anxiety, fear Knowledge deficit Anticipatory grieving
Evaluation	Uncertainty Doubt Stress over finances	Knowledge deficit Anxiety, fear Ineffective coping
Awaiting a donor	Vigilance and hope Fear of death Guilt over being a burden Out of control	Anxiety Fear Ineffective coping Powerlessness, hopelessness
Perioperative	Fear and anxiety Lack of knowledge	Anxiety, fear Knowledge deficit
Postoperative	Joy and hope of a rebirth Loss of family and work roles Anxiety	Disturbance in body image Loss of self-esteem, grieving Anxiety
Complications/ possible death	Fear of death Fatigue	Helplessness, guilt Fatigue
Discharge	Lack of knowledge Family conflicts, role changes Poor compliance	Knowledge deficit Alteration in family process Noncompliance Impaired adjustment
Postdischarge	Anxiety and depression Inability or lack of motivation to follow through with medical regimen and change in lifestyle Attempts to stabilize family roles and finances	Anxiety, depression Impaired adjustment Ineffective management of therapeutic regimen Ineffective family coping

ness, dependency and regression during the long waiting and rehabilitation periods, family conflicts, and financial stresses as bills mount up for the expensive surgery and immunosuppressive drugs. During periods of organ deterioration before transplant or during the immediate post-transplant phase when the patient is first placed on high doses of steroids and antirejection medications, the patient may experience organic brain dysfunction, psychotic states, cognitive and attention deficits, and even suicidal ideations. In addition, patients may have psychotic reactions after surgery that are related to sensory overload and sleep deprivation, metabolic disturbances, medications, or emotional events.

Although most patients seem to adjust fairly well both physically and psychologically to their new organ, others seem to need to work through a psychologic integration in which the organ from the donor is accepted into their new body image. This "psychologic transplant" occurs in stages. In the initial stage the patient reacts to the transplanted organ as a "foreign body," reporting that the organ "feels funny." They may worry that the organ will "stop working" or "get loose and fall out." During the next phase, the patient is less preoccupied with the functioning of the organ. Finally when the patient begins to accept the organ as part of his or her body, the organ is completely assimilated.

Distinct psychologic features characterize the various types of transplants. For example, response to the transplant may be quite different depending on whether the organ came from a living-related donor or a cadaveric donor. Unlike heart and liver transplants in which only minimal donor-recipient histocompatibility testing is necessary, extensive testing is required to identify a compatible kidney donor. A family member may volunteer for testing but once determined to be "a good match" may feel ambivalent about donating. He or she may fear his or her own kidney failure of the one remaining kidney later in life or the pain of surgery and may wonder whether the risk of graft rejection is worth the donation.

Unlike kidney transplant patients, patients awaiting heart transplant cannot be maintained on artificial life support indefinitely. Also, the heart is the most symbolic of our internal organs, and patients seem to respond more emotionally to the personal characteristics of the heart donor. For example, patients may express concern that their new heart came from a "kind, good-hearted" person, not from a "mean or bad-hearted" person. Unlike other patients with end-stage organ disease, patients in need of a liver transplant often bear a social stigma: they are often assumed to be alcoholic or drug addicted. The physical changes accompanying liver disease, such as ascites, jaundice, and bruising, are more obvious. The patient may exhibit cognitive changes from hepatic encephalopathy earlier than would be the case in other organ failures.

In general, patients who have experienced organ deterioration over a long period of time adjust to the idea of transplantation more readily than patients who develop an acute organ failure and have not had the time to consider the changes in their body functions or body image.

Related Clinical Concerns

The most commonly encountered psychiatric problems seen in transplant patients are anxiety, depression, delirium, and psychosis. These reactions may represent a more serious psychiatric condition or an adjustment disorder related to the patient's medical condition and the stress of dealing with the transplant. Liver and bone marrow transplant patients have more psychiatric complications than kidney or heart recipients, probably due to the increased medical and surgical complications related to these types of transplants.

Increase in psychiatric symptoms at any time during the transplant process may herald the onset of neurologic or infectious complications. Because of the high doses of corticosteroids, transplant patients are at risk for viral and fungal infections, such as candidiasis and aspergillosis, which are associated with metastatic brain abscesses with meningeal involvement. Many patients with early infections have mild signs of cognitive impairment. If these mental status changes are blamed on metabolic encephalopathy or "ICU psychosis," diagnosis of a life-threatening infection may be delayed.

Lifespan Issues

INFANTS AND CHILDHOOD

There is no lower age limit on most transplants. Life-saving transplants have been performed on neonates within the first few days of life.

For the chronically ill child, facing a transplant may present few changes for the child as he or she may be used to long hospitalizations, complications, and pain. For the parents, however, transplants often produce a euphoria as their prayers are answered and at the same time they must face tremendous financial burdens, long hospital stays, strains on the marriage and relationships with other children, and even relocation in some cases to be near a transplant center. Parents who are potential donors or are rejected as donors must face tremendous emotional turmoil and guilt. Parents may also be faced with decisions about using a sibling as a donor. Studies also show that some children receiving transplants may be more prone to learning disabilities, impaired growth, and even malignancies in the future due to complications and long-term immunosuppressive therapy.

ADOLESCENCE

The need for a transplant forces the teen to face potential imminent death. The teen is also confronted with appearance, body, and self-esteem changes that influence his or her body image. The teen may also be more likely to struggle with compliance with posttransplant regimens as part of his or her struggle for independence.

ADULTHOOD

Many transplants occur in adults who are at the prime of their productive lives. The impact of the illness and treatment will significantly influence family relationships, obligations, career, and financial commitments.

ELDERLY

Many transplant programs have upper age limits on potential recipients. This is due not only to the higher risk for complications but also to the dilemma of who should receive the scarce resource of a donated organ. Many transplant programs, however, do accept appropriate patients in their sixties and seventies.

Nurses may question the ethics or morality of transplantation and the allocation of scarce resources, especially if more than one transplant is needed, for instance, if the first transplant is rejected or if patient has lifestyle risks the nurse finds unacceptable such as substance abuse.

Possible Nurses' Reactions

- May feel uncomfortable caring for a patient whom the nurse believes is an unsuitable organ recipient.
- May feel conflict over continuing to prepare the patient for transplant and holding out hope, while at the same time fearing that a donor will not be found in time.
- May feel guilt about the death of the donor especially if the donor was a patient in the same institution or same unit.
- May be concerned over the increasing dependency of the patient on the staff or individual nurse. Family members may not be available to continually support the patient through the long transplant process.
- May have difficulty adjusting quickly and always responding appropriately to the up-and-down emotional changes the patients and family members frequently go through.
- May be upset about being the recipient of the anger from the patient or family should the transplant fail. This often happens because of the intense relationships that often develop between the transplant patient and certain care providers.
- May resent taking care of an angry ungrateful patient that may make the nurse feel frustrated and inadequate.
- May have difficulty confronting their own mortality and ambivalent feeling about transplants.
- May become enmeshed in conflicts with other members of the transplant team if not provided with opportunities to deal with these emotionally laden issues as a group.
- May fear approaching families of potential donors because they feel they are intruding on the family, are unprepared, or do not know what to say.
- May have the difficult task of helping patients adjust emo-

tionally to almost certain death if they do not receive an organ in time while at the same time helping them prepare for their surgery and subsequent recovery after transplantation.

Assessment

Behavior and/or Appearance

- Verbalizes nonacceptance or denial of end-stage disease, the need for transplant, and health status change
- Verbalizes difficulty or lack of desire to learn new behaviors
- Lack of interest in learning new regimens, medications, and other health maintaining behaviors
- Behaviors indicative of failure to adhere to transplant protocols
- Inaccurate or incomplete follow-through of instruction
- Unable or unwilling to increase self-care activities
- Failure to show up for teaching sessions or appointments

Mood and/or Emotions

- Mild to severe anxiety or depression
- Fearful of transplant outcome or death
- Grieving over loss of diseased organ
- Guilty over burden on family
- Extended period of emotional shock

Thoughts, Beliefs, and Perceptions

- Impaired cognition
- Poor judgment
- Unable to be involved in decision making, problem solving, or goal setting
- Unable or unwilling to recall or repeat new information
- Lack of future-oriented thinking
- Misinterpretation of information

Relationships and Interactions

- Increased dependence on family and caregivers
- Fears changes in family or marital relationships and work roles

- Increased financial stressors
- Inadequate support systems

Physical Responses

- Too tired to participate in learning
- Symptoms of organ failure
- Evidence of side effects from antirejection medications
- Failure to progress or improve physically
- Evidence of development of multiple and varied complications
- Evidence of exacerbation of old symptoms
- Evidence of infection

Pertinent History

- History of chronic illness
- History of behaviors that could jeopardize transplant, such as substance abuse, noncompliance

Collaborative Management

Multidisciplinary Team Communication

Because of the prevalence of psychiatric problems seen during transplant, the availability of a psychiatrist, psychologist, or psychiatric clinical nurse specialist to evaluate and follow transplant patients and their families is very important. Medical social workers and hospital chaplains are also vital in providing comprehensive services. A dietitian and admission-discharge coordinator are also invaluable in helping the medical team plan effectively.

Because of the complex interactions among the many drugs transplant patients must take to stabilize their medical conditions, maximize the success of their transplant, and minimize infections, a pharmacist is an essential addition to the transplant team.

Pharmacologic

Almost all the major pharmacologic agents for treatment of psychiatric symptoms, such as antidepressant, antipsychotic, and antianxiety drugs, can have adverse effects on transplant patients. For example, benzodiazepines used to treat anxiety, which are protein bound, depend on liver metabolism for degradation and excretion by the kidney. Metabolites can accumulate in patients with renal or hepatic insufficiency, so they should be used with caution in patients with these conditions. Benzodiazepines also reduce the ventilatory response to hypoxia, so they should be used cautiously in patients with cardiac or pulmonary disease. Tricyclic antidepressants are often contraindicated in liver and heart transplant patients because of decreased liver metabolism or the risk of congestive heart failure and dysrhythmias. Analgesics may also be needed to treat incisional pain or pain from treatment side effects like mucositis (mouth sores after chemotherapy in bone marrow transplants).

If the patient is delirious, careful attention must be paid to the diagnosis, cause, and treatment of the delirium. In transplant patients, etiologic factors are many: a metabolic disruption such as uremia or encephalopathy, a physiologic disturbance such as cardiogenic shock or infection, rejection, drug reaction, or neurologic events. First and foremost, the underlying cause must be found and treated. Haloperidol is effective for agitation and can be given intravenously for emergencies or intramuscularly or orally to maintain its effect. This medication is especially useful in heart transplant patients because it has almost no pulmonary or cardiovascular side effects. It should be used cautiously with liver failure patients because it is metabolized by the liver.

For acute psychosis, again the underlying cause must be identified and eliminated. Sleep deprivation, medication side effects from steroids, and alterations in the patient's metabolic and physical condition are possible causes. Sometimes treatment must be instituted while the cause is still undetermined. Pharmacologic intervention is indicated if the patient becomes disruptive or out of control. The risks associated with undermedicating and inadequately supervising the patient are greater than the potential for overdosing the patient. Haloperidol is the drug of choice for acute psychosis in transplant patients.

Many patients receiving organ transplants must remain on immunosuppressive medications for the rest of their lives to prevent rejection. The most common drug is cyclosporine. Side effects include nephrotoxicity, hypertension, tremors, and burning hands and feet. This drug along with other immunosuppressives are extremely expensive, often costing the patient at least $10,000 per year, and they may not be covered by insurance.

Nursing Management

KNOWLEDGE DEFICIT EVIDENCED BY ANXIETY OR INACCURATE PERCEPTIONS RELATED TO ABSENCE OR DEFICIENCY OF COGNITIVE INFORMATION ABOUT THE TRANSPLANT PROCESS.

Patient Outcomes

- Demonstrates interest in education process
- Verbalizes knowledge of treatment, medications, signs and symptoms of infection and rejection, and other transplant-related information
- Demonstrates successful self-care skills

Interventions

- Assess patient's and family's knowledge and skill level. Monitor their readiness to learn, and identify barriers to learning. Modify the teaching plan as needed.
- Provide opportunity for patient and family to discuss their learning needs. Actively listen to patient's and family's description of their learning needs.
- Develop patient's and family's trust in your teaching skills through planned consistent interactions and positive reinforcement of participation.
- Encourage return demonstrations and repetition of new information.
- Include family and caregivers in teaching sessions when possible.
- Provide realistic information yet at same time encourage hope.
- Teach stress-reducing techniques to get through waiting periods.
- Prepare for emotional changes of waiting for a donor including anxiety and/or loss of control.
- Prepare patient for need to increase self-monitoring as part of post-transplant care.
- Refer to other services and agencies for further educa-

tion as needed such as pharmacy, dietary, social services, and home health.
- Review discharge teaching immediately before discharge to reinforce earlier education and resolve any remaining questions.
- Make sure family members have adequate living arrangements and other needed support to reduce their stress.

IMPAIRED ADJUSTMENT EVIDENCED BY INABILITY TO MODIFY HIS OR HER LIFESTYLE AND BEHAVIOR AND RELATED TO HEALTH STATUS AND TRANSPLANT.

Patient Outcomes

- Will participate in goal setting and problem solving
- Assumes responsibility for self-care
- Verbalizes acceptance of health status change

Interventions

- Assess pretransplant lifestyle and coping style. If problems are identified, assist the patient to learn more effective coping strategies.
- Assess the patient's and family's responses to situation, fears and concerns about adapting to transplant, and fears about death. Assist them in facing these fears and finding effective ways to deal with them.
- Encourage patient to talk about feelings of accepting a new organ. Prepare patient for feelings of anxiety, guilt, and concerns about changes in body image and sexuality.
- Reinforce adaptive coping mechanisms for long hospitalization with possible periods of isolation.
- Identify any beliefs or values that the patient and family hold that may affect adjustment to transplant.
- Discuss with patient and family their knowledge about the transplant process and lifestyle or behavior changes. Provide educational materials about the transplant process and needed lifestyle or behavior changes.
- Assess possible adverse effects of medication, and consult physician regarding dosage adjustments, as appropriate.
- Monitor for signs of rejection or infection. Prepare patient for what symptoms to report.

- If signs of rejection are present, avoid criticizing or condemning the patient. Maintain hope and point out that rejection does not necessarily mean death and can be treated but that he or she must be prepared for the return of the previous symptoms. Allow grieving loss of new organ and provide support.
- Reinforce independent decisions to reduce dependency on staff and caregivers.
- Provide reality orientation to the confused patient.
- Reinforce need to grieve loss of diseased organ and previous lifestyle.

ALTERNATE NURSING DIAGNOSES

Alteration in family process
Anxiety
Depression
Disturbance in body image
Fatigue
Fear
Grieving, anticipatory
Guilt
Ineffective individual coping
Ineffective management of therapeutic regimen

WHEN TO CALL FOR HELP

- ✔ Any changes in cognitive functioning such as attention deficit, recall of recent events, change in mental status
- ✔ Onset of mood change, especially severe depression or anger, suicidal thoughts
- ✔ Any indication of delirium, paranoid thinking, or psychotic behavior
- ✔ Patient's and family's changing their mind about transplant
- ✔ Increased staff concern or conflict over management of patient care
- ✔ Increased staff reactions over caring for patient or complaints about patient's behavior
- ✔ Patient's and family's refusing to participate in planning discharge, learning about post-transplant medications, or other treatment plans

Patient and Family Education

- Review signs and symptoms of infection and rejection.
- Review side effects of medications. Stress the importance of taking immunosuppressive drugs as ordered. Remind patient to report all side effects to the doctor and to never change dose without checking with physician.
- Prepare patient and family for the emotional changes of accepting a new organ and changes in lifestyle after the transplant.
- Educate the patient's family and friends about the critical need for organ donation.

Charting Tips

- Use objective, nonjudgmental terms to describe behavior.
- Document patient's and family's responses to information and teaching about transplant procedures. Document any changes in patient's and family's attitude or decision about transplantation and how questions were resolved.
- Document patient's and family's ability to follow postdischarge medication orders before discharge.
- Document use of psychotropic medications and patient's response to them.
- Document patient's psychologic integration of new organ into body image.

Discharge Planning

- Provide support and information regarding resuming active life, returning to work, or other significant issues.
- Refer to available support group or counseling as needed.
- Encourage patient and family participation in discharge planning. Communicate plan of care to all involved in discharge planning.
- Inform all appropriate agencies of patient's progress, current status and medication requirements, and projected needs, for instance, for home health care or rehabilitation services.

- Ensure that follow-up appointments are made according to the post-transplant discharge protocols.
- Make sure patient has access to obtain needed medications. Refer to social worker if patient needs financial assistance to obtain these medications or assistance with meeting other financial obligations.

Nursing Outcomes

- Staff cares for patient throughout transplant process consistently to provide for patient's physical and emotional needs.
- Staff selects interventions appropriate to patient's physical and emotional abilities and suitable to transplant stage.
- Staff collaborates with other transplant team members to provide consistent, coordinated treatment throughout transplant process.

Suggested Learning Activities

- Plan to meet with a group of post-transplant patients and their family members. Ask what was most helpful and not helpful from their healthcare providers during their transplant experience.
- Arrange for an inservice from a local transplant specialist to discuss how to approach families of potential donors.
- Send for the most recent statistics on tissue and organ transplants in the United States from your local organ procurement center or from UNOS—United Network for Organ Sharing (1-800-666-1884).
- Find out what is being done in your community to educate the public about the shortage of donor organs.
- Ask to observe or participate in a transplant unit's staff support meeting. Prepare questions you would like to ask about dealing with the issues and concerns they experience with transplant patients and their families.

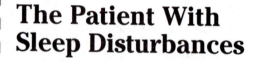

The Patient With Sleep Disturbances

LEARNING OBJECTIVES

▼ *Differentiate among mild, moderate, and severe sleep pattern disturbances.*
▼ *Identify factors leading to poor sleep and fatigue.*
▼ *Select the most appropriate interventions for dealing with sleep pattern disturbance.*

Sleep is unconsciousness from which the person can be awakened by sensory stimuli such as sound, light, and touch. Sleep disorders put an individual at risk for experiencing a change in the quantity or quality of rest and sleep as related to biologic and emotional needs. Adverse physical, mental, and emotional changes may occur if needed or normal rest and sleep patterns are interrupted. Most people have suffered from at least transient sleep

---

Glossary

Sleep disorders—Chronic disturbance of sleep patterns affecting the amount, quality, or timing of sleep or events occurring during sleep such as nightmares.

Insomnia—Abnormal wakefulness, an inability to fall asleep easily or to remain asleep during night.

Somnolence—Abnormal drowsiness or sleepiness during usual waking hours.

Sleep apnea—Sleep-induced respiratory impairment.

Obstructive sleep apnea—A serious sleep-related breathing disorder manifested by daydream sleepiness or excessive loud snoring. Frequently associated with cardiac dysrhythmias.

Sleep deprivation—Periods without normal sleep pattern, resulting in irritability, fatigue, difficulty in concentrating and memory, poor muscle coordination, and sometimes hallucinations and illusions.

Narcolepsy—An infrequent but serious disorder consisting of recurrent episodes of uncontrollable sleep.

Hypersomnia—Sleeping more than normal amount of the time; may occur after some CNS damage.

Sleep walking (somnambulism)—Repeated acts of rising from bed during sleep and ambulating. Generally occurs in stages 3 and 4 of sleep and in the time phase of 30 to 200 minutes after onset of sleep.

Sleep drunkenness—Exaggerated transition from sleep to waking, with confusion state lasting 1 to 2 hours or more, during which perception and judgment are compromised.

Fatigue—An overwhelming sustained sense of exhaustion or lack of energy and decreased capacity for physical or mental work.

disturbances. Many factors lead to poor sleep, such as the environment of the sleeping area (levels of sound, light and temperature), the age and general physical and psychologic condition of the patient, as well as recent stressful events.

Sleep had been considered a homogeneous quiet period with minimal brain activity until the discovery of the electroencephalographic (EEG) record. With this technology, the description of rapid eye movement (REM) and non-REM (NREM) periods during sleep and their association with dreaming has provided better understanding of sleep physiology and sleep disorders.

Sleep research has shown that there are two types of sleep during a sleep period: sleep when the brain is very active (REM) and sleep with slow brain waves (NREM). The reason these two types of sleep exist is unknown. The sleep center is located in the pons and the medulla. Most sleep at night is NREM sleep; it occurs when a person first falls asleep and is a deep and restful sleep.

On the basis of EEG studies, NREM sleep is divided into four stages:

- *Stage 1:* Very drowsy, musculature relaxes.
- *Stage 2:* Muscles relax further; cerebral activity decreases.
- *Stage 3:* Physiologic changes evident; vital signs decrease; gastrointestinal functions and venous dilation increase to facilitate cellular metabolism and exchange.
- *Stage 4:* Deep sleep with lowest level of body function.

During NREM sleep, pulse and respirations drop 20 to 30 percent, blood pressure decreases, muscles relax, skin vessels dilate (increasing heat loss), metabolic rate decreases by 10 to 30 percent, and body temperature decreases.

Episodes of REM sleep occur about every 90 minutes, last about 5 to 30 minutes, and are associated with dreaming that is remembered. During REM sleep heart rate and respirations often become irregular, and metabolism and temperature increase.

The need for sleep decreases with age: Newborns sleep 18 or more hours a day, school-age children sleep about 10 to 12 hours a day, adults sleep 7 to 9 hours, and the elderly,

TABLE 19–5. **Classifying Sleep Disorders**

DSM-IV Classification	Association of Sleep Disorders Centers Classification
• *Dyssomnias*: Primary insomnia, primary hypersomnia, narcolepsy, breathing-related sleep disorder such as results from shift work • *Parasomnias*: Nightmare disorder, sleep terror disorder, sleepwalking disorder • *Sleep disorder related to another mental disorder*: Depression, psychosis • *Other sleep disorders due to medical condition*: substance related disorder	• Disorders of initiating and maintaining sleep (DIMS) • Disorders of excessive sleepiness (DOES) • Disorders of the sleep-wake cycle • Dysfunctions associated with sleep, sleep stages, or partial arousals (parasomnias)

about 6 hours per night with additional napping during the day. Sleep needs increase during illness. Lack of sleep results in progressive deterioration of mental functioning, physical fatigue, discomfort, and emotional instability.

Both the American Psychiatric Association and the Association of Sleep Disorders have developed a system for classifying sleep disorders (see Table 19–5, Classifying Sleep Disorders).

Etiology

There are many medical and psychiatric conditions that may affect the patient's ability to maintain normal sleep pattern. Patients with respiratory conditions, Alzheimer's, and chronic pain frequently complain of sleep problems. Anxiety, depression, mania, and delirium are also often accompanied by inability to sleep satisfactorily.

Evaluating a complaint of insomnia requires a thorough history that first considers medical, toxic, and environmental conditions, as well as drug and alcohol use. If tolerance to or excessive use of drugs or alcohol is the likely cause of the insomnia, the patient must undergo withdrawal under careful supervision. Insomnia is associated with a long list of drugs, including stimulants and alcohol. Hypnotics used over a long period of time can also cause insomnia due to the development of tolerance and suppression of REM sleep.

Sleep lab studies reveal that some patients with obstructive sleep apnea have between 30 episodes of upper airway obstruction each night resulting in inability to achieve deep sleep state. Hyperventilation, carbon dioxide retention, and severe hypoxemia occurs. Treatment possibilities include weight loss for obese patients and positive-pressure respiratory treatments to keep airway open. Surgical intervention (a procedure to remove excess tissue in the pharynx or a tracheotomy) may be required for more serious cases.

Narcolepsy is sometimes accompanied by cataplexy (partial or complete loss of muscle tone), presleep hallucinations, and sleep paralysis. These symptoms are more debilitating than the sleepiness. Specific treatment includes short daytime napping and prescription of a central nervous system stimulant.

Conditions most frequently associated with excessive daytime sleepiness include:

- Regularly sleeping 10 to 14 hours
- Psychophysiologic causes: Transient and situational sleepiness due to stress, boredom, or depression
- Nocturnal myoclonus, also known as "restless legs" or leg jerking
- Idiopathic CNS hypersomnolence not due to head trauma
- Sleep drunkenness
- Menstrual cycle–associated syndrome: Increased daytime sleepiness around period
- Self-induced insufficient sleep: Related to increased work hours, pressured deadlines, or other self-imposed behavior

Related Clinical Concerns

Hospital routines and policies, such as how late sleeping medication may be given or how late patients can watch TV, can actually restrict nurses in effectively intervening with the more common sleep disturbance problems. Patients often complain that hospital rules and routines are disturbing to their normal sleep patterns. After just a few days in an unfamiliar environment with multiple sleep interruptions, a patient's usual sleep routine can be almost totally reversed, with the patient sleeping most of the day and awake most of the night.

If the patient's physical condition requires intense nursing care, sleep needs will be secondary until physical stability is achieved. However, the need for sleep and its role in a patient's care plan must not be overlooked even during acute care periods. Sleep deprivation is a major contributor to ICU psychosis. Anything that can be done by the staff, patient, or family to attain and maintain a better sleep pattern will be beneficial to the patient.

Many medications used to treat medical conditions can contribute to sleep problems including many asthma medications, cortisone, levadopa, thyroxine, and some chemotherapies.

Lifespan Issues

CHILDHOOD

Sleep terrors, enuresis, and bedtime fears are more common in toddlers and in 7 to 12-year-olds. Sleepwalking and tooth grinding (bruxism) are considered childhood sleep disorders because they are probably developmentally related and usually disappear before or during adolescence.

Children can develop distress at bedtime because of fears of separation and other anxieties. Providing a calm, reassuring routine is important.

ELDERLY

Age is the single most powerful determinant of a person's sleep physiology. Sleep disturbances increase with age and change in type during the aging process. The elderly typically have more trouble falling asleep and awaken frequently throughout the night and early in the morning. They are more easily awakened by noise or other stimuli.

The elderly are especially prone to drug toxicity with hypnotics because of reduced renal function. Antihistamines are frequently used as safe alternatives.

Possible Nurses' Reactions

- May experience patient-staff conflict because patient states that he or she was awake all night and the nurses reported that the patient had slept.
- May be unwilling to or feel incapable of doing anything about patients' sleep problems.
- May feel hospital rules cannot be changed and patients will just have to tolerate frequent interruptions.
- May become frustrated because patients who are awake all night require more care. This problem is compounded when staffing is short.

Assessment

Behavior and/or Appearance

- Tired, lethargic, depressed, agitated, even delirious depending on cause and duration of sleep disturbance
- Drawn and pale, with puffy dark circles under eyes
- Frequent yawning, dozing during the day
- Forgetting appointments or responsibilities
- Minor accidents, such as dropping things, hitting self on cupboard or table corners, not being able to complete or misdoing routine tasks

Mood and/or Emotions

- Changes in mood
- Less tolerance for even minor problems
- More frustrated at difficult tasks
- Severe anxiety
- Irritable
- Angry and hostile
- Depressed

Thoughts, Beliefs, and Perceptions

- Minor errors in memory or ability to calculate
- Confusion
- Inability to retain information
- Inattention and lack of concentration

- Hallucinations, paranoia, or psychotic thinking

Relationships and Interactions

- Spouse or partner complaints about patient's sleep problems
- Changes in sexual relationships
- Change in relationship due to patient's irritability and fatigue

Physical Responses

- Decreased energy for usual activities
- Daytime sleepiness and napping
- Increased fatigue
- Sleep apnea
- Cardiac dysrhythmias
- Low arterial oxygen levels
- Morning headache
- Less pain tolerance
- Injuries due to sleep walking, narcolepsy, or sleep deprivation

Pertinent History

- History of sleep disturbance
- Medical diagnosis associated with sleep disturbances
- Situational or lifestyle events that affect sleep pattern:
  ○ Immobility due to casts or traction
  ○ Pain, illness
  ○ Pregnancy
  ○ Anxiety
  ○ Depression
- Lifestyle disruptions, such as changes in occupation, finances, or relationships
- Environmental changes, such as hospitalization or travel
- Use of medication or other chemical substances, such as alcohol, caffeine, tranquilizers, sedatives, hypnotics, antidepressants, antihypertensives, amphetamines, anesthetics, barbiturates, or steroids
- Alternative work schedules such as evening or night shift work

Collaborative Management

Pharmacologic

Pharmacologic treatment of insomnia generally includes hypnotics and sedatives used for short periods of time. Effective management of pain and other symptoms will enhance sleep as well.

Using sedatives to induce sleep confounds the sleep stages and may actually lead to worsening of the sleep disturbance and to depression if used for more than a few days or weeks. They inhibit other mental and physical activities, such as respiration, cognition, circulation, digestion, and elimination.

Tricyclic antidepressants, MAO inhibitors, and diazepam, all used at times to enhance sleep, may cause sleep disturbances when discontinued or reduced. With antidepressants and some hypnotics, REM sleep is actually suppressed and, when these medications are discontinued, the REM rebound can cause agitation and frightening dreams.

Nursing Management

SLEEP PATTERN DISTURBANCE EVIDENCED BY DIFFICULTY FALLING ASLEEP, FREQUENT AWAKENINGS, AND/OR EARLY MORNING RISING RELATED TO SLEEPING IN UNFAMILIAR ENVIRONMENT, POST-OPERATIVE CARE, OR HOSPITAL CARE ROUTINES THAT INTERRUPT SLEEP PATTERN.

Patient Outcomes

- Able to sleep a satisfactory amount of time and awaken feeling rested
- Able to rest between disturbances for required care
- Has enough rest to participate in activities ordered, including pre- and postoperative care and rehabilitation

Interventions

- Assess the patient's sleep for quantity and quality. Ask about patient's normal sleep habits. Determine what is promoting or inhibiting patient's sleep in the new environment.

- To help establish a sense of security, familiarize patient with environment; walk around unit, and describe building.
- Establish a sleep routine for the patient using familiar sleep habits if possible, such as special activities in preparation for sleep, fixing the bedding, or playing music.
- Allow the patient some personal comfortable bedding and pajamas and other personal possessions if available.
- Encourage the use of presleep relaxation measures including back rub, medication, prayer, soft music, reading, or bedtime snack if patient desires.
- Position patient comfortably; assist in turning and using bathroom as needed.
- Minimize use of caffeine or other stimulants in afternoon or evening.
- Provide a quiet, undisturbed period of sleep with comfortable room temperature and nonglaring, dim lighting if needed.
- Use hypnotics or sedatives only as a last resort or if patient is experiencing unusually stressful events. Do not use more than a few days as sleep patterns can be further disturbed by frequent or chronic use of sleep medication.
- Teach the causes and interventions for sleep disturbance provoked by new environment. If sleep-rest pattern continues to be disturbed after a reasonable amount of time for adjustment, reassess for other possible problems, such as depression or anxiety.
- If possible, assess patient's sleep habits before surgery and after surgery and observe for behavior changes that may indicate sleep deprivation, such as confusion or agitation. Plan nursing care activities with patient to limit number of disturbances and to increase sleep periods within patient safety and postoperative care requirements.
- Plan as many activities between sleep periods as can be arranged.
- Inform other caregivers when patient's sleep periods are planned.
- Be prepared to reassess patient's needs and necessity of care routines as patient's condition changes. Move pa-

TABLE 19–6. **Suggestions for Better Sleep Hygiene**

- Sleep as much as needed to feel refreshed and energetic the next day, but no more. Curtailing time spent in bed enhances the quality of sleep. Too much time in bed may actually promote fragmented and shallow sleep.
- A regular arousal time strengthens circadian cycles and helps to establish a regular time of sleep onset.
- A steady amount of physical exercise probably deepens sleep. Occasional exercise will not improve sleep the following night.
- Occasional loud noises will disturb people even if they are not awakened by it or do not remember it later. Decreasing sounds will help some people sleep better.
- Although excessively warm rooms disturb sleep, there is no evidence that an excessively cold room improves sleep. Try to set room temperature to patient's desired level.
- Hunger may interrupt sleep. A light snack before bed may help sleep. If patient cannot eat, offer back or foot rub.
- Caffeine can disturb sleep cycles, even in those who feel it does not. Avoid caffeine several hours before bedtime.
- Alcohol may help tense people fall asleep more easily, but the resultant sleep will probably be fragmented.
- Chronic use of tobacco can disturb sleep.
- People who feel frustrated or angry about their sleep problems should not try harder to fall asleep. Instead, they should get out of bed if possible and do something different, such as reading, watching TV, or doing light housework, until they feel tired.
- An occasional sleeping pill may be beneficial to those with a short-term sleeping problem. However, chronic use of hypnotics is ineffective for most insomniacs.

tient to a quieter area of ICU or to a more private room as soon as medically safe to encourage more effective sleep-rest periods.

- Inform family or caregivers about interventions and goals to improve sleep (see Table 19–6, Suggestions for Better Sleep Hygiene).
- Have staff on night shift provide the patient with feedback on his or her sleep pattern.

IMPAIRED REST-ACTIVITY PATTERN EVIDENCED BY PACING, AGITATION, INABILITY TO REGULATE ONE'S OWN BEHAVIOR RELATED

TO HYPERACTIVITY, HALLUCINATIONS, OTHER PSYCHOTIC SYMPTOMS.

Patient Outcomes

- Remains awake during the day
- Sleeps at least 4 hours every night
- Demonstrates appropriate nighttime behavior.

Interventions

- Identify factors that increase stimulation to patient, and attempt to reduce or eliminate these factors.
- Provide a calming environment.
- Limit coffee and other caffeine-containing foods and drinks such as tea, cola, or chocolate especially after 4:00 p.m. Encourage use of decaffeinated products.
- Establish a contract with the patient to lie down and remain quiet for a specified period of time at night.
- Discourage daytime naps. During the day encourage patient to keep drapes open and remain active. Provide structured activities during the day if needed.
- Avoid reinforcing behaviors that encourage being awake at night such as not allowing eating, television, or socializing.
- Administer ordered medications as indicated. Discuss with physician and pharmacist the changing of doses or timing of medications.

ALTERNATE NURSING DIAGNOSES

Anxiety
Fear
Hopelessness
Impaired gas exchange
Ineffective breathing pattern
Ineffective individual coping

WHEN TO CALL FOR HELP

✔ Increased complaints of inability to rest or sleep to the point of physical or mental fatigue affecting patient's ability to participate in treatment or rehabil-

itation or safely perform daily activities such as driving a car or operating mechanical equipment
✔ Onset of delirium, paranoid thinking, or hallucinations related to sleep deprivation
✔ Long-term or episodic misuse or abuse of sedatives or hypnotics
✔ Idiosyncratic response to sleep medication
✔ Evidence of serious complications of sleep apnea, such as cardiac dysrhythmias or dyspnea

Patient and Family Education

• Teach patient and/or family about improving sleep hygiene.
• If the patient is using sleep medications, review the potential adverse effects and problems with long-term use.
• Review negative effects of poor sleep habits, especially irregular bedtimes and use of stimulants before bedtime.

Charting Tips

• Document the patient's reports of poor sleep, increased tiredness, or fatigue.
• Document the patient's sleep history and bedtime routines that help improve sleep.
• Document the patient's response to sleep interventions.
• Document the use and effects of or response to sleep medications.

Discharge Planning

• Educate the patient and family about general benefits of a regular sleep schedule and suggestions for better sleep.
• Provide referrals, as indicated, to sleep disorder center for patients with obstructive sleep apnea, narcolepsy, or other serious disorders.
• Encourage the patient to minimize use of sedatives and/or hypnotics.
• Provide information about sleep problems to other staff if patient is transferred to another unit or facility.

Nursing Outcomes

- Staff acknowledges sleep pattern disturbance induced by their treatments and patient care activities and plans care to limit the effects to the patient.
- Interventions selected to minimize sleep disturbances are carried out consistently.
- Staff encourages the patient to use his or her own personal bedtime routines as much as possible in the care setting.

Suggested Learning Activities

- Arrange for a presentation on sleep disorders by a local sleep disorder center expert.
- Do a survey of patients, ask them what is helpful or not helpful in the environment related to getting sleep and/or rest.
- Assess the environment of your facility for factors that may lead to sleep pattern disturbance. Check for bright lights in patient areas at night, staff activities and conversations too loud near patient rooms, or unpleasant odors or temperatures. Compare what you found with patient survey data.

20 PSYCHO-PHARMACOLOGY

Pharmocologic Interventions

LEARNING OBJECTIVES

▼ *Identify the indications and clinical uses for antipsychotic, antidepressant, antianxiety, and antimanic medications.*
▼ *List safe administration practices for patients taking these drugs.*
▼ *Select appropriate nursing interventions and patient education strategies for patients on these drugs.*

Not all inappropriate patient behaviors require pharmacologic intervention. It is important to differentiate psychiatric problems that respond to medication from patient behaviors that are personality and coping maladaptations. The latter can become difficult for nursing management but do not require and do not respond to pharmacologic intervention. Those requiring pharmacologic intervention generally respond to one or more of the following classifications of drugs: antipsychotics, antidepressants, monoamine oxidase inhibitors, antianxiety agents, and antimania agents that include lithium and some anticonvulsants.

Antipsychotic Medications

Antipsychotic medications, also known as *neuroleptics* or *major tranquilizers*, are prescribed for psychotic patients whose thinking is disordered and who have abnormalities of feeling and behavior. These medications regulate and control psychotic symptoms but do not cure the underlying cause. While all psychotic patients have thought disorders, they may exhibit varying types of behaviors. For instance, the patient may be hyperactive or totally inert (catatonic) or he or she many be belligerent and combative.

Antipsychotics can be effective for acute psychotic reactions in patients who have a chronic schizophrenia and in those who have no prior history of psychosis. Between acute episodes of psychosis, patients with schizophrenia are usually maintained on lower doses of the same medication. If the patient stops taking the antipsychotic medication, a dramatic escalation of psychosis usually follows, requiring readmittance to a psychiatric hospital. Patients who have had a psychotic episode but who are not schizophrenic and can resume previous functional levels may be kept on lower doses of antipsychotics for a number of months (up to a year), depending on their condition. Antipsychotics do not produce dependency.

With adequate dosage, the patient can show response within the first few days. This is especially true for anxiety, agitation, hyperactivity, belligerence, combativeness, and sleep problems. Hallucinations may take longer to resolve. Delusions may also disappear in time, but some delusions, particularly the long-standing ones, may be more resistant. There may be only a slight modification in the delusion, such as becoming less intense, less disturbing, or less pre-occupying for the patient, but this may take weeks or even longer.

In our current emphasis on brief hospitalizations, a pa-tient may be medically ready for discharge before all psy-chiatric symptoms have fully abated. The patient needs to be assessed for his or her ability to obtain or maintain basic safe living arrangements, clothing, and food, as well as his or her ability to continue treatments for health problems and psychiatric follow-up.

Antipsychotics are available in long-acting forms, called *enanthates* or *decanoates*. An injection of a long-acting an-tipsychotic remains active in the patient for several weeks, sometimes up to a month. For instance, fluphenazine (Pro-lixin) deconoate administered intramuscularly lasts several weeks, while fluphenazine HCL intramuscularly lasts only several hours.

Different antipsychotics provide different degrees of sedation: a more sedating drug should be used with more agitated patients. Once stabilized, the patient may be given most or all of the dose at bedtime unless poten-tial adverse effects require that the drug be given in di-vided doses.

New on the scene are the so-called atypical antipsychot-ics risperidone and clozapine. While all previous anti-psychotics have their major action as potent inhibitors of the neurotransmitter dopamine, this new class presents with a more pronounced effect on inhibiting serotonin re-ceptors. The result of this chemical change includes success in some "treatment-resistant" schizophrenias, a much lower incidence of extrapyramidal effects, and a proven effect on some of the negative symptoms of psy-chosis, including loss or diminution of normal function-ing, flat affect, apathy, and social withdrawal. These new neuroleptics have a different group of adverse effects in-cluding agranulocytosis with clozapine and adverse cardiovascular effects, primarily hypotension, with ris-peridone.

Pharmacology

Mechanism of Action

Most inhibit dopamine. This is also the cause of one of the major adverse effects—extrapyramidal symptoms. Some of the new antipsychotics inhibit serotonin.

Indications

- Psychosis: Schizophrenia, schizoaffective disorder, post-operative psychosis, behavioral disorders, dementia, and delirium
- Psychotic episodes in acute mania
- Antiemetic effect (Chlorpromazine)
- Intractable hiccoughs (Chlorpromazine)

Clinical Effects

- Improvement is seen in psychotic symptoms.
  - *Thought:* General disorganized thinking, acute delusions, and hallucinations
  - *Feeling:* Extreme tension, negativism, and inappropriateness of feelings (in degree or in response to a situation)
  - *Behavior:* Hyperactivity; hostility and combativeness; sleep disturbance; poor self-care, social withdrawal
- *Rapid tranquilization*: Intramuscular administration of potent antipsychotics at frequent intervals can rapidly control an acute psychotic episode. For instance, 5 mg of haloperidol lactate can be administered intramuscularly every hour until the patient is calm to a maximum of 6 doses.

Adverse Effects

- These will vary depending on the drug used.

EXTRAPYRAMIDAL SIDE EFFECTS (EPS)

- Pseudoparkinsonism (virtually indistinguishable from classic parkinsonism)
  - Loss of facial movements, akinesia, shuffling gait, mask-like facies, monotonous speech

- *Incidence:* 15 percent
- *Treatment:* Can be effectively treated with an antiparkinson agent such as benzatropine, trihexyphenidyl, or diphenhydramine.

- *Akathisia:* Subjective desire to be in constant motion; pacing, shifting weight from one foot to the other, or rocking
  - *Incidence:* 21 percent
  - *Treatment:* Lowering dosage of neuroleptic or changing drugs is not always effective. Diphenhydramine, diazepam, amantadine, or beta blockers like propranolol may be of benefit but using antiparkinson drugs is questionable.

- Acute dystonic reactions (muscle stiffness; muscle spasms in neck, eyes, face)
  - More common in young men
  - *Incidence:* 2 percent
  - *Treatment:* Dramatic response with antiparkinson drugs, such as benztropine, 2 mg intramuscularly, or diphenhydramine, 50 mg intramuscularly. If these are helpful, they can be continue orally to prevent further attacks.

- Tardive dyskinesia (involuntary chewing movements, lip smacking, jaw and tongue movements, facial tics, and grunting, which continues indefinitely)
  - Higher incidence in elderly women
  - May be result of using higher doses over long periods
  - *Incidence:* 0.5 to 40 percent depending on reporting criteria
  - *Treatment:* None are reported to be effective. Prevention includes using the smallest dose of antipsychotic possible for the shortest amount of time.

SEDATION

- Tolerance develops after several weeks and the sedative effects are lessened.

ANTICHOLINERGIC

- Dry mouth, blurred vision, urinary retention, and constipation.
- Use with caution in patients with narrow-angle glaucoma and benign prostatic hypertrophy.

CARDIOVASCULAR
- Orthostatic hypotension
  - Elderly are more susceptible.
  - More common with parenteral administration.
  - May be seen with initial dose titration of risperidone.
- ECG changes
  - Elderly may be predisposed.
  - Possible conduction abberancies include increased QT interval, depression of QT segment, and flat or inverted T waves.

ENDOCRINE
- Weight gain: Seen with most antipsychotics.
- Loxapine and molindone may not cause weight gain (may even promote weight loss).
- Amenorrhea.

SEXUAL DYSFUNCTION
- Not seen with all drugs
  - *Men:* Failure to achieve or maintain erection and ejaculatory disturbances (more common with thioridazine)
  - *Women:* May have difficulty in achieving orgasm

ANTICHOLINERGIC
- Blurred vision
- Dry mouth
- Urinary retention
- Constipation

CENTRAL NERVOUS SYSTEM
- May lower seizure threshold and precipitate seizures in some patients
  - Patients well controlled on anticonvulsants can be safely treated with antipsychotics in most cases

DERMATOLOGIC
- Four types of reactions:
  - *Hypersensitivity reaction:* Urticarial, maculopapular, petechiae, and edema
  - *Contact dermatitis:* More common with chlorpromazine
  - *Photosensitivity reaction:* Appears like severe sunburn
  - *Abnormal pigmentation:* More common with chlor-

TABLE 20-1. Comparing Antipsychotic Drugs

Drug	Acute Dose, mg/day	Maintenance Dose, mg/day	Adverse Effects			
			Sedation	Extrapyramidal	Anticholinergic	Cardiovascular
Chlorpromazine (Thorazine)	400–1000	200–800	High	Moderate	Moderate	High
Promazine (Sparine)	40–1200	40–1200	Moderate	Moderate	High	Moderate
Tifluopromazine (Vesprin)	60–150	60–150	High	Moderate	High	Moderate
Thioridazine (Mellaril)	400–800	200–800	High	Low	High	High
Mesoridazine (Serentil)	200–400	100–400	High	Low	High	High
Acetophenazine (Tindal)	80–120	60–120	Moderate	High	Moderate	Low
Perphenazine (Trilafon)	12–64	12–64	Low	High	Moderate	Low

Drug						
Prochlorperazine (Compazine)	15–150	15–150	Moderate	High	Low	Low
Fluphenazine (Prolixin)	20–60	10–40	Low	High	Low	Low
Trifluoperazine (Stelazine)	20–80	10–40	Low	High	Low	Low
Thiothixene (Navane)	20–80	10–40	Low	High	Low	Low
Haloperidol (Haldol)	20–60	10–40	Low	High	Low	Low
Molindone (Moban)	50–200	20–80	Low	High	Low	Low
Loxapine (Loxitane)	50–250	20–80	Low	High	Low	Low
Clozapine (Clorzaril)	300–900	300–600	High	Low	Low	Low
Risperidone (Risperdal)	2–8	2–6	High	Low	High	High

promazine, after long-term use; may see gray-blue pigmentation in sun-exposed areas

HEMATOLOGIC
- Agranulocytosis (especially seen with clozapine)
  - Rare, but can be fatal
  - Symptoms include sore throat and fever

HEPATIC
- Cholestatic jaundice

Dosage

Varies with individual drugs (see Table 20–1, Comparing Antipsychotic Drugs).

Drug Interactions

- Sedative-hypnotics: May cause excessive additive sedation with other sedating drugs, such as some alcohol, antidepressant, benzodiazepines, and antihistamines. Patients should avoid alcohol.
- Anticholinergic drugs, such as some antidepressants, antiparkinson drugs, some antipsychotics, and atropine: Possible additive anticholinergic effects.
- Antihypertensives: May cause additive hypotension.
- Levodopa and dopamine antagonists: May antagonize the effects of neuroleptics.

Toxicity

- Acute overdose:
  - Possible enhanced adverse effects, such as increased sedation, severe extrapyramidal symptoms, hypotension, and central nervous system depression
  - Treatment is mostly supportive and symptomatic
- Chronic toxicity:
  - Possible cholinergic rebound, such as sweating, salivation, and diarrhea, with some antipsychotics
  - Usually seen when drug has been abruptly discontinued after prolonged use
  - Prevented by titrating patient off the antipsychotic

Nursing Management

Administration

ORAL
- Avoid contact with skin as contact dermatitis can occur with liquid dosage forms.
- Avoid mixing liquids with juice or water. Some of these preparations can have a very bad taste.
- Avoid mixing liquids with other liquid medications, such as lithium citrate.

INTRAMUSCULAR
- Very irritating to tissues. May cause sloughing of skin at injection site.
- Orthostatic hypotension more likely.

SUPPOSITORIES
- Erratic absorption.
- Adult suppositories are not to be given to children.

LONG-ACTING FORMS (FLUPHENAZINE DECANOATE, FLUPHENAZINE ENANTHATE, HALOPERIDOL DECANOATE)
- *Onset of action:* Several days after injection.
- *Duration of action:* Up to 1 month, depending on the individual patient and the drug used.
- Long-acting forms are in a sesame seed oil base and should be given deep intramuscularly.
- *Haloperidol decanoate:* Should be given by Z-track injection.

INTRAVENOUS
- None are approved for intravenous use, though some drugs, such as haloperidol and chlorpromazine, have been given by this route.

Food Interactions

- Food slows the rate, but not the extent, of absorption.
- May take with food, milk, or water to minimize GI distress.

Nursing Considerations

- Monitor patient carefully for side effects, especially sedation, orthostatic hypotension, and extrapyramidal symptoms. As indicated, administer ordered medications to treat presence of extrapyramidal symptoms (see Table 20–2, Drugs Used to Treat Extrapyramidal Reactions).
- Remember that the elderly, the debilitated and the critically ill, and those with kidney and liver disease are especially susceptible to adverse reactions.
- Avoid giving large intramuscular doses (more than 2 to 3 mL) in one site. Rotate sites if repeated injections are necessary.
- Take baseline blood pressure before administering intramuscular injections of these medications. This is especially important with chlorpromazine and mesoridazine and before each injection with rapid tranquilization.
- Keep patient recumbent for at least 30 minutes after an intramuscular injection. Then, slowly elevate his or her head and observe for tachycardia, fainting, or dizziness. To prevent falls, be sure the side rails are in the up position when administering this drug.
- Observe patient for paradoxical agitation.
- As needed, treat the anticholinergic effects of the medications (see Table 20–3, Managing Anticholinergic Effects).
- Assess for the presence of adverse effects in noncompliant patients, particularly the presence of sexual dysfunc-

TABLE 20–2. **Drugs Used to Treat Extrapyramidal Reactions**

Generic Name	Trade Name
Amantadine	Symmetrel
Benztropine	Cogentin
Biperiden	Akineton
Diphenhydramine	Benadryl
Ethopropazine	Parsidol
Procyclidine	Kemadrin
Trithexyphenidyl	Artane

TABLE 20–3. **Managing Anticholinergic Effects**

Anticholinergic drugs have some very troublesome adverse effects. Instituting measures to treat these can improve the patient's level of comfort and, possibly, improve compliance.

Adverse Effect	Treatment
Sedation	Administer the doses at regular intervals throughout the day so that patient receives a smaller amount each time, or, if possible, give the bulk of the daily dose at bedtime.
Dry mouth	Offer frequent sips of water or sugarless candy (to prevent caries and oral infection). Rinse with mouthwash or ice chips.
Urinary retention	May need to treat with cholinergic drugs, such as bethanecol.
Constipation	Provide stool softeners, high-fiber diet, and plenty of fluids.
Blurred vision	No satisfactory treatment. If mild, may use magnifying glass while reading.

tion, which patients may be reluctant to mention. Often patients stop taking the medications because they cannot tolerate the adverse effects.

- Hold medication and call physician immediately if:
  ○ Patient voids brown urine (this may be a sign of cholestatic jaundice).
  ○ Patient has fever and sore throat (this may be a sign of agranulocytosis).
- Monitor complete blood count in long-term patients.
- For patients taking clozapine, monitor the following at least weekly: complete blood count with differential, temperature, pulse, respirations, blood pressure, and signs of infection. Notify the physician if:
  ○ White blood count is less than 3000/mm^3
  ○ White blood count decreases more than three times
  ○ Granulocyte count is less than 1500/mm^3
  ○ White blood count drops more than 3000/mm^3 from last reported value

Patient and Family Education

- Alert family that the patient is sedated but that this will not last long and is not a sign of mental deterioration.
- Warn patient not to change positions abruptly, such as quickly going from a sitting to standing position or getting out of bed, and to avoid hot showers. Sudden position changes can cause lightheadedness, dizziness, and possibly fainting.
- Instruct the patient to use a sunblock with an SPF of 10 or greater when prolonged exposure to the sun is anticipated.
- Warn patient to expect that the medication may turn his or her urine pink but to notify physician should urine turn dark brown.
- Instruct the patient to notify physician immediately if he or she develops sore throat and fever.
- Instruct women of childbearing age to continue to use contraception.
- Prepare patients that sexual dysfunction is a potential adverse effect of the medication. If this occurs, notify the physician, who may order alternative medications. Symptoms will reverse when medication is discontinued.
- Instruct the patient to report any extrapyramidal symptoms.
- Provide information in dealing with the anticholinergic effects of the medications (see Table 20–3, Managing Anticholinergic Effects).

Antidepressant Medications

Antidepressant medications, also called "mood elevators" or "psychic energizers," are used to alleviate the symptoms of depression. The tricyclic and second-generation antidepressants exert their antidepressant action on the neurotransmitters norepinephrine or serotonin in brain cells. The newest class of antidepressants, the selective serotonin reuptake inhibitors (SSRIs), act by selectively affecting serotonin. Because their mechanisms of actions differ, the newer antidepressants do not cause the same types of adverse reactions that made taking the tricyclic and second-generation drugs so problematic.

Antidepressants help the patient achieve a normal, rather than an elevated, mood. Occasionally, however, antidepressants will trigger a manic response in a patient with bipolar disease. Antidepressants are not addictive although some may cause anticholinergic "rebound" symptoms if they are withdrawn abruptly.

Antidepressants are most effective for more severe depression when patients have a distinctly different quality in the severity of the moods, for instance, in those patients who cannot respond with improved mood to events or persons previously enjoyed and demonstrate loss of interest and pleasure in all or almost all activities. They may also show deeper depression in the morning, have early morning wakening, marked anorexia, weight loss, or excessive inappropriate guilt. They are now often prescribed when depression shows no signs of improvement after several months. However, in patients who have depression of 2 years or longer duration and a depressive personality style, they may have only a minimal effect. Antidepressants should not be prescribed for normal grief reactions to a stress or blow to self-esteem. For less severe forms of depression, psychotherapy would be the treatment of choice.

The most common error in using antidepressants has been prescribing doses that are too low to reach therapeutic levels. Once antidepressants are prescribed, it is important to monitor the patient's response to determine the drug's effectiveness. The sequence of improvement is:

1. A lag of about 5 days before any improvement is seen.
2. Sleep improves.
3. Appetite and increased psychomotor activity follow.
4. Characteristic ups and downs in mood are noted.
5. Increased socialization occurs.
6. Consistent improvement in mood occurs.

Note that the patient's subjective sense of relief and improved mood is often the last to occur. That is because the patient may not realize earlier improvements that may seem obvious to others. It is often both necessary and helpful to point out to the patient the improvements he or she has made in sleep, appetite, and activity.

Anxiety that accompanies depression may be reduced in time by antidepressants. If additional medication is prescribed for anxiety, be aware that benzodiazepines may deepen and exacerbate the depression. Antidepressants may be used with antipsychotics in patients with coexisting depression and thought disorders. They should not be used with barbiturates.

Pharmacology

Mechanism of Action

- Tricyclics and second-generation drugs increase concentrations of serotonin and/or norepinephrine in the brain cells.
- Selective serotonin reuptake inhibitors affect only the reuptake of serotonin by the brain cells.

Indications

- Depression
- Panic attacks, particularly fluoxetine and sertraline
- Childhood enuresis (imipramine)
- Chronic pain
- Neuropathic pain
- Prophylaxis for cluster or migraine headaches
- Duodenal ulcers
- Eating disorders
- Obsessive compulsive disorders

Clinical Effects

- Requires full therapeutic trial of 3 to 4 weeks for antidepressant effect.

Adverse Effects

- These will vary dependent on the drug used. Geriatric patients may be especially susceptible.

ANTICHOLINERGIC
- Blurred vision
- Dry mouth
- Urinary retention
- Constipation

CARDIOVASCULAR
- Orthostatic (postural) hypotension
- Sinus tachycardia
- Antidysrythmic (Quinidine-like) effect
- Ventricular irritability with trazodone

GASTROINTESTINAL
- Nausea
- Heartburn

CENTRAL NERVOUS SYSTEM
- Sedation (varies according to drug)
- Extrapyramidal symptoms (only amoxapine)
- Tremors or twitching
- Lowering of seizure threshold (especially maprotilene)
- Insomnia, agitation, headache (SSRIs)

SEXUAL DYSFUNCTION
- Priapism (involuntary erection) reported with trazodone; low incidence
- *Impotence:* Incidence about 1 percent

ENDOCRINE
- *Weight gain or weight loss:* Most can cause either.
  - Fluoxetine, paroxetine may cause weight loss.
  - Venlafaxine may cause weight gain.
- Galactorrhea and amenorrhea seen with amoxapine.

Dosage

Varies with individual drugs (see Table 20–4, Comparing Antidepressant Drugs).

Drug Interactions

- Antihypertensive (clonidine, guanethidine): The antidepressant blocks the antihypertensive effect and adversely affects blood pressure.
- Monoamine oxidase inhibitors (MAOIs): Can cause dizziness, agitated delirium progressing to hypertonicity seizures, hyperpyrexia, and cardiovascular instability. The combination of a tricyclic or second-generation antidepressant and an MAOI can be used safely in some patients with refractory depression as long as the patient is carefully monitored.

TABLE 20–4. Comparing Antidepressant Drugs

Drug	Acute Dose, mg	Maintenance Dose, mg	Adverse Effects			
			Sedation	Anticholinergic	Cardiovascular	Other
Amitriptyline (Elavil)	150–300	50–150	High	Very high	High	
Imipramine (Tofranil)	150–300	50–150	Moderate	Moderate	Moderate	
Doxepin (Sinequan)	150–300	50–150	High	High	Moderate	
Trimipramine (Surmontil)	150–300	50–150	High	Moderate	Moderate	
Nortriptyline (Aventyl)	100–150	50–100	Moderate	Moderate	Moderate	
Desipramine (Norpramin)	150–300	50–150	Low	Low	Moderate	
Protriptyline (Vivactil)	40–60	10–30	Very low	Low	Moderate	
Amoxapine (Asendin)	150–300	50–150	Moderate	Moderate	Moderate	

Maprotilene (Ludiomil)	100–225	75–150	Moderate	Moderate	Moderate	
Trazodone (Desyrel)	150–600	75–150	High	Low	Moderate	
Buproprion (Wellbutrin)	200–450	244–450	Low	Very low	Very low	Anorexic effect
Fluoxetine (Prozac)	20–60	48–96	Very low	None	None documented	
Nefazodone (Serzone)	200–600	300–500	Low to moderate	Low to moderate	Low	Nausea, constipation, asthenia
Paroxetine (Paxil)	20–50	20–50	Low to moderate	Low	Very low	Nausea, headache, dry mouth
Sertraline (Zoloft)	50–200	50–200	Low	Very low	Very low	Nausea, headache, dry mouth, diarrhea, male sexual dysfunction
Venlafaxine (Effexor)	75–375	75–225	Low to moderate	Low	Low	Asthenia, sweating, nausea, constipation, transient high BP

- Benzodiazepines, barbiturates, alcohol, other sedating drugs, such as antihistamines: May cause additive sedation.
- SSRIs and MAOIs should not be used together as severe or even fatal reactions have occurred.
- Sympathomimetics, such as phenylephrine (seen in many over-the-counter cough and cold remedies and diet preparations, and isoproterenol), amphetamines: May see additive effects such as vasoconstriction and increased blood pressure possibly leading to hypertensive crisis.

Toxicity

- *Acute:* Very toxic
  - Signs and symptoms appear in 1 to 2 hours after ingestion and include seizures, coma, respiratory depression, tachycardia, and hypotension.
  - Treat symptomatically as medical emergency.
- Chronic.
- Possible cholinergic rebound, such as sweating, salivation, and diarrhea, with abrupt withdrawal.
- No treatment usually required.
- Avoid abrupt withdrawal.
- SSRIs have a better safety profile in overdoses

Nursing Management

Administration

ORAL

- May give with food and milk. Trazodone should be given with food and milk to reduce gastrointestinal effects.
- May administer smaller doses at regular intervals to minimize side effects.

INTRAMUSCULAR

- Amitriptyline and imipramine are available for intramuscular use.
- Switch to oral as soon as possible.

Food Interactions

- Food does not affect the absorption of these drugs and may be given to alleviate gastrointestinal distress.

Nursing Considerations

- Monitor carefully for adverse effects, especially sedation, orthostatic hypotension, and anticholinergic effects, such as dry mouth, constipation, and blurred vision. As needed, treat the anticholinergic effects of the medications (see Table 20–3, Managing Anticholinergic Effects).
- Remember that the elderly are especially susceptible to troublesome adverse effects and may require smaller doses when drug is started.
- Monitor carefully patients with urinary retention, constipation, benign prostatic hypertrophy, narrow angle glaucoma, or cardiovascular disease. These conditions may be aggravated by anticholinergic effects of tricyclic and second-generation antidepressants.
- Know that maprotilene may cause seizures even at therapeutic doses and trazodone may cause gastrointestinal upset.
- Administer fluoxatine in morning to prevent insomnia.
- Symptoms of toxicity include cardiac dysrhythmias, confusion, and delirium.
- Monitor susceptible patient for suicide risk. As energy level increases, patient may have more energy to act on suicide plan before depressed mood improves.

Patient and Family Education

- Inform the patient and family that it may take up to 1 month until the full effects of the antidepressant are evident. However, adverse effects may begin within the first few days. The patient may need support to maintain hope and to continue to pursue activities to the highest degree possible while waiting for the drug effect to occur.
- The patient should continue taking the medication unless severe adverse effects appear. Instruct the patient to notify the physician should any adverse effects occur that are intolerable.

- Inform the patient to check with his or her physician before taking any over-the-counter medications, especially cold remedies.

Monoamine Oxidase Inhibitors

Monoamine oxidase inhibitors (MAOIs) are also used to relieve symptoms of depression but are usually reserved as second- or third-line agents when tricyclics or second-generation antidepressants are ineffective.

MAOIs do have a significant risk of adverse reactions, particularly if they are not taken carefully and the patient monitored routinely. Hypertensive crisis can prove a potentially lethal drug interaction of MAOIs. The dangerously high blood pressure can lead to cerebrovascular accidents and bleeding, which can be triggered by the patient's eating foods containing tyramine or taking certain other medications. MAOIs should be given only to patients who, after discharge, can responsibly monitor diet or who will be supervised for medication and diet.

There are documented cases of seriously adverse drug interactions between tricyclic antidepressants and MAOIs. For some patients who have not responded to conventional approaches, however, this combination has proved beneficial; however, it requires close medical supervision.

MAOIs can either be sedating or stimulating. Sedating medications can be given at bedtime. If the patient is experiencing insomnia, more or all of the dose may be given early in the day. MAOIs are neither habituating nor addicting.

Pharmacology

Mechanism of Action

Inhibition of enzyme known to inactivate norepinephrine and serotonin.

Indications

- Atypical depression

- Depression refractory to other antidepressants or when conventional medications are contraindicated
- Panic attacks and phobic anxiety states

Clinical Effects

- Improvement is seen gradually over several weeks.
- Drug and diet precautions should be maintained while the patient is taking the drug and for approximately 2 weeks after the drug is discontinued to allow monoamine oxidase enzymes to resynthesize (1 week for tranylcypromine).

Adverse Effects

ANTICHOLINERGIC

- Dry mouth
- Blurred vision
- Urinary retention
- Constipation
- Not as severe as with tricyclic antidepressants

CARDIOVASCULAR

- Orthostatic hypotension especially with phenelzine

TABLE 20–5. **Comparing Monoamine Oxidase Inhibitors**

Drug	Dosage Range, mg/day	Onset of Action	Comments
Phenelzine (Nardil)	15–90	3–4 weeks	Most sedating, most anticholinergic, most hypotensive Useful for phobic and obsessive symptoms
Tranylcypromine (Parnate)	20–30	10 days	Most stimulating, least hypotensive

TABLE 20–6. **Drug Interactions With Monoamine Oxidase Inhibitors**

Drug	Interactions
Insulin Oral antidiabetic agents: Acetohexamide Chlorpropamide Glipizide Glyburide Tolazamide Tolbutamide	May increase hypoglycemic effects, such as lightheadedness, diaphoresis, and tachycardia
Levodopa	May increase flushing and headache Possibility of hypertensive crisis
Sympathomimetics: Dopamine Ephedrine Mephentermine Metaraminol Phenylephrine Phenypropanolamine Pseudoephedrine	May increase headache and hyperpyrexia Possibility of hypertensive crisis
Meperidine	Cardiovascular instability Hyperpyrexia Restlessness Agitation Seizures Coma
Tricyclic antidepressants (may be used together with very close monitoring)	Nausea Dizziness Agitated delirium progressing to hypertonicity Seizures Hyperpyrexia Dyspnea Cardiovascular instability

CENTRAL NERVOUS SYSTEM
- Sedation or simulation, depending on drug
- Nightmares: Usually when abruptly discontinued, especially with tranylcypromine

SEXUAL DYSFUNCTION
- Delayed or inhibited ejaculation in men
- Failure to achieve orgasm in women
- Low incidence of sexual dysfunction

Dosage

- Varies with individual drugs (see Table 20–5, Comparing Monoamine Oxidase Inhibitors).

Drug Interactions

See Table 20–6, Drug Interactions with Monoamine Oxidase Inhibitors.

Toxicity

ACUTE
- Possible drowsiness, dizziness, ataxia, headache, restlessness, mental confusion, tachycardia
- Treatment is usually supportive

CHRONIC
- No physical dependence, but patient may experience nightmares if abruptly withdrawn. If these occur, taper patient off medication gradually.

Nursing Management

Administration

ORAL
- All doses should be titrated up slowly.
- When withdrawn, doses should be tapered off over several days.

Food Interactions

- Food and beverages containing high amounts of tyramine (see Table 20–7, Dietary Restrictions With Monoamine Oxidase Inhibitors).
- Interaction results in hypertensive crisis.

Nursing Considerations

- Remember that *hypo*tension is a side effect for some

TABLE 20–7. **Dietary Restrictions With Monoamine Oxidase Inhibitors**

Foods to Avoid
Beer
Wine, particularly Chianti wine
Cheese, except cottage cheese and cream cheese
Smoked or pickled fish (herring)
Beef or chicken liver
Summer (dry) sausage
Fava or broad bean pole pods (Italian green beans)
Yeast vitamin supplements (brewer's yeast)
Questionable Foods (Unlikely to Cause Problems Unless Consumed in Large Quantities)
Other alcoholic beverages
Ripe avocados
Ripe fresh bananas
Sour cream
Soy sauce (possible individual sensitivity to monosodium glutamate)
Yogurt
Foods That May Be Used (Insufficient Evidence to Support Exclusion)
Chocolate
Figs
Meat tenderizers
Raisins
Yeast breads
Coffee, tea, caffeine-containing beverages

Source: McCall, B: Dietary considerations for MAOI regimens. J Clin Psychiatry 43:178, 1982, reprinted with permission.

MAOIs, and that *hyper*tension is the result of a drug or food interaction.
- Monitor carefully for the presence of sedation and orthostatic hypotension. If hypertensive crisis occurs, be prepared to initiate treatment. Treatment for hypertensive crisis includes:
  - Phentolamine (Regitine), 5 mg, slow intravenous push
  - Chlorpromazine (Thorazine), 25 to 50 mg, intramuscularly
  - Nifedipine (Procardia), 10 mg, sublingual; may be prescribed to treat or prevent hypertensive crisis. Instruct

patient to bite into the capsule once and then place it under the tongue. Some responsible outpatients may carry this with them.

- Be aware of the many food interactions, and ensure that the patient receives an MAO diet.
- Be aware of drug interactions, and be especially alert to orders for narcotic analgesics (especially meperidine), antiasthmatics (such as ephedrine), and certain cough and cold remedies (such as pseudoephedrine).

Patient and Family Education

- Warn patients on phenelzine about sedation and additive effects when taking with alcohol and other sedating drugs.
- Instruct the patient not to take any over-the-counter drugs without first checking with the physician or pharmacist. Many cough and cold medications contain a drug that can interact with MAOIs.
- Instruct patient to call physician immediately if throbbing headache, diaphoresis, stiff neck, chest pains, rapid heartbeat, or nausea and vomiting occur.
- Instruct patient to take last dose of isocarboxazid or tranylcypromine before 6:00 p.m. These drugs may have a stimulating effect that can interfere with sleep.

Antianxiety Medications

Antianxiety medications, also called *minor tranquilizers* or *anxiolytics*, act as tranquilizers and can reduce thought and behavior symptoms caused by anxiety, fear, and tension. They are not effective for psychotic symptoms. The most common antianxiety agents are benzodiazepines. Two newer nonbenzodiazepine drugs, buspirone and zolpidem, are also effective. These drugs are chemically and pharmacologically different and do not produce the sedative and euphoric effects commonly seen with the benzodiazepines. They also do not have the potential for dependency.

There are multiple indications for short-term use of antianxiety medications. They are helpful when the patient's level of anxiety is great enough to disturb usual thinking or functional patterns including activities of daily living. A patient may experience aspects of illness or hospitalization as a personal crisis and react with intense anxiety. Reducing anxiety leads to better coping and problem solving and, if required, allows the patient to participate in psychotherapy. The patient's medical condition may necessitate reduced tension, for example, patients with a recent myocardial infarction; preoperative patients, and patients being treated for pain when anxiety is contributing to the pain cycle. Reducing tension may also be necessary to obtain the patient's full cooperation during medical procedures and treatments.

Antianxiety medications are both physiologically and psychologically addicting. If taken in large doses for long periods of time, ever higher dosages may be needed to obtain relief, which may result in chronic intoxication. Withdrawal symptoms, including seizures and delirium, can occur if these drugs are stopped abruptly. Withdrawal symptoms may not emerge until 7 to 10 days following the last ingestion, although benzodiazapines have a low lethality potential as a single-drug overdose.

The specific indications and expected outcomes of giving antianxiety medications need to be thoughtfully and judiciously assessed. In our pill-oriented, quick-answer culture, these drugs are often abused by patients hoping to feel better immediately and stay that way. This leads to dependency on drugs to cope with the inevitable tensions of everyday living. Healthcare professionals often respond too quickly to patients' emotional distress by offering antianxiety medications so that the actual cause of distress is never directly addressed and resolved. As a result the medications tend to perpetuate the condition rather than treat it. A more thorough assessment may reveal that the patient needs to experience painful feelings, such as what occurs in a normal grief reaction, to resolve a situation and to then move on with his or her life. This means that psychosocial interventions, rather than strictly pharmacologic ones, may provide the best outcome for the patient. The patient may need to be encouraged to use more adaptive coping mechanisms, and may need assistance in problem solving, anxiety reduction techniques, and reassurance and possibly, referrals to appropriate sources for assistance.

The symptoms of anxiety are similar to the presenting symptoms of some physical illnesses, such as hyperthyroidism and angina pectoris, as well as drug interactions and withdrawal. These conditions should be ruled out and a psychosocial assessment performed before antianxiety medications are administered.

Usually the smallest amount of the drug for the shortest amount of time is the most constructive approach. The patient who uses these drugs periodically only when needed is able to benefit from the full effect of the medication without concerns of dependency and habituation.

The nurse's role includes encouraging appropriate use when the need is indicated, discouraging use when not indicated, teaching the patient alternative coping methods, and helping the patient differentiate levels of anxiety including anticipatory fear of anxiety.

Pharmacology

Mechanism of Action

- Most depress the central nervous system.
- The nonbenzodiazepines alter interaction of neurotransmitters.

Indications

- Short-term treatment of anxiety, fear, and tension
- Preoperative sedation (lorazepam, midazolam)
- Insomnia (zolpidem)
- Skeletal muscle relaxants (diazepam)
- Treatment of withdrawal symptoms from sedatives or hypnotics and ethanol
- Anticonvulsants (diazepam IV, lorazepam IV, clonazepam PO)
- Antidepressant (alprazolam)
- Panic attacks (alprazolam)
- Adjunctive medication to reduce symptoms of acute exacerbation of schizophrenia or mania

Clinical Effects

- Choice of drug depends on age of patient, reason for use, length of time action is desired, and hepatic function.
- These drugs should be used at the lowest effective dose for the shortest time possible to avoid dependency.

Adverse Effects

CENTRAL NERVOUS SYSTEM

- *Sedation:* Dose related; wide variation among patients
- Impaired concentration, confusion, disorientation, depression, psychomotor retardation, and paradoxical rage
- Amnesia for recent events sometimes seen with IV administration and with some oral use such as triazolam and lorazepam
- May exacerbate depression

Dosage

- Varies with individual drugs (see Table 20–8, Comparing Antianxiety Medications).

Drug Interactions

- *Alcohol and other sedating drugs:* Possible additive sedation, additive psychomotor impairment. Combination drug overdoses can be fatal.
- *Cimetidine (Tagamet):* May interfere with clearance of some benzodiazepines from the body, such as diazepam and chlordiazepoxide, leading to prolongation of some effects, such as sedation.

Toxicity

ACUTE

- Fatal overdose from benzodiazepines as *sole* drug is rare.

CHRONIC

- May result from large doses used over long periods.
- Withdrawal symptoms from abrupt discontinuation include tremulousness, sweating, difficulty sleeping, delirium, and seizures.

TABLE 20–8. **Comparing Antianxiety Medications**

Drug	Usual Dose, mg/day	Major Uses
Alprozolam (Xanax)	0.75–4	Anxiety
Chlordiazepoxide (Librium)	15–100	Anxiety
Clonazepam (Klonopin)	1.5–4	Mania, schizoaffective disorders
Clorazepate (Tranxene)	15–60	Anxiety
Diazepam (Valium)	15–60	Anxiety, anticonvulsant (IV)
Estrazolam (Prosom)	0.5–2	Hypnotic
Flurazepam (Dalmane)	15–30	Hypnotic
Lorazepam (Ativan)	2–6	Anxiety, preoperative sedation, anticonvulsant (IV)
Midazolam (Versed)	1–5	Preoperative sedation
Oxazepam (Serax)	30–120	Anxiety
Quazepam (Doral)	7.5–30	Hypnotic
Temazepam (Restoril)	15–30	Hypnotic
Triazolam (Halcion)	0.25–0.5	Hypnotic
Buspirone (Buspar)	1.5–60	Anxiety
Zolpidem (Ambiem)	5–10	Hypnotic

- Avoid abrupt withdrawal by titrating dose down slowly over time.
- Treatment of withdrawal symptoms done symptomatically and with titration of drug or with other adequate substitute, such as using a long-acting benzodiazepine when a short-acting benzodiazepine is the offending agent.

Nursing Management

Administration

ORAL
- May give with food and milk.
- Lorazepam tablets may be given sublingual in patients who cannot swallow or for whom a faster onset of action is desired.

INTRAMUSCULAR
- *Diazepam, lorazepam:* No dilution necessary
- *Chlordiazepoxide:* Should be diluted with special diluent supplied by manufacturer

INTRAVENOUS
- Diazepam:
  - No dilution necessary.
  - Administer at a rate no greater than 5 mg/min.
- Chlordiazepoxide:
  - Must be diluted.
  - Use 5 mL powdered vial with 5 mL of sterile water for injection or physiologic saline.
  - Should be given slowly over 1 minute.
- Lorazepam:
  - Must be diluted with equal volume of diluent.
  - May use sterile water for injection USP, sodium chloride injection USP, or 5% dextrose injection USP.
  - Should not be given at rate higher than 2 mg/min.

Food Interactions
- May be given with food.

Nursing Considerations
- Monitor for sedation, dizziness, confusion, respiratory depression, and unsteadiness, especially in the elderly.
- Expect patient to experience some degree of amnesia (may be desired effect) when given prior to surgery.
- If the hospitalized patient is suspected of using these drugs over a long time and suddenly discontinues them

when admitted, monitor for signs of physical withdrawal, such as anxiety, restlessness, tremor, and insomnia.
- Be aware of additive sedation when used with other sedating drugs, such as phenothiazines, antidepressants, and antihistamines.
- If a patient appears more sedated than the current medication regime warrants, the nurse should question if the patient has brought a personal supply and is taking extra doses.
- Buspirone should be administered on a regular closing schedule and not prn.

Patient and Family Education

- Warn patient about overdose and addictive potential. These drugs should be taken only as prescribed.
- Warn that sleep disorder may not improve for several nights.
- Tell patient that these drugs should not be abruptly discontinued after prolonged use without consulting a physician.
- Instruct patient to avoid driving or operating machinery while under the influence of the drug.
- Instruct patient not to use any over-the-counter medications without consulting with the pharmacist or physician. Many cough and cold remedies contain medications that can increase central nervous system depression.
- Instruct the patient not to drink alcohol while using these drugs.

Antimania Medications

Lithium carbonate has traditionally been the drug of choice for the treatment of bipolar disorder. Lithium can help regulate both the manic and depressive phases; however, during the depressive phase additional use of an antidepressant is common. Lithium alleviates mania by affecting neurotransmitters. It may increase norepinephrine reuptake and increase serotonin receptor sensitivity.

Lithium is used for long-term treatment, and the patient will usually take it for many years. It is not addictive. High dosages will usually manage acute phases of mania and depression; lower dosages are maintained between episodes to reduce the frequency and intensity recurrence of the acute phases. Lithium can be used for patients who manifest only depression without mania.

Lithium can take 7 to 10 days to begin to influence behavior. If a patient is in an acute manic episode and lithium therapy has just been started, it may be beneficial to use an antipsychotic to control behaviors until the lithium takes effect. The antipsychotic may or may not be continued at that time depending on the patient's response to lithium.

The anticonvulsants carbemazepine and valproic acid are also used to treat mania.

Patient compliance in taking medication, both in the hospital and after discharge, is often a problem. The patient may deny having manic depression or its serious consequences. Also, some patients miss their former elevated moods. Patient and family teaching during hospitalization should focus on the necessity for follow-up treatment and medication. Transfer to a psychiatric hospital or unit may be necessary if the patient refuses medications, is totally unmanageable, and the medical condition allows.

Pharmacology

Mechanism of Action

- Increases norepinephrine reuptake and increases serotonin receptor sensitivity

Indications

- Manic-depressive illness
- Schizoaffective states

Clinical Effects

- 7 to 10 days required before clinical improvement seen.
- Full therapeutic effect seen after several weeks.
- Improves euphoric mood, irritability, hallucinations,

rapid speech, excessive energy, insomnia, paranoid ideation, acute delusions, flight of ideas, grandiosity, distractibility, and attention span.

Adverse Effects

CARDIOVASCULAR
- Mild, benign ECG changes

ENDOCRINE
- Mild, transient hypothyroidism in some patients

GASTROINTESTINAL
- Nausea, vomiting, diarrhea especially when starting
  drug; however, tolerance develops in most patients after
  a few days.

CENTRAL NERVOUS SYSTEM
- Sedation, lethargy, mild hand tremor, dizziness, muscle
  weakness, mild disorientation
- *Severe:* Nystagmus, hyperactive deep tendon reflexes

HEMATOLOGIC
- *Blood:* Mild, transient, reversible leukocytosis

RENAL
- Some nephropathies seen in some patients; predisposing
  factors uncertain
- Increased thirst and increased urination
- Weight gain

Dosage

- 900 to 2400 mg/day

Drug Interactions

- Additive sedation with other sedating drugs, such as antipsychotics, antidepressants, and benzodiazepines.
- Potassium-depleting drugs, such as thiazide diuretics,
  may predispose patient to toxicity.
- Lithium clearance may be reduced by some nonsteroidal
  anti-inflammatory drugs, such as phenybutazone and in-
  domethacin.
- Interactions may occur with naprosyn and ibuprofen.

Toxicity

- Lithium toxicity is life-threatening; toxicity can occur even at therapeutic blood levels in some patients.
- Patients with renal failure and hyponatremia have the greatest risk.
- Early signs of toxicity include:
  - Appearance of sedation or gastrointestinal disturbances, such as nausea and vomiting, in a patient who has not previously experienced such complications
  - Reappearance of sedation or gastrointestinal disturbances in a patient who had become tolerant to such complications
  - Tremor in a patient who has not previously experienced one
  - Tremor
  - Reappearance or worsening of tremor
- Signs of moderate toxicity include gross tremors and muscular irritation or twitching.
- Signs of severe toxicity include coma, seizures, or death.
- Treatment is supportive.
- To prevent toxic reactions in patients being started or having dosages increased, monitor serum lithium blood levels frequently.
- Therapeutic blood levels are 0.5 to 1.5 mEq/L for most patients.
- Maintain adequate hydration and sodium intake in patients with diarrhea.
- Avoid diuretics because of the reduction in fluid, sodium, and potassium levels.

Nursing Management

Administration

ORAL

- Available for oral use only in capsules, liquid, and sustained-release tablets.
- Do not mix liquid with other liquid medications, such as liquid antipsychotics.
- May mix liquid in juice, water, or soup.

Food Interactions

- Lithium may be given with food, juice, or soup.

Nursing Considerations

- May give drug with food or milk if gastrointestinal upset occurs, or administer doses at regular intervals throughout the day.
- Ensure that blood levels are monitored regularly. Blood for lithium levels should be obtained 12 hours after last dose. This is best done by holding the morning dose until the level is taken.
- Know that low potassium levels may predispose patient to toxicity.
- Maintain adequate sodium intake.
- Call physician immediately for intolerable gastrointestinal effects, feelings of oversedation or lethargy, or appearance or worsening of tremors.
- Monitor for the signs and symptoms of lithium toxicity as well as common adverse effects. Toxicity should be suspected if previous adverse effects suddenly reappear. If any signs of toxicity are present, lithium should be stopped immediately and the physician notified.
- If patient is NPO, monitor behavior closely and make sure lithium is resumed as soon as patient is able to take oral medications.

Patient and Family Education

- Emphasize need to take medication regularly.
- Emphasize need to keep appointments to monitor blood levels.
- Inform the patient that he or she is able to dilute medication in beverages but should not mix it with other liquid medications.
- Inform the patient that medication can be taken with food or milk if gastrointestinal upset occurs.
- Warn patient to avoid saunas, hot baths, overexertion in hot weather, and any activities that may cause profuse perspiration as these may predispose toward toxicity, as will excessive vomiting and diarrhea.

- Instruct patient to drink an adequate amount of fluids.
- Warn patient to avoid caffeine-containing liquids which promote diuresis and loss of sodium.
- Instruct patient to notify physician at once for intolerable gastrointestinal effects, feelings of over sedation or lethargy, appearance or worsening of tremors, or profuse diarrhea or vomiting.
- Instruct women of childbearing age to avoid pregnancy.
- Encourage patient to make an agreement with family members to ensure that he or she takes medication. The patient should know that the family will notify the physician if he or she ceases to take the medication or if symptoms of mania occur.

Anticonvulsant Medications Pharmacology

Mechanism of Action

- Unclear but may influence nerve cell membrane

Indications

- Manic-depressive illness
- Seizures

Clinical Effects

- Mania (carbamazepine, clonazepam, and valproic acid)
- Reduction or elimination of seizures
- Chronic pain
- Neuropathic pain

Adverse Effects

GASTROINTESTINAL
- Primarily nausea, vomiting, indigestion (carbamazepine and valproic acid)

CENTRAL NERVOUS SYSTEM
- Sedation, dizziness, drowsiness, unsteadiness
- Tremor, ataxia, headache (valproic acid)

HEMATOPOETIC
- Leukopenia (carbamazepine)
- Agranulocytosis, aplastic anemia: Rare, but life threatening (carbamazepine)
- Easy bruising (valproic acid)

HEPATIC
- Minor increase in hepatic enzymes, jaundice, and hepatitis (carbamazepine)
- Minor increase in hepatic enzymes (valporic acid)

DERMATOLOGIC
- Skin rash

Dosage

- Varies with individual drugs (see Table 20–9, Comparing Anticonvulsant Medications).

Drug Interactions

- Warfarin and oral contraceptives: May decrease effectiveness of carbemazepine.
- Phenytoin may decrease effectiveness of carbamazepine and valproic acid.
- Added central nervous system depression may occur when clonazepam or valproic acid are used with other central nervous system depressants.

TABLE 20–9. **Comparing Anticonvulsant Medications**

Drug	Acute Dose, mg/day	Maintenance Dose, mg/day	Desired Blood Level, µg/mL
Carbamazepine (Tegretol)	200–1200	Up to 1200	4–10
Clonazepam (Klonopin)	1.5–20	Up to 20	N/A
Valproic acid (Depakene; Depakote)	750–2000	750–1500	50–100

Toxicity

ACUTE

- Carbamazepine: Nausea, vomiting, somnolence, nystagmus, ataxia
- Clonazepam: Excessive sedation and lethargy
- Valproic acid: Motor restlessness, visual hallucinations, deep coma, and death

CHRONIC

- Clonazepam: physical dependence develops with prolonged use, the drug should not be abruptly discontinued.

Nursing Management

Administration

ORAL

- All are available in only an oral form.
- Be aware that Depakene is an immediate-release valproic acid and that Depakote is a sustained-release valproic acid.
- Carbamazepine 100-mg tablets are chewable, while 200-mg tablets are to be swallowed whole.

Food Interactions

- All three may be taken with food or milk to alleviate gastrointestinal upset.

Patient and Family Education

- Emphasize the need for complying with obtaining blood levels to monitor carbamazepine and valproic acid.
- Patient may take medications with food or milk if gastrointestinal upset occurs.
- Instruct patient to swallow, and not chew, valproic acid capsules.
- Instruct patient to notify physician if excessive drowsiness and sedation, bleeding, bruising, or voiding dark urine occurs.

- Instruct patient to notify physician if he or she is placed on other medications by another physician.
- Inform patient not to take any over-the-counter medications without first checking with the pharmacist or physician. Many cough and cold preparations contain medications that could increase central nervous system effects.
- Warn patient not to drive or operate machinery if drowsiness occurs.

Nursing Considerations

- May give dose with food or milk if gastrointestinal upset occurs, or may divide dose and administer smaller doses at regular intervals throughout the day.
- Ensure that blood levels of carbamazepine and valproic acid are monitored regularly. Blood for analysis should be obtained 12 hours after last dose. This is best done by holding the morning dose until the level is taken.
- Monitor for signs of additive sedation when drug is taken with other central nervous system depressants.
- A complete blood count with differential should be monitored periodically in patients on carbamazepine.

Initial Screening Assessment for Symptom and/or Behavior Change

Patient: _____   Date: _____

Describe change: _____
_____
_____
_____

Vital signs: Today _____
    Last vital signs taken (note date): _____
Recent change in medications?   Yes _____   No _____
    If yes, describe: _____
Current abnormal lab values?   Yes _____   No _____
    If yes, describe: _____
Recent change in daily routine?
    Hygiene habits _____   Diet _____
    Sleep _____   Activity level _____
    Other _____   None _____
    If changed, describe: _____
Other recent changes in behavior, mood?
    Communication _____   Agitation _____
    Aggressiveness _____   Confusion _____
    Depression _____   Other _____   None _____
    If changed, describe: _____

Recent change in support systems?

     Family visits _____   Staff interaction patterns _____

     Other _____   None _____

     If changed, describe: _____

Signature _____

Mini-Mental State Examination

Maximum score 30. Score <20 suggests significant cognitive impairment.

I. ORIENTATION (MAXIMUM SCORE 10)

Ask "What is today's date?" Then ask specifically for parts omitted; e.g., "Can you also tell what season it is?"

Ask "Can you tell me the name of this hospital?"

"What floor are we on?"

"What town (or city) are we in?"

"What county are we in?"

"What state are we in?"

Date (e.g., January 21)	1	_____
Year	2	_____
Month	3	_____
Day (e.g., Monday)	4	_____
Season	5	_____
Hospital	6	_____
Floor	7	_____
Town/City	8	_____
County	9	_____
State	10	_____

II. REGISTRATION (MAXIMUM SCORE 3)

Ask the subject if you may test his/her memory. Then say "Ball," "Flag," "Tree," clearly and slowly, about one second for each. After you have said all 3 words, ask subject to repeat them. This first repetition determines the score (0–3) but keep saying them (up to 6 trials) until the

"Ball"	11	_____
"Flag"	12	_____
"Tree"	13	_____

subject can repeat all 3 words. If he/she does not eventually learn all three, recall cannot be meaningfully tested.

Record number of trials _____

III. ATTENTION AND CALCULATION (MAXIMUM SCORE 5)

Ask the subject to begin at 100 and count backward by 7. Stop after 5 subtractions (93,86,79,72,65). Score one point for each correct number.

"93"	14 _____
"86"	15 _____
"79"	16 _____
"72	17 _____
"65"	18 _____

If the subject cannot or will not perform this task, ask him/her to spell the word "world" backwards (D,L,R,O,W). The score is one point for each correctly placed letter, e.g., DLROW = 5, DLORW = 3. Record how the subject spelled "world" backwards:

IV. RECALL (MAXIMUM SCORE 3)

Ask the subject to recall the three words you previously asked him/her to remember (learned in Registration).

"Ball"	19 _____
"Flag"	20 _____
"Tree"	21 _____

V. LANGUAGE (MAXIMUM SCORE 9)

Naming: Show the subject a wristwatch and ask "What is this?" Repeat for pencil. Score one point for each item named correctly.

Watch	22 _____
Pencil	23 _____

Repetition: Ask the subject to repeat, "No ifs, ands, or

Repetition	24 _____

buts." Score one point for correct repetition.

3-Stage Command: Give the subject a piece of blank paper and say, "Take the paper in your right hand, fold it in half and put it on the floor." Score one point for each action performed correctly.

Takes in right hand	25 _____
Folds in half	26 _____
Puts on floor	27 _____

Reading: On a blank piece of paper, print the sentence, "Close your eyes" in letters large enough for the subject to see clearly. Ask the subject to read it and do what it says. Score correctly only if he/she actually closes his/her eyes.

Closes eyes   28 _____

Writing: Give the subject a blank piece of paper and ask him/her to write a sentence. It is to be written spontaneously. It must contain a subject and verb and make sense. Correct grammar and punctuation are not necessary.

Writes sentence   29 _____

Copying: On a clean piece of paper, draw intersecting pentagons, each side about an inch, and ask subject to copy it exactly as it is. All 10 angles must be present and two must intersect to score 1 point. Tremor and rotation are ignored (example).

Draws pentagons   30 _____

Score: Add number of correct responses.(Maximum total score 30)

**Rate subject's level of
  consciousness:** (a) coma, (b)
  stupor, (c) drowsy, (d) alert   Total score _____

From Folstein, MF, Folstein, FE, and McHugh, PR: Mini-mental state: A practical method for grading the cognitive state of patients for the clinician. J Psychiatric Research 12:189, 1975. Reprinted with permission from Pergamon Press, Ltd.

Relaxation Techniques

Relaxation Techniques can include any of the following:

1. Deep breathing: Take in several slow deep breaths by inhaling through your nose and exhaling slowly through your mouth. As you exhale focus on relaxing your shoulders. Each time you take a deep breath, repeat a calming word to yourself like peace or one.
2. Muscle Relaxation: After taking two slow deep breaths, raise up your shoulders for 2 to 3 seconds and then let go. Do this 2 to 3 times. Then make a fist, hold it for 2 to 3 seconds then let go. Each time you let go, think of another part of your body becoming more relaxed. Imagine yourself going limp like a ragdoll. You can continue to tense and relax other muscle groups in your body.
3. Imagery: After taking several slow deep breaths and relaxing your muscles, create a pleasant image in your mind that you associate with relaxation. It can be a comforting memory or a pleasant image like a garden or floating on a raft in the sunshine. Let your mind wander to what ever you find relaxing.

Tips on enhancing relaxation
- Create a quiet environment
- Get in a comfortable chair
- Every time your mind wanders to distracting thoughts, focus on your breathing
- Practice regularly (relaxation is not always easy)
- Consider the use of audio or video relaxation tapes, headsets

REFERENCES

Abramowicz, M (ed): Drugs for psychiatric disorders. Med Letter Drug Therapy 36(933):89, 1994.

Agency for Health Care Policy and Research: Acute Pain Management: Operative or Medical Procedures and Trauma. Clinical Practice Guideline. Public Health Service, US Department of Health and Human Services (DHHS), Rockville, MD, February 1992.

Agency for Health Care Policy and Research: Management of Cancer Pain. Clinical Practice Guideline. Public Health Service, US Department of Health and Human Services (DHHS), Rockville, MD, March 1994.

Agency for Health Care Policy and Research: Depression in Primary Care, vol 1 and 2. Public Health Service, US Department of Health and Human Services (DHHS), Rockville, MD, 1993.

Aguilera, DC: Crisis Intervention Theory and Methodology, ed 7. Mosby, St Louis, 1994.

Aiken, TD: Legal, Ethical and Political Issues in Nursing. FA Davis, Philadelphia, 1994.

Albert, PL: Overview of the organ donation process. Crit Care Nurs Clin North Am 6(3):553, 1994.

Alcoholics Anonymous: Twelve Steps and Twelve Traditions. New York, 1953.

Allen, T: Understanding Alzheimer's disease: An overview. Nurseweek 7(25):8, 1994.

Alston, MH, and Robinson, BH: Nurses' attitudes toward suicide. Omega 25(3):205, 1992.

American Hospital Association: A Patient's Bill of Rights. Chicago, 1972.

American Nurses Association: Compendium of Position Statements on the Nurse's Role in End-of-Life Decisions. Washington, DC, 1992.

American Pain Society: Principles of Analgesic Use in Treatment of Acute Pain and Cancer, ed 3. Skokie, IL, 1992.

American Psychiatric Association (APA): Diagnostic and Statistical Manual of Mental Disorders, ed 4. Washington, DC, 1994.

American Society of Hospital Pharmacists: Drug Information 1994. American Hospital Formulary Service, Bethesda, 1994.

Antai-Otong, D: Psychiatric Nursing: Biological and Behavioral Concepts. WB Saunders, Philadelphia, 1995.

Atkinson, JH, and Grant, I: Natural history of neuropsychiatric manifestations of HIV disease. Psychiatr Clin North Am 17(1):29, 1994.

Barnhart E (ed): Physician's Desk Reference, ed 49. Medical Economics, Philadelphia, 1995.

Barry, PD: Mental Health and Mental Illness, ed 5. JB Lippincott, Philadelphia, 1994.

Barry, PD: Psychosocial Nursing Assessment and Intervention, ed 2. JB Lippincott, Philadelphia, 1989.

Bauer, B, and Hill, S: People who defend against anxiety through aggression toward others. In Varcarolis, EM (ed): Foundations of Psychiatric Mental Health Nursing. WB Saunders, Philadelphia, 1994.

Beattie, M: Codependent No More. Harper-Collins, New York, 1992.

Beck, A: Cognitive Therapy and Emotional Disorder. New American Library, New York, 1979.

Belcaster, A: Caring for the alcohol abuser. Nurs 24(2):56, 1994.

Berkow, R. et al: Merck Manual. Merck Research Laboratories, Rahway, NJ, 1992.

Bernstein, SB: Breaking the vicious cycle of noncompliance. Nursing 19(1):74, 1989.

Black, C: It Will Never Happen to Me. Ballantine, New York, 1987.

Blair, DT, and New, SA: Assaultive behavior: Know the risks. J Psychosoc Ment Health Serv 29:25, 1991.

Blair, DT, and New, SA: Patient violence in psychiatric settings: Risk identification and treatment as provocation. In Smoyak, SA, and Blair, DT (eds): Violence and Abuse. Slack, Thorofare, NJ, 1992.

Blumenreich, PE, and Lewis, S (eds): Managing the Violent Patient. Brunner/Mazel, New York, 1993.

Bowen, M: Family Therapy in Clinical Practice. Aronson, New York, 1978.

Breitbart, W, and Holland, JC (eds): Psychiatric Aspects of Symptom Management in Cancer Patients. American Psychiatric Press, Washington, DC, 1993.

Brentin, L, and Sieh, A: Caring for the morbidly obese. Am J Nurs 91(8):40, 1991.

Bruch, H: The Golden Cage: The Enigma of Anorexia Nervosa. Harvard University Press, Cambridge, MA, 1978.

Burke, MM, and Walsh, MB: Gerontologic Nursing: Care of the Frail Elderly. Mosby, St Louis, 1992.

Butler, BM: When the nurse and patient battle for control. RN 49(9):67–69, 1986.

Caine, RM, and Bufalino, PM: Nursing Care Planning Guides for Adults. Williams & Wilkins, Baltimore, 1991.

Caltin, G: The role of culture in grief. J Soc Psychol 133(2):173, 1993.

Campbell, J, and Humphreys, J: Nursing Care of Survivors of Family Violence. Mosby, St Louis, 1993.

Campinha-Bacote, J: Transcultural psychiatric nursing: Diagnostic and treatment issues. J Psychosoc Ment Health Serv 32(8):41, 1994.

Caregivers say alternatives to restraints must be found. Medical Ethics Advisor 10(5):57, 1994.

Carnegie Council on Adolescent Development: Turning Points: Preparing American Youth for the 21st Century. Carnegie Corporation of New York, Washington, DC, 1989.

Carpenito, L: Nursing Diagnosis: Application to Clinical Practice, ed 6. JB Lippincott, Philadelphia, 1995.

Carr, VH: Managing the psychosocial responses of the transplant patient. In Sigardson-Poor, KM, and Haggerty, LM (eds): Nursing Care of the Transplant Recipient. WB Saunders, Philadelphia, 1990.

Carroll, DL: When Your Loved One Has Alzheimer's. Harper & Row/ Perennial Library, New York, 1990.

Carson, VB: Spiritual Dimensions of Nursing Practice. WB Saunders, Philadelphia, 1989.

Centers for Disease Control and Prevention: HIV/AIDS Surveillance Report. US Department of Health and Human Services, Atlanta, 1995.

Chenevert, M: STAT: Special Techniques in Assertiveness Training for Women in Health Professions, ed 4. Mosby, St Louis, 1994.

Cherny, NI, and Portenoy, RK: The management of cancer pain. CA: A Cancer Journal for Clin 44(5):262–303, 1994.

Chez, N: Helping the victim of domestic violence. Am J Nurs 94(7):33, 1994.

Chochinov, HM, et al: Desire for Death in the Terminally Ill. Am J Psychiatry 152(8):1185, 1995.

Christ, G: Psychosocial tasks throughout the cancer experience. In Stearns, NM, Lauria, MM, Hermann, JF, and Fogelberg, PR: Oncology Social Work: A Clinician's Guide. American Cancer Society, Atlanta, 1993.

Clark, J: Psychosocial dimensions: The patient. In Groenwald, SL, Frogge, MH, Goodman, M, and Yarbro, CH (eds): Cancer Nursing Principles and Practice, ed 3. Jones & Bartlett, Boston, 1993.

Collins, CE: Interventions with family caregivers of persons with Alzheimer's disease. Nurs Clin North Am 29(1):195, March 1994.

Collins, GB: Contemporary issues in the treatment of alcohol dependence. Psychiatr Clin North Am 16(1):33, 1993.

Copeland, LG: Caring for children with chronic conditions: Model of critical times. Holistic Nurse Pract 8(1):45, 1993.

Coyle, N: The euthanasia and physician-assisted suicide debate: Issues for nursing. Oncol Nurs Forum 19(7 suppl):41, 1992.

Cruzan v. Director, Missouri Department of Health 58 U.S.L.W.4916 (June 25 1990).

Curl, A: When family caregivers grieve for the Alzheimer's patient. Geriatric Nursing, 13(6):305, 1992.

DeLaune, SC: Effective limit setting: How to avoid being manipulated. Nurs Clin North Am 26:3, 1991.

Devlin, BK, and Reynolds, E: Child abuse. Am J Nurs 94(3):26, 1994.

Deykin, EY, and Buka, SL: Suicide ideation and attempts among chemically dependent adolescents. Am J Pub Health 84(4):634, 1994.

Dreyfus, JK: Depression assessment and interventions in the medically ill frail elderly. J Gerontol Nurs 14(9):27, 1988.

Drug facts. Facts and Comparisons. JB Lippincott, Philadelphia, 1994.

Fincannon, JL: Analysis of psychiatric referrals and interventions in an oncology population. Oncol Nurs Forum 22(1):87, 1995.

Finke, LM: Nursing interventions with children and adolescents experiencing substance abuse. In West, P, and Evans, CS (eds): Psychiatric and Mental Health Nursing with Children and Adolescents. Aspen, Gaithersburg, MD, 1992.

Fitchett, G: Assessing Spiritual Needs: A Guide for Caregivers. Augsburg Fortress, MN, 1993.

Fitton, A, and Heel, RC: Clozapine: A review of its pharmacological properties and therapeutic use in schizophrenia. Drugs 40:722, 1990.

Flaskerud, JH, and Ungvarski, PJ: HIV/AIDS: A Guide to Nursing Care, ed 3. WB Saunders, Philadelphia, 1995.

Folstein, MF, Folstein, FE, and McHugh, PR: Mini-mental state: A practical method for grading the cognitive state of patients for the clinician. J Psychiatric Research 12:189, 1975.

Fontaine, KL: The conspiracy of culture. Nurs Clin North Am 26(3):669, 1991.

Forrester, DA, and Murphy, PA: Nurses' attitudes toward patients with AIDS and AIDS-related risk factors. J Adv Nurs 17(2):1260, 1992.

Fraser, K, and Gallop, R: Nurses' confirming/disconfirming responses to patients diagnosed with borderline personality disorder. Arch Psychiatr Nurs 7(6):338–341, 1993.

Friedman, MM: Family Therapy: Theory and Practice, ed 3. Appleton & Lange, Norwalk, CT, 1992.

Friersdon, RL, and Lippmann, SB: Suicide and AIDS. Psychosomatics 29(2):226, 1988.

Galanter, M, and Kleber, HD: Textbook of Substance Abuse Therapy. American Psychiatric Press, Washington, DC, 1994.

Galanti, G: Caring for Patients from Different Cultures. University of Pennsylvania Press, Philadelphia, 1991.

Galazis, RS, and Kempe, A: Therapy with clients with eating disorders. In Beck, CK, Rawlins, RP, and Williams, SR (eds): Psychiatric Nursing. CV Mosby, St Louis, 1988.

Geary, SM: Intensive care unit psychosis revisited: Understanding and managing delirium in the critical care unit. Crit Care Nurs Q 17(1):51, 1994.

Gerner, RF: Treatment of acute mania. Psychiatr Clin North Am 16(3):443, 1993.

Glod, CA: Long-term consequences of childhood physical and sexual abuse. Arch Psychiatr Nurs 7(3):163, 1993.

Glod, CA, and Mathieu, J: Expanding use of anticonvulsants in the treatment of bipolar disorder. J Psychosoc Nurs Ment Health Serv 31(5):37, 1993.

Goldenberg, I, and Goldenberg, H: Family Therapy: An Overview, ed 3. Brooks/Cole, Pacific Grove, CA, 1991.

Goodwin, FK, and Jamison, KR: Manic-Depressive Illness. Oxford University Press, New York, 1990.

Gorman, L, Sultan, D, and Luna-Raines, M: Psychosocial Nursing Handbook for the Nonpsychiatric Nurse. Williams & Wilkins, Baltimore, 1989.

Grossman, D: Enhancing your cultural competence. Am J Nurs 94(7):58, 1994.

Haber, J, McMahon, AL, Price-Hoskins, P, and Sideleau, BF: Comprehensive Psychiatric Nursing, ed 4. Mosby-Year Book, St Louis, 1992.

Haffner, L: Translation is not enough. Western Journal of Healthcare 157(3):255, 1992.

Hanna, VM, and Smith, JA: Helping a dependent patient help himself. Nursing '92 22(6):32c, 1992.

Harvard School of Public Health: Highlights of Public Attitudes Toward Organ Donation and Transplantation. Conducted by the Gallup Organization for the Partnership for Organ Donation, March 1993.

Harvath, TA, et al: Dementia-related behaviors. J Psychosoc Nurs Ment Health Serv 33(1):35, 1995.

Hatton, C, and Valente, S: Suicide: Assessment and Interventions. Appleton-Century-Crofts, Norwalk, CT, 1984.

Haven, E, and Piscitello, V: The patient with violent behavior. In Lewis, S, et al (eds): Manual of Psychosocial Nursing Interventions. WB Saunders, Philadelphia, 1989.

Hoffman, NG, and Miller, NS: Perspectives of effective treatment for alcohol and drug disorders. Psychiatr Clin North Am 16(1):127, 1993.

Hogarty, SS, and Rodaitis, CM: A suicide precautions policy for the general hospital. J Nurs Admin 17(10):36, 1987.

Houpt, JL, and Brodie, HKH: Psychiatry, Vol 3, Consultation-Liaison Psychiatry and Behavioral Medicine. JB Lippincott, Philadelphia, 1986.

Huart, S, and O'Donnel, M: The road to recovery from grief and bereavement. Caring, 12(11):71, 1993.

Hudelson, E: Points to remember when caring for an obese patient. Nurs 22(10):62, 1992.

Humphrey, JH: Stress in the Nursing Profession. Charles C Thomas, Springfield, IL, 1988.

Husted, GL: Ethical Decision Making in Nursing, ed 2. Mosby, St Louis, 1995.

Jacob, SR: An analysis of the concept of grief. J Adv Nurs 18(11):1787, 1993.

Jacox, A, Ferrell, B, Heidrich, G, Hester, N, and Miaskowski, C: A guideline for the nation: Managing acute pain. Am J Nurs, 92(5):49–55, 1992.

Janicake, P, et al: Principles and Practice of Psychopharmaco-therapy. Williams & Wilkins, Baltimore, 1993.

Jensen, DP, and Herr, KA: Sleeplessness. Nurs Clin North Am 28(2):385–405, 1993.

Johnston, JE: Sleep problems in the elderly. J Am Acad Nurse Pract 6(4):161–166, 1994.

Joint Commission on Accreditation of Health Care Organizations (JCAHO): Accreditation Manual for Hospitals. Chicago, 1995.

Kane, JM, and Lieberman, JA (ed): Adverse Effects of Psychotropic Drugs. Guilford, New York, 1992

Kane, JM: Newer antipsychotic drugs: A review of their pharma-cology and therapeutic potential. Drugs 46(4):585, 1993.

Kaplan, HI, and Sadock, BJ: Synopsis of Psychiatry. Williams & Wilkins, Baltimore, 1991.

Kashani, J, et al: Family violence: Impact on children. J Am Acad Child and Adol Psychiatr 31(2):181, 1992.

Kelly, GL: Childhood depression and suicide. Nurs Clin North Am 26(3):545, 1991.

Keltner, NL, Schwecke, LH, and Bostrom, CE (eds): Psychiatric Nursing, ed 2. Mosby, St Louis, 1995.

Keltner, NL, and Folks, DO: Psychotropic Drugs. Mosby, St Louis, 1993.

Kemp, C: Terminal Illness: A Guide to Nursing Care. JB Lippincott, Philadelphia, 1995.

Kerfoot, K: Keeping spirituality in managed care: The nurse man-ager's challenge. Nurs Econ 13(1):49, 1995.

King, CJ, et al: Diagnosis and assessment of substance abuse in older adults: Current strategies and issues. Addictive Behaviors 19(1):41, 1994.

Kohut, A: Guidelines for using interpreters. Hosp Progress 56(4):39, 1975.

Krach, P: Nursing implications: Functional status of older persons with schizophrenia. J Gerontol Nurs 19(8):21, 1993.

Kreisman, JJ, and Straus, H: I Hate You—Don't Leave Me: Under-standing the Borderline Personality. Avon Books, New York, 1989.

Kubler-Ross, E: On Death and Dying. MacMillan, New York, 1969.

Kupfer, DJ: Long-term treatment of depression. J Clin Psychiatry 52(suppl):28, 1991.

Lachman, VD: Stress Management: A Manual for Nursing. Grune & Stratton, New York, 1983.

Larson, DG: The Helpers Journey: Working with People Facing Grief, Loss and Life-threatening Illness. Research Press, Champaign, IL, 1993.

Ledray, LE, and Arndt, S: Examining the sexual assault victim: A new model for nursing care. J Psychosoc Nurs Ment Health Serv 32(2):7, 1994.

Lego, S: Borderline personality disorders. In Varcarolis, E: Foundations in Mental Health Nursing. WB Saunders, Philadelphia, 1994.

Levenkron, S: The Best Little Girl in the World. Warner Books, New York, 1978.

Lewis, A, and Levy, J: Psychiatric Liaison Nursing. Reston Publishing, Reston, VA, 1982.

Lewis, S: Verbal intervention. In Blumenreich, PE, and Lewis, S, (eds): Managing the Violent Patient. Brunner/Mazel, New York, 1993.

Liken, MA, and Collins, CE: Grieving: Facilitating the process for dementia caregivers. J Psychosoc Nurs Ment Health Serv 31(1):21, 1993.

Lindemann, E: Symptomatology and management of acute grief. Am J Psychiatry 101:141, 1944.

Lomax, JW: Obesity. In Kaplan, HI, and Sadock, BJ (eds): Comprehensive Textbook of Psychiatry. Williams & Wilkins, Baltimore, 1989.

Mace, NL: Dementia: Patient, Family and Community. Johns Hopkins University Press, Baltimore, 1991.

Mace, NL, and Rabins, PV: The 36-Hour Day, rev ed. Johns Hopkins University Press, Baltimore, 1991.

Madden, DJ, Lion, JR, and Penna, MW: Assaults on psychiatrists by patients. Am J Psychiatry 133:422, 1976.

Marks, RM, and Sachar, EJ: Undertreatment of medical inpatients with narcotic analgesics. Annals of Internal Medicine, 78:173–181, 1973.

Maslow, A: Motivation and Personality. Harper & Row, New York, 1954.

Massie, MJ, Gagnon, P, and Holland, JC: Depression and suicide in patients with cancer. J Pain Sympt Manage 9:325–340, 1994.

Matheny, KB, and Riordan, RJ: Stress—And Strategies for Lifestyle Management. Georgia State University Business Press, Atlanta, 1992.

Matthiesen, V, Sivertsen, L, and Foreman, MD: Acute confusion:

Nursing intervention in older patients. Orthopaedic Nursing 13(2):21, 1994.

Mayfield, D, McLeod, G, and Hall, P: The CAGE questionnaire: Validation of a new alcoholism screening instrument. Am J Psychiatry 131:121, 1974.

McAndrew, M: People who depend on substances other than alcohol. In Varcarolis, EM (ed): Foundations of Psychiatric Mental Health Nursing, ed 2. WB Saunders, Philadelphia, 1994.

McCaffery, M, and Beebe, A: Pain in Children. In Pain: Clinical Manual for Nursing Practice. CV Mosby, St Louis, 1989.

McCaffery, M, and Ferrell, BP: Understanding opioids and addiction. Nurs 94(8):56, 1994.

McCall, B: Dietary considerations for MAOI regimens. J Clin Psychiatry 43:178, 1982.

McCray, ND: Psychosocial issues. In Otto, SE (ed): Oncology Nursing, ed 2. Mosby, St Louis, 1994.

McFarland, GK, and McFarlane, EA: Nursing Diagnosis and Intervention. Mosby, St Louis, 1993.

McFarland, GK, and Thomas, MD: Psychiatric Mental Health Nursing. JB Lippincott, Philadelphia, 1991.

McFarland, GK, Wasli, E, and Gerety, EK: Nursing Diagnoses and Process in Psychiatric Mental Health Nursing. JB Lippincott, Philadelphia, 1992.

McGee, RF: Overview of psychosocial dimensions. In Groenwald, SL, Frogge, MH, Goodman, M, and Yarbro, CH (eds): Cancer Nursing Principles and Practice, ed 3. Jones & Bartlett, Boston, 1993.

McKenry, LM, and Salernoe, E: Mosby's Pharmacology in Nursing, ed 19. Mosby, St Louis, 1995.

McMahan, AL: Substance abuse among the elderly. Nurs Practitioner Forum 4(4):231, 1993.

McNeil, J: US Bureau Report. US Census Bureau, Washington, DC, February 21, 1992.

Med Letter: Drugs that cause psychiatric symptoms. Med Let 35:65, July 23, 1993.

Medved, R: Strategies for handling angry patients and their families. Nursing '90, 20(4):66, 1990.

Melzack, R, Abbott, FW, Zackon, W, Mulder, DS, and Davis, MWL: Pain on a surgical ward: A survey of the duration and intensity of pain and the effectiveness of medication. Pain 29:67–72, 1987.

Miller, A: Drama of the Gifted Child. Basic Books, New York, 1990.

Miller, CA: Interventions for sleep pattern disturbances. Geriatric Nursing 14(5):235–236, 1993.

Miller, JF: Coping with Chronic Illness. ed 2. FA Davis, Philadelphia, 1992.

Millison, M, and Dudley, JR: Providing spiritual support: A job for all hospice professionals. Hospice Journal 8(4):49, 1992.

Morrison, EF: The evolution of a concept: Aggression and violence in psychiatric setting. Arch Psych Nurs 8(4):245, 1994.

Morrison, EF: Toward a better understanding of violence in psychiatric settings: Debunking the myths. Arch Psych Nurs 7(6):328, 1993.

Myer, SA: Multisystem complications of bulimia: A critical care case. Dimens Crit Care Nurs 12(4):194, 1993.

National Crisis Prevention Institute: Art of Setting Limits: Participant Manual. Brookfield, WI, 1991.

North American Nursing Diagnosis Association (NANDA): Nursing Diagnoses: Definitions and Classifications 1995–1996. Philadelphia, 1995.

Novello, AC, and Soto-Torres, LE: Women and the Hidden Epidemic. The Female Patient 17:17, 1992.

Odell, TM: Organ Donations: What Families Need to Know. Nurs 24:321, 1994.

Oncology Nursing Society: Current issues in pain management: Leadership through expert nursing care. Oncol Nurs Forum 19(suppl):3–48, 1992.

Patterson, W. et al: Evaluation of Suicidal Patients. Psychosomatics. 24:343, 1983.

Peet, M, and Pratt, JP: Lithium: Current status in psychiatric disorders. Drugs 46:7, 1993.

Perkins, K, and Tice, C: Suicide in Older Adults. J Appl Gerontol, 13:438, 1994.

Pronsky, ZM: Powers and Moore's Food Medication Drug Interactions, ed 9. Powers & Moore, Pottstown, PA, 1995.

Rando, T: Treatment of Complicated Mourning. Research Press, Champaign, IL, 1993.

Raudsepp, E: Six steps to becoming more assertive. Nursing 21(3):112, 1991.

Rawlins, RP, Williams, SR, and Beck, CK: Mental Health–Psychiatric Nursing. A Holistic Life-Cycle Approach, ed 3. Mosby, St Louis, 1993.

Redman, BK: The Process of Patient Education, ed 7. Mosby, St Louis, 1993.

Rodgers, SB: Legal framework for organ donation and transplantation. Nurs Clin North Am 24(4):837–850, 1989.

Sales, E: Psychosocial impact of the phase of cancer on the family: An updated review. J Psychosocial Oncology 9:1–17, 1991.

Schneider, JM: Clinically significant differences between grief, pathological grief, and depression. Patient Counseling and Health Education. Fourth quarter: p 276, 1980.

Schooler, NR: Negative symptoms in schizophrenia: Assessment of the effects of risperidone. J Clin Psychiatry 55(suppl):22, 1994.

Schultz, JM, and Videbeck, SD: Manual of Psychiatric Nursing Care Plans. JB Lippincott, Philadelphia, 1994.

Seligman, M: Helplessness: On Depression, Development and Death. WH Freeman, New York, 1975.

Selnes, OA, et al: The multicenter AIDS cohort study. HIV-1 infection: No evidence of cognitive decline during asymptomatic stages. Neurology 40:204, 1990.

Selzer, JA, and Lieberman, JA: Schizophrenia and substance abuse. Psychiatr Clin North Am 16(2):401, 1993.

Sisney, KF: The relationship between social support and depression in recovering chemically dependent nurses. Image 25(2):107, 1993.

Smith, SL: Tissue and Organ Transplantation: Implications for Professional Nursing Practice. Mosby, St Louis, 1990.

Smith-Dijulio, K, and Holzapfel, SK: Families in crisis: Family violence. In Varcarolis, EM (ed): Foundations of Psychiatric Mental Health Nursing, ed 2. WB Saunders, Philadelphia, 1994.

Smythe, E: Surviving Nursing. Addison-Wesley, Menlo Park, CA, 1984.

Stanhope, M, and Lancaster, J: Community Health Nursing, ed 3. Mosby, St Louis, 1992.

Stanley, M, and Beare, PG: Gerontological Nursing. FA Davis, Philadelphia, 1995.

Stephens, ST: Patient education materials: Are they readable? Oncol Nurs Forum 19(1):83, 1992.

Stepnick, A, and Perry, T: Preventing spiritual distress in the dying client. J Psychosoc Nurs and Ment Health Serv 30(1):17, 1992.

Stolley, JM, et al: Managing the care of patients with irreversible dementia during hospitalization for comorbidities. Nurs Clin North Am 28(4):7, 1993.

Stone, TM: Schizophrenia in the elderly: What nurses need to know. Arch Psychiatr Nurs 3(1):47, 1989.

Strauss, AL, et al: Chronic Illness and the Quality of Life, ed 2. CV Mosby, St Louis, 1984.

Stuart, GW, and Sundeen, SJ: Principles and Practices of Psychiatric Nursing, ed 5. CV Mosby, St. Louis, 1995.

Sullivan-Marx, EM: Delirium and physical restraint in the hospitalized elderly. Image 26(4):295, 1994.

Sundeen, SJ, et al: Nurse-Client Interaction, ed 5. Mosby, St Louis, 1994.

Tatro, DS (ed): Drug interaction facts. Facts and Comparisons. JB Lippincott, Philadelphia, 1993.

Taylor, EJ, Amenta, M, and Highfield, M: Spiritual care practices of oncology nurses. Oncol Nurs Forum 22(1):31, 1995.

Townsend, MC: Psychiatric/Mental Health Nursing: Concepts of Care. FA Davis, Philadelphia, 1993.

Turnbill, J, et al: Turn it around: Short-term management of aggression and anger. J Psychosoc Nurs Ment Health Serv 28(6):1, 1990.

United Network of Organ Storing (UNOS). Annual Report, Richmond, VA, 1992.

UNOS Ethics Committee. 1991 Report on Organ Allocation and Living Donors. Transplantation Proceedings 24(5):2226–2237, 1992.

US Food and Drug Administration (FDA): Safety Alert: Potential Hazards with Restraint Devices. Department of Health and Human Services, Washington, DC, 1992.

US Public Health Service: Vital and Health Statistics: Current Estimates from the National Health Interview Study. US Department of Health, Education, and Welfare, Washington, DC, 1989.

Valente, SM: Recognizing Depression in the Elderly. Am J Nursing 94(12):18, 1994.

Valente, SM, et al: Understanding grief after suicide. Nurseweek 6:10, 1993.

Valente, SM, Saunders, JM, and Cohen, MZ: Evaluating depression among patients with cancer. Cancer Practice 2:65–71, 1994.

Varcarolis, EM: Foundations of Psychiatric Mental Health Nursing, ed 2. WB Saunders, Philadelphia, 1994.

Walker, L: The Battered Woman. Harper & Row, New York, 1979.

Wasserberger, J, et al: Violence in the emergency department. Top Emerg Med 14(2):71, 1992.

Webb, C (ed): Living Sexuality: Issues for Nursing & Health. Scutari Press, London, 1994.

White, GB (ed): Ethical Dilemmas in Contemporary Nursing Practice. American Nursing Publications, Washington, DC, 1992.

Wong, DL: Whaley and Wong's Essentials of Pediatric Nursing, ed 3. Mosby, St Louis, 1993.

Woods, NF (ed): Human Sexuality in Health and Illness. CV Mosby, St Louis, 1984.

Worden, JW: Grief Counseling and Grief Therapy. Springer, New York, 1991.

INDEX

A "t" following a page number indicates a table.